Adel E. Ahmed Ganaw
Nissar Shaikh • Nabil A. Shallik
Marco Abraham E. Marcus
Editors

Management of Subarachnoid Hemorrhage

Springer

Editors
Adel E. Ahmed Ganaw
Anesthesia, Perioperative Medicine and Critical Care Department
Hamad General Hospital
Hamad Medical Corporation
Doha, Qatar

Nissar Shaikh
Department of Anesthesia
Perioperative Medicine
and Critical Care
Surgical Intensive Care Unit
Hamad Medical Corporation
Doha, Qatar

Nabil A. Shallik
Faculty of Medicine
Tanta University
Tanta, Egypt

Marco Abraham E. Marcus
Department of Anesthesiology
University of Muenster
Muenster, Germany

ISBN 978-3-030-81332-1 ISBN 978-3-030-81333-8 (eBook)
https://doi.org/10.1007/978-3-030-81333-8

This Springer imprint is published by the registered company Springer Nature Switzerland AG
The registered company address is: Gewerbestrasse 11, 6330 Cham, Switzerland

Preface

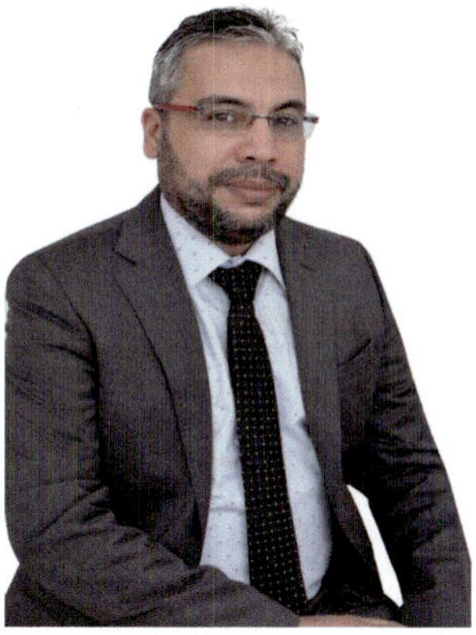

When a person dies, his deeds are cut off except for three: Continuing charity, knowledge that others benefited from, and a righteous son who supplicates for him.—Prophet Mohammad

Aneurysmal subarachnoid hemorrhage (aSAH) is considered one of the most devastating neurosurgical emergencies affecting healthy individuals in the most productive stage of their life. Less than 16% of patients will return to their premorbid status.

This book is designed by the authors to be a comprehensive description of aneurysmal subarachnoid hemorrhage. The book discusses different workup modalities, investigations, and both pharmacological and interventional approaches to managing this condition.

The fourteen chapters cover the fundamentals of aSAH and relevant patient-related information. The initial section/part of this book consists of an overview of relevant vascular anatomy, neurophysiology, and neuroprotection. Acquisition of this knowledge is the keystone for the rational practice of clinical neurosurgery.

Early chapters then focus on diagnosis including history, clinical examination, and various radiological modalities. A very useful chapter discusses the grading of aSAH, exploring the different scoring systems used to assess the severity and to predict complications from this condition. Subsequent chapters cover perioperative management, including the different techniques employed to secure cerebral aneurysms, as well as neurological and non-neurological complications. Critical care management is also discussed in detail. The final chapters cover traumatic subarachnoid hemorrhage, brain death, and ethics.

In summary, I strongly recommend this superb book to all medical students, residents, specialists, and fellows of emergency medicine, neurology, neurosurgery, neuroanesthesia, internal medicine, intensive care, and trauma.

The authors' broad training in basic science and their extensive clinical experience provide them with a unique background enabling them to develop invaluable insights in this subject. They have been successful in presenting the vast expanse of basic and clinical knowledge necessary for the management of aSAH in the twenty-first century, in a coherent manner.

Undoubtedly, all will enjoy reading this book. I would like to congratulate all of the authors and editors for their efforts in producing this book.

I dedicate this book to my father's immaculate soul and my mother, both of whom have taught me over the years and gave me the opportunity to succeed.

I am very much thankful to my wife and my kids for their patience, continuous support, and encouragement while writing this book.

Doha, Qatar Adel E. Ahmed Ganaw

Preface

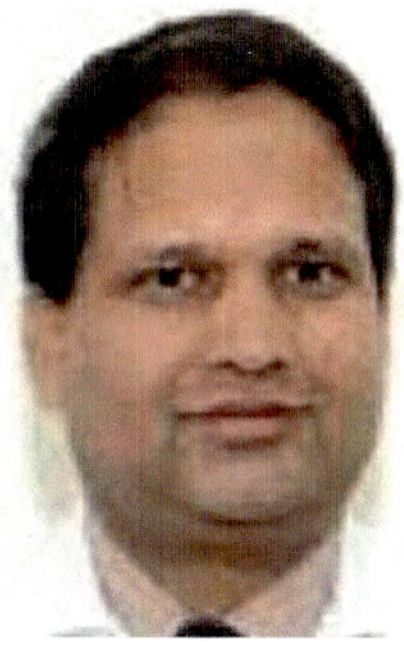

Aneurysmal subarachnoid hemorrhage (aSAH) is a dreaded disease, which is a challenge to manage and requires a multidisciplinary team approach for better patient outcome. The authors have been taking care of these patients for more than two decades and are up-to-date with the developments in the field from diagnosis with improved imaging to the endovascular management of aSAH patients; hence we decided to write this book.

This book includes chapters from applied anatomy to updated management of aSAH and its complications written in a simple scientific language, which will be equally beneficial to specialists, fellows, residents, students, and paramedical staff in neurology, neurosurgery, anesthesiology, and intensive care department involved in the management of aSAH.

We are certain that the reader will find this book useful and interesting. Also the book will provide a comprehensive updated knowledge about aSAH as chapters have been written by a team of multidisciplinary experts in intensive care, neurosurgery, neurology, and anesthesiology from a reputed tertiary care university hospital.

I am thankful to my fellow editors, authors, and colleagues as well as to my wife Dr. Firdous and daughters Dr. Amara and Jaza for their patience, constant support, and encouragement to write this book.

Doha, Qatar
May 19, 2021

Nissar Shaikh

Preface

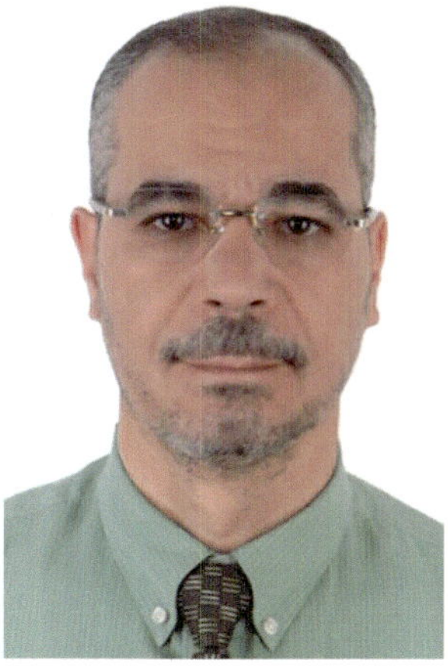

We strongly believe that sharing knowledge is beneficial for humanity and so we are thrilled to introduce our new book titled *Management of Subarachnoid Hemorrhage*.

As you discover the exciting world of anesthesiology and critical care management, we hope that you will find our book up to date in the management of subarachnoid hemorrhage during your studies and practice.

We have used our experience and feedback from multiple delegates to guide the creation of this book. I am extremely proud to have welcomed contributions from colleagues around the world who are among the highest-ranked physicians and researchers in the field of subarachnoid hemorrhage. The content of this book is the result of a mixture of compiled clinical experience, author opinion, allied expert opinion, best practice guidance, and up-to-date evidence base as practiced in modern medicine as on the date of publication of this book.

While every effort has been made to provide accurate and up-to-date information, which is in accord with accepted standards and practice at the time of publication, nevertheless, the authors, editors, and publishers would like to caution the reader that medical practice keeps changing and therefore we cannot make any warranties that the information contained herein is totally free from error.

This volume is intended to be a practical book, not just to be read and placed on a shelf, but hopefully one that will be taken into the workplace and used as an aid during clinical practice.

Hopefully, all will read this book with pleasure. I congratulate every author for the effort they have put in and the other editors, especially Dr. Adel E. Ahmed Ganaw, for their patience and endurance.

I would like to dedicate this book to my father and my mother who have taught me over the years and given me the opportunity to succeed and to my wife for her support and my children for their smiles, which keep me going.

Doha, Qatar Nabil A. Shallik

Contents

Abbreviations

3-D	Three-Dimensional
99mTc-HMPAO	Technetium-99m Hexamethyl Propylene Amine Oxime
μmol	Micromole
ABC	Airway, Breathing, and Circulation
ACA	Anterior Cerebral Artery
ACEP	The American College of Emergency Physicians
ACOM	Anterior Communicating Artery Aneurysm
ACT	Activated Clotting Time
ACTH	Adrenocorticotrophic Hormone
ADH	Antidiuretic Hormone
AHA	American Heart Association
AICA	Anterior Inferior Cerebellar Artery
APACHE II Score	Acute Physiology and Chronic Health Evaluation II Score
aPTT	Activated Partial Thromboplastin Time
ASA	American Stroke Association
aSAH	Aneurysmal Subarachnoid Hemorrhage
ATP	Adenosine Triphosphate
$AVDO_2$	Arterio-Venous Difference of Oxygen
BAC	Balloon-Assisted Coiling
BBB	Blood-Brain Barrier
BCI	Bicaudate Index
BIS	Bispectral Index
BNP	Brain Natriuretic Peptide
BPS	Behavioral Pain Scale
CBF	Cerebral Blood Flow
CIN	Contrast-Induced Nephropathy
CK-BB	Creatinine Kinase BB
CKD	Chronic Kidney Disease
CMR	Cerebral Metabolic Rate
$CMRO_2$	Cerebral Metabolic Rate of Oxygen Consumption
CNIII	Cranial Nerve 3
CNS	Central Nervous System
CONSCIOUS-1 study	Clazosentan to Overcome Neurological Ischemia and Infarction Occurring After Subarachnoid Hemorrhage study

COPD	Chronic Obstructive Pulmonary Disease
COW	Circle of Willis
CPOT	Critical-Care Pain Observation Tool
CPP	Cerebral Perfusion Pressure
CRP	C-Reactive Protein
CSF	Cerebrospinal Fluid
CSW	Cerebral Salt Wasting
CSWS	Cerebral Salt Wasting Syndrome
CT	Computerized Tomography
CTA	Computerized Tomographic Angiography
CTP	Computed Tomogram Perfusion
CVA	Cerebrovascular Accidents
CVD	Cerebrovascular Diseases
CVP	Central Venous Pressure
DAI	Diffuse Axonal Injury
DCI	Delayed Cerebral Ischemia
DSA	Digital Subtraction Angiography
DVT	Deep Venous Thrombosis
ECG	Electrocardiogram
ECMO	Extra-Corporeal Membrane Oxygenation
ECSB	Extracellular Space of the Brain
EEG	Electroencephalogram
ESO	European Stroke Organization
ETT	Endotracheal Tube
EVD	External Ventricular Drainage
FDA	Food and Drug Administration
FLAIR	Fluid Attenuated Inversion Recovery
GA	General Anesthesia
GABA	Gamma-Aminobutyric Acid
GCS	Glasgow Comma Scale
GDC	Guglielmi Detachable Coils
GI	Gastrointestinal
GLUT	Glucose Transporters
GRE	Gradient Reversal Echo
H&H score	Hunt and Hess score
HICP	High Intracranial Pressure
HIT	Heparin-Induced Thrombocytopenia
HTN	Hypertension
ICA	Internal Carotid Artery
ICAM	Intercellular Adhesion Molecule
ICP	Intracranial Pressure
ICU	Intensive Care Unit
IL	Interleukin
INR	Interventional Neuroradiology
IR	Interventional Radiology
ISAT	International Subarachnoid Aneurysm Trial
IU	International Unit
IV	Intravenous

IVH	Intraventricular Hemorrhage
LMA	Laryngeal Mask Airway
LMWH	Low Molecular Weight Heparin
LP	Lumbar Puncture
LV	Left Ventricle
MAC	Minimum Alveolar Concentration
MAP	Mean Arterial Pressure
MCA	Middle Cerebral Artery
MDA	Mondial Dehydrate
MHC	Major Histocompatibility Complex
MRA	Magnetic Resonance Angiography
MRI	Magnetic Resonance Imaging
MTT	Mean Transit Time
mV	millivolt
NCS	Neurocritical Care Society
NDMR	Non-depolarizing Muscle Relaxant
NIBP	Noninvasive Blood Pressure
NIRS	Near-Infrared Spectroscopy
NMDA	N-Methyl-d-Aspartate
NMT	Neuromuscular Transmission
NO	Nitric Oxide
NORA	Non-operating Room Anesthesia
NRS	Numerical Rating Score
NSAIDs	Non-steroidal Anti-inflammatory Drugs
NSM	Neurogenic stunned myocardium
OA	Ophthalmic Artery
ONSD	Optic Nerve Sheath Diameter
OP	Opening Pressure
OR	Operating Room
PAASH	Prognosis On Admission of Aneurysmal Subarachnoid Hemorrhage
$PbtO_2$	Brain Tissue Oxygen
PCA	Posterior Cerebral Artery
PCI	Percutaneous Coronary Intervention
PEEP	Positive End Expiratory Pressure
PET	Positron Emission Tomography
PICA	Posterior Inferior Cerebellar Artery
PiCCO	Contour Cardiac Output
PMSA	Perimesencephalic Subarachnoid Hemorrhage
PT	Partial Thromboplastin Time
PTCA	Percutaneous Transluminal Balloon Angioplasty
PTV	Post-traumatic Vasospasm
RBCI	Relative Bicaudate Index
RBCs	Red Blood Cells
RCTs	Randomized Control Trials
REM	Rapid Eye Movement
SAC	Stent-Assisted Coiling
SAH	Subarachnoid Hemorrhage

SBP	Systolic Blood Pressure
SCA	Superior Cerebellar Artery
SH	Sentinel Headache
SIADH	Syndrome of Inappropriate Antidiuretic Hormone
SIRS	Systemic Inflammatory Response Syndrome
$SjvO_2$	Cerebral Venous Oxygen Saturation
SPECT	Single Photon Emission Computed Tomography
SSEP	Somatosensory Evoked Potential
STASH	Simvastatin in Aneurysmal Subarachnoid Hemorrhage
SWI	Susceptibility Weighted Imaging
TBI	Traumatic Brain Injury
TCD	Transcranial Doppler Ultrasonography
TD-CBF	Cerebral Blood Flow Thermal Diffusion
TIA	Transient Ischemic Attack
TIVA	Total Intravenous Anesthesia
TMD	Tympanic Membrane Displacement
TMPG	Transmural Pressure Gradient
TNF	Tumor Necrosis Factor
tPA	Tissue Plasminogen Activators
tSAH	Traumatic Subarachnoid Hemorrhage
UDDA	Uniform Determination of Death Act
UNOS	United Network for Organ Sharing
VA	Veno-Arterial
VAS	Visual Analog Scale
VOR	Vestibulo-ocular Reflex
VP Shunt	Ventriculoperitoneal Shunt
VT	Ventricular Tachycardia
VV	Veno-Venous
WFNS	World Federation of Neurological Surgeons Scale

Aneurysmal Subarachnoid Haemorrhage: Epidemiology, Aetiology, and Pathophysiology

1

Nissar Shaikh, Arshad Chanda, Shoaib Nawaz, Alisha Alkubaisi, Abdulnasser Alyafei, Adel E. Ahmed Ganaw, and Mohammad Faisal Malmstrom

1.1 Introduction and Epidemiology

The aneurysmal subarachnoid haemorrhage (aSAH) accounts for 5% of all strokes. 85% of the spontaneous subarachnoid haemorrhages are due to rupture of the cerebral aneurysm hence termed as aneurysmal subarachnoid haemorrhage (aSAH). Worldwide, the overall incidence of aneurysmal subarachnoid haemorrhage (aSAH) shows a decreasing trend. Globally, the incidence of aSAH decreased from 10.2/100,000 in the 1980s to the 6.1/100,000 population in 2010. Furthermore, the incidence of aSAH varies according to geographic location. (Fig. 1.1). In Australia and New Zealand, the incidence is 7.4/100,000, in the United States of America 6.9/100,000, in Central America 5.1/100,000, in Asia except Japan 3.7/100,000 while in Qatar is 2.3/100,000. The lowest rate of aSAH is reported in China, 2.2/100,000 population, whereas the highest rates are reported from Japan and Finland 28 and 37/100,000 population respectively. These low and higher incidences of aSAH may be related to the higher age of survival and genetic aetiology [1, 2].

At a younger age, the aSAH is common in males, while in the elderly population, females have a higher incidence of aSAH [1, 2]. There is an increase in the chances of cerebral aneurysm bleeding by 1.03 folds with each year increase in age after the age of 35 years.

Despite improvement in diagnosis, medical and surgical management of stroke patients, aSAH ends up with significantly higher mortality, morbidity, and disease burden. The mortality is approximately 40% in 30 days, and the functional outcome is less than 25% in survivors [1].

A variant of SAH is the perimesencephalic SAH (PMSAH) is defined by the absence of an aneurysmatic bleeding and blood's classic presence within the perimesencephalic and prepontine cisterns. Computed tomography angiogram (CTA) and magnetic resonance angiography (MRA) have high sensitivity of excluding aneurysmal bleedings in PMSAH. PMSAH has fewer complications and a better prognosis than aneurysmal SAH [3].

N. Shaikh (✉)
Department of Anesthesia, Perioperative Medicine and Critical Care, Hamad Medical Corporation, Doha, Qatar

Surgical Intensive Care Unit, Hamad Medical Corporation, Doha, Qatar
e-mail: Smahemoob@hamad.qa

A. Chanda · S. Nawaz · A. E. A. Ganaw
M. F. Malmstrom
Department of Anesthesia, Perioperative Medicine and Critical Care, Hamad Medical Corporation, Doha, Qatar
e-mail: achanda@hamad.qa; snawaz1@hamad.qa; aganaw@hamad.qa; mmalmstrom@hamad.qa

A. Alkubaisi · A. Alyafei
Department of Neurosciences, Neurosurgery Section, Hamad Medical Corporation, Doha, Qatar
e-mail: aalkubaisi8@hamad.qa; athabet@hamad.qa

A. E. A. Ganaw et al. (eds.), *Management of Subarachnoid Hemorrhage*,
https://doi.org/10.1007/978-3-030-81333-8_1

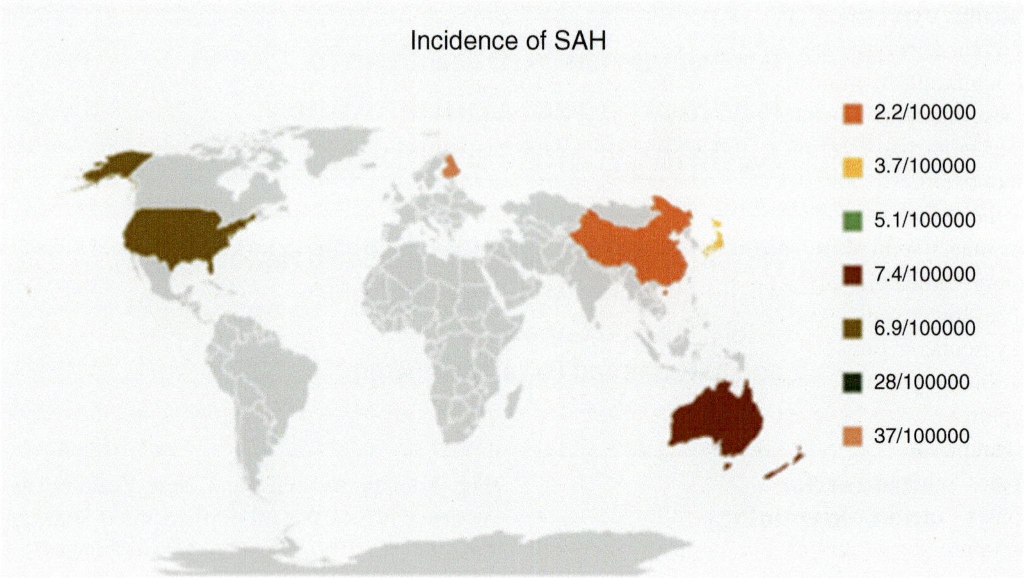

Fig. 1.1 Incidence of aSAH varies according to geographic location (courtesy of Dr. Arshad Chanda)

1.2 Aetiology and Risk Factors for aSAH

There are many clinically diverse aetiological factors and associated diseases in developing a cerebral aneurysm and their rupture, causing aSAH. The aetiologies and associated disease conditions are listed in Table 1.1.

The modifiable risk factors in the development and rupture of cerebral aneurysms, such as hypertension, smoking, alcohol abuse, dyscholesterolemia recreational drug abuse, and low body mass index. Whereas the non-modifiable risk factors for increased aSAH are gender, familial, and connective tissue disorders.

Table 1.1 Aetiological factors and Diseases associated with cerebral aneurysm and SAH [3]

Infectious arterial vasculitis	Mycotic (infectious) aneurysm
	Meningovascular lues
	Lyme disease
	Gnathostomiasis (Gnathostoma spinigerum)
Immune vasculitis	Primary CNS angiitis
	Polyarteritis nodosa
	Wegener's vasculitis
	Churg-Strauss syndrome
	Behçet's disease
Other cerebrovascular diseases	Arteriovenous angioma
	Dural arteriovenous fistula
	Spinal arterial aneurysm
	Intracranial arterial dissection
	Venous sinus thrombosis
	Cerebral amyloid angiopathy
	Moyamoya disease
Tumour	Intracranial and intraspinal tumour
Haematology	Sickle cell anaemia
Drugs	Anticoagulants and thrombolytic therapy
Substance abuse	Cocaine and amphetamine

1.2.1 Modifiable Risk Factors for Aneurysmal Subarachnoid Haemorrhage (aSAH)

1.2.1.1 Cigarette Smoking

It is a significant modifiable risk for aSAH and remains one of the important preventable causes for aSAH. It is attributed to the formation, progression, and rupture of cerebral aneurysms. Approximately 29% of the attributable risk of aSAH is due to smoking, and its cessation decreases its risk. The risk is higher in current smokers than the ex-smokers. The fundamental mechanisms by which cigarette smoking causes vascular dysfunction and the formation of the cerebral aneurysm are unclear. Cigarette smoke is a mixture of more than 4000 chemicals [4]. These chemical generates excess reactive oxygen species, increase oxidative stress on the vascular smooth muscle cell. They also cause an alteration in the inflammatory pathways and the cerebral immune system, thus resulting in direct vascular injury, endothelial dysfunction, and production of reactive oxygen species. These changes result in vascular smooth cell injury [5].

Smoking is associated with a younger age of rupture of cerebral aneurysms. Paradoxically cigarette smoking was associated with better outcomes on many measures, reduced poor outcomes in poor-grade patients. The recent literature shows that nicotine replacement therapy among smokers with aSAH was associated with better outcomes [4, 6]. There is a strong correlation between smoking and hypertension which considered as a second most common risk factor of SAH.

1.2.1.2 Hypertension

Hypertension (HTN) is the second most common preventable cause of aSAH. Hypertensive patients have a nearly seven-fold higher risk of aSAH. The cerebral aneurysm secondary to hypertension occurs mainly (90%) in the anterior circulation, in constant positions like anterior communicating, internal carotid, and middle cerebral arteries. Only 10% of aneurysms seen in the posterior circulation in hypertensives.

The main three mechanisms by which hypertension causes aneurysm formation and rupture are (a). Occlusion of vasa vasorum (b). Endothelial damage, causing endothelial dysfunction and smooth muscle phenotypic changes (c). Elevations in wall shear stress for prolonged duration results in elastin and collagen synthesis abnormalities in the vascular smooth muscles and setting in of the inflammatory response and release of the matrix metalloproteinases, which degrades collagen and elastin. Once the aneurysm is formed, low wall shear stress due to intra-aneurysmal recirculation will promote inflammation and growth in the aneurysm's size. In combination with these three mechanisms, hypertension increases the hemodynamic stress on the cerebral arteries, contributing to the increased formation and rupture of cerebral aneurysms. This is seen mostly at the branching points where the blood flow is turbulent and develops high shear stress. If the vessels are hypoplastic, branching at sharper angles or taking complex curvatures may further increase hemodynamic stress. A disruption in the balance between hemodynamic stresses and vascular wall strength causes rupture of the aneurysm [7–9].

1.2.1.3 Alcohol Consumption

It is another modifiable risk factor for aSAH. There is a dose-dependent relationship between alcohol consumption and the occurrence of aSAH. It has a protective effect in small doses, whereas heavy alcohol consumption damages the vascular endothelium by generating reactive oxygen species, oxidative stress, and increased nitric oxide (NO) production [7, 10].

1.2.1.4 Recreational Drug Abuse

Cocaine and Amphetamine Abuse

These are associated with significant risk for cerebral aneurysms and aSAH. These are the commonly used illicit drug all over the globe. Up to 4%of cocaine, abusers have an aSAH [2, 11].

These drugs have a sympathomimetic effect. The cocaine-related aneurysms are usually located in the anterior circulation. aSAH due to cocaine-related aneurysms are seen with small aneurysms and in younger age patients. Usually, the outcome is poor in cocaine-related aneurysms because of the cocaine-related cardiovascular complication, CVAs, higher incidence of vasospasm, and delayed cerebral ischemia [11].

Cocaine increases blood pressure, thus increasing the risk for aSAH. The sympathomimetic effect of cocaine is mediated by the potentiation of monoamines. This potentiation of monoamines is rendered by blocking of the reuptake of norepinephrine. Cocaine also increases catecholamine receptor sensitivity. The combination of the potentiation of monoamines and increased catecholamine receptors sensitivity leads to sympathetic hyperactivity-induced transient hypertension. Hypertension is one of the significant risk factors in the development and rupture of intracranial aneurysms as mentioned earlier. Cocaine can evoke, aggravate, or sustain hypertension.

Furthermore, cocaine causes cerebral vasoconstriction and increase of intraluminal pressure, facilitating both the formation and rupture of the aneurysms. The aneurysmal sacs, which are deficient in functional elastin and collagen, are relatively non-distensible. The rise in intraluminal pressure increases the stress on the aneurysmal wall leading to rupture of cerebral aneurysm [12].

Marijuana

The literature suggests that the use of recreational marijuana to be independently associated with an 18% increased likelihood of aSAH. Marijuana may cause reversible cerebral vasoconstriction syndrome. Hence marijuana abuse not only increases the incidence of aSAH but also has a poor outcome due to more frequent delayed cerebral ischemia.

The estimated incidence of multifocal intracranial stenosis and stroke secondary to marijuana abuse was 21%, the intracranial stenosis may recover if marijuana abuse is stopped [13, 14].

1.2.1.5 Oral Contraceptives and Hormonal Replacement Therapy

The use of oral contraceptives with higher oestrogen content was described to increase the aSAH. The possible mechanism is that the high doses of oestrogen induced hypertension. Nevertheless, low doses of oestrogen have a protective effect on the vascular endothelium by lowering nitric oxide production, TNF. Thus, protects the vascular endothelium from inflammation and maintains their integrity [15].

1.2.1.6 Hypocholesterolemia

Hypocholesterolemia is inversely related to the risk of aSAH. The low serum cholesterol levels increases the risk of haemorrhagic stroke, as the lipids are required by cells to maintain their membrane. An experimental study reported that high cholesterol level inhibits smooth muscle necrosis. However, a recent study contradicts this finding and concludes that elevated triglycerides levels may increase the risk for aSAH among men; therefore, lipid profile should be taken into account when assessing risk for aSAH in men [16, 17].

1.2.1.7 Atherosclerosis

Atherosclerosis is considered a risk factor in the formation of a cerebral aneurysm. Smoking and hypertension are also risk factors for atherosclerosis and aSAH. Both formation of cerebral aneurysm and atherosclerosis might have same pathophysiology. There were some histologic and biochemical resemblance noticed between the aneurysmal wall and the atherosclerotic plaques.

Noteworthy, high serum level of lipoprotein which is commonly observed in aSAH patients is considered as risk factor for atherosclerosis. The lipid accumulation initiates the oxidative stress and free radicals generation in the atherosclerotic wall and sets in a pro-inflammatory response. This culminates in apoptosis and proteolysis by cytokines and matrix metalloproteinases [18, 19].

1.2.1.8 Diabetes Mellitus

Type I diabetes mellitus promotes the formation of cerebral aneurysm [20]. Diabetes mellitus with insulin resistance causes endothelial dysfunction and increases oxidative stress, thus increasing the risk of cerebral aneurysms. The role of diabetes mellitus in cerebral aneurysm formation and rupture has not been thoroughly investigated. But diabetes mellitus induces micro- and macroangiopathy complications. It causes vascular endothelial damage, the intima and media thickening, atherosclerotic changes, decreases the expression of cerebral tight junction protein. These changes, especially the reduced expression of tight junction protein and endothelial damage, may contribute to the formation of the cerebral aneurysm. Degradation of the Type IV collagen, a constituent of the basement membrane by the pro-inflammatory mediators and the matrix metalloproteinase 9, contributes to the vascular lesions [20].

Type 2 diabetes mellitus does not increase the risk of aSAH. Type 2 diabetic population showed a lower prevalence of aneurysmal subarachnoid haemorrhage when compared to the general population. The mechanisms for this lower prevalence are unknown. The oral antihyperglycaemic agents may exert several anti-inflammatory actions and inhibit the production of the matrix metalloproteinase 9. This hypothesis could explain the possible mechanism in the prevention of aneurysmal rupture as well [21, 22].

1.2.1.9 Low and High Body Mass Index (BMI)

Individuals with low body mass index (BMI) or lean body mass index are at a higher risk for strokes, including aSAH. However, Kawate et al. reported that a high BMI was directly associated with SAH [23].

1.2.1.10 Socioeconomic Status and Occupational Stress

Low socioeconomic status and educational status are reported to be independent risk factors for the increased occurrence of aSAH. The mechanism is not fully understood [24].

1.2.2 Non-modifiable Risk Factors for Increased aSAH

1.2.2.1 Gender

A unique epidemiological feature of aSAH is that it is more common in females (2:1); the risk of aSAH increases significantly after menopause. Ghods et al. described that up to 72% of aSAH occurs in females [25].

The proposed mechanism for increasing aSAH in female post-menopause is the loss of vessel endothelium and compromised vascular remodelling secondary to decreasing oestrogen levels. Oestrogen by their pleiotropic effects on vascular endothelial cells, collagen, and nitric oxide promotes normal vascular function. This hypothesis can be substantiated by a reduction in the rate of aneurysm formation and rupture by hormone replacement therapy.

Moreover, vascular geometry and wall stress differ between the genders. Females have narrow cerebral blood vessels and asymmetric branch angles, which results in greater blood flow velocity and higher wall shear stress at the arterial bifurcations. This also explains why internal carotid artery aneurysms are the most common in females in contrast to males in whom the anterior communicating artery aneurysms are common. Females tend to have multiple aneurysms [25, 26].

1.2.2.2 Familial or Connective Tissue Disorders

The familial occurrence of aSAH is well described. Twenty percent of patients with aSAH have a positive family history. First-degree relatives of patients with aSAH have up to sevenfold increased risk of having aSAH. Onda et al. found that the formation and rupture of intracranial aneurysms were related to chromosome 7q11 in families [27]. In another genome linkage study in a Finnish population, a country where aSAH is common showed a stronger correlation of aSAH and chromosome 19q13-2 in families (Table 1.2). Keun-Hwa. et al. confirmed the familial occur-

Table 1.2 Hereditary disorders with susceptibility to an intracranial aneurysm [28]

Disorder	Pathophysiology
mTOR signalling	
Polycystic kidney disease	Phospho-mTOR was downregulation
Tuberous sclerosis	mTOR signalling
Neural crest development	
Bicuspid valve	Neural crest development
Alagille syndrome	Neural crest development
Marfan syndrome	Transforming growth factor-β signalling, extracellular matrix integrity
Transforming growth factor-β signalling	
Loeys-Dietz syndrome	
Hereditary haemorrhagic telangiectasia	
Collagen metabolism, extracellular matrix integrity	
Osteogenesis imperfecta	Collagen metabolism, extracellular matrix integrity
Ehlers-Danlos syndromes	Collagen metabolism, extracellular matrix integrity
Other aetiologies	
Neurofibromatosis	Ras-Raf-MEK-ERK pathway)
Familial thoracic aortic aneurysm	Smooth muscle development
Turner syndrome	Unknown

rence of aSAH, more commonly affected MCA aneurysms in relatives, and the interesting finding was that the aSAH age was similar in all relatives [28–30]. Connective tissue disorders are a rare cause of aSAH. It accounts for 2% of all aSAH, commonly in association with polycystic kidney disease [31].

1.3 Pathophysiology of Cerebral Aneurysms

The pathogenesis and shape form the basis of classification for cerebal aneurysms. The commonest form is a saccular aneurysm, also called berry aneurysm, as they are berry-shaped or multilobed outpouchings. The saccular aneurysms are formed spontaneously. They are the cause of aSAH in 85% of the patients.

Trauma, tumour, and infection may contribute in formation of cerebral aneurysm. The bacterial or fungal infection may cause focal necrosis of an arterial wall resulting in an aneurysm. Fusiform aneurysms are usually spindle-shaped bulging of the artery, often due to atherosclerosis. Dissecting aneurysms results from dissection of the vessel wall usually occur from traumatic injury or can occur spontaneously. (Fig. 1.2).

While discussing the pathophysiology of a cerebral aneurysm, there are three important processes to be considered. These are the formation, the growth, and the rupture of the aneurysm. (Fig. 1.3).

The precise mechanism of cerebral aneurysm formation is unknown, but pathological changes in the vessel wall composition and structural changes

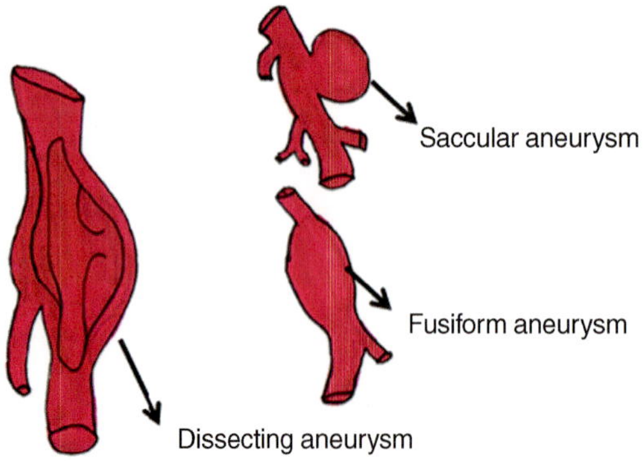

Fig. 1.2 Different types of aneurysm

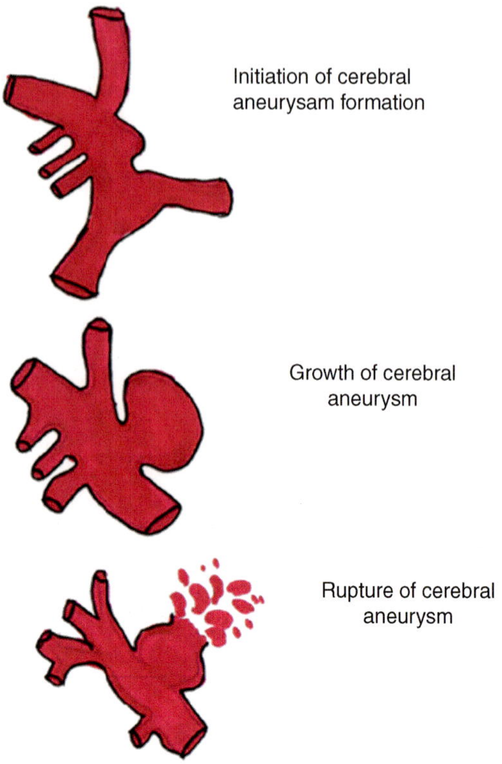

Fig. 1.3 Showing the formation, growth, and rupture of cerebral aneurysm (courtesy of Dr. Arshad Chanda)

are the initiating factors. The presence of predisposing genetic factors, environmental factors, and epidemiological factors will contribute further to the cerebral aneurysm formation. (Fig. 1.2).

Around 85% of aneurysms occur in the anterior circulation, and 20% of the patients will have multiple aneurysms. Most of the multiple aneurysms are located at the mirror site bilaterally. As the aneurysm development progresssses and forms neck and dome typically. Typical aneurysm rupture occurs at the dome as the dome wall is thinned and tears (Fig. 1.4). Various factors that increase the risk of rupture of aneurysms are (a) aneurysms size more than 7 mm in diameter (b) aneurysms at the tip of the basilar artery (c) aneurysm at bifurcations or at the origin of posterior communicating arteries. With the initial rupture of the aneurysms, a small amount of blood is leaked into the subarachnoid space causing headaches, but blood cannot be detected in computerised tomography (CT). The patient gets

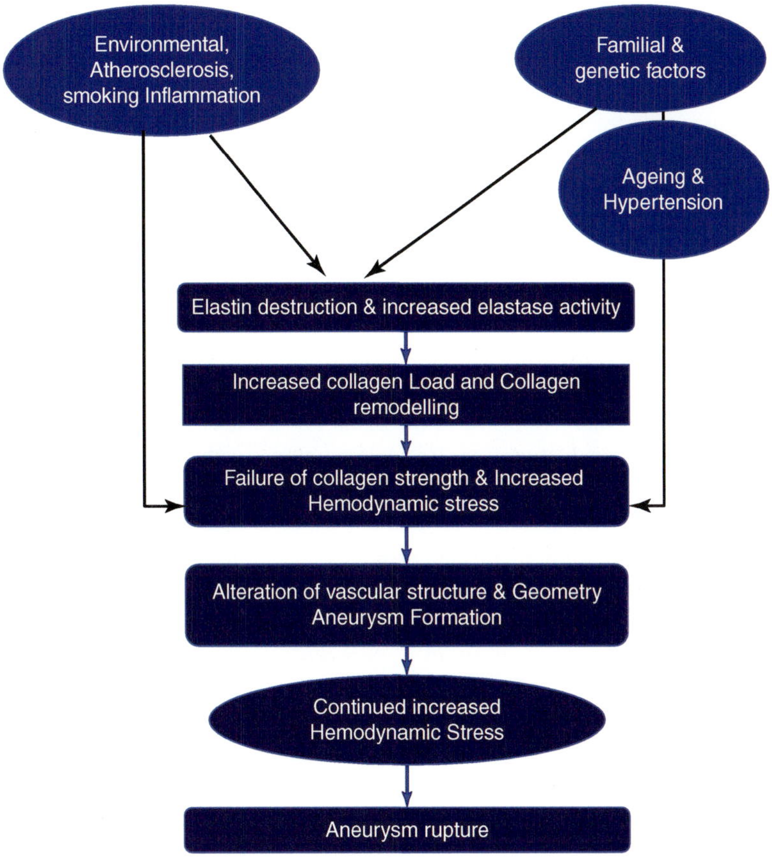

Fig. 1.4 Mechanism of cerebral aneurysm formation and rupture (Courtesy of Dr. Nisssar Shaikh)

discharged from the hospital to be admitted later with significant SAH and usually with a severe grade of aSAH and severe symptoms. Hence the initial headache is called a sentinel headache. Ruptured cerebral aneurysms cause the signs and symptoms either due to mass effect or blood in the subarachnoid and ventricular space [32].

Anterior communicating artery (ACom) or middle cerebral artery (MCA) bifurcation aneurysm rupture causes bleeding into the surrounding brain tissues causing intracerebral haemorrhage (ICH). This causes pressure symptoms like hemiparesis, aphasia, and abulia. The presence of blood in subarachnoid and ventricular space causes hydrocephalus, cerebral vasospasm, and cerebral ischemia (Fig. 1.5) [32].

The chances of rebleeding from the ruptured aneurysm are maximal during the initial 7 days, as the natural thrombolysis will displace the clot plug from the site of rupture. The rebleed in these patients with aSAH had higher morbidity and mortality [32].

Acute hydrocephalus can occur in the first hours after aSAH due to obstruction to the flow of CSF (obstructive and non-communicating), whereas late hydrocephalus occurs around 2 weeks of aSAH due to the blood in subarachnoid and ventricular space causing blockage of CSF (cerebrospinal fluid) absorption in the subarachnoid villi leading to the normal pressure communicating hydrocephalus (Fig. 1.4). The risk of cerebral vasospasm is highest from the day of ictus to the 14th day after the ictus, with the highest incidence on day seven post-ictus. Spasm of the major cerebral arteries will cause increasing headache, fluctuating level of consciousness, and focal neurological deficits. If the spasm persists, it can lead to cerebral ischemia and infarctions, brain oedema, with raised intracranial pressure [32].

Apart from primary and secondary brain injuries due to a ruptured aneurysm, it also causes distal non-neurological organ injuries and dysfunction, which are increasingly recognised cause for higher morbidity and mortality [32]. Various theories are proposed for the occurrence of distal organ dysfunction in aSAH. For more details please refer to Chap. 10.

1.3.1 Catecholamine Induced Injury

There is a surge of catecholamine after a rupture of a cerebral aneurysm that leads to a significant increase in serum renin, angiotensin II, adrenaline, and noradrenaline levels, resulting in cardiopulmonary injuries, multiorgan vasospasm, and organ dysfunction. It is documented that there is a threefold increase in the renin-angiotensin secretion in immediate post-experimental aSAH. Simultaneous occurrence of the cerebral salt wasting syndrome will cause natriuresis and diuresis. The diuresis is proved to potentiate the vasospasm in experimental animals [32, 33].

1.3.2 The Systemic Inflammatory Response Syndrome (SIRS) and Metabolic Derangements

Systemic inflammatory response syndrome (SIRS) and metabolic derangements in aSAH patients cause tachycardia, fever without any signs and symptoms of infections. It is reported in the literature that as high as 87% of aSAH patients may have SIRS and metabolic derangements. The severity of the SIRS and metabolic derangements are associated with the increase in morbidity and mortality in SAH patients [34]. SIRS response following SAH is associated with an increased incidence of delayed ischemic, neurological deficit, cerebral infarction, and poor neurological outcome, according to exploratory analysis of data from 413 patients of CONSCIOUS-1 database. (Fig. 1.5) Systemic inflammatory markers like C-reactive protein and IL-6 levels are elevated early following SAH; higher levels are associated with poor neurological outcome [34].

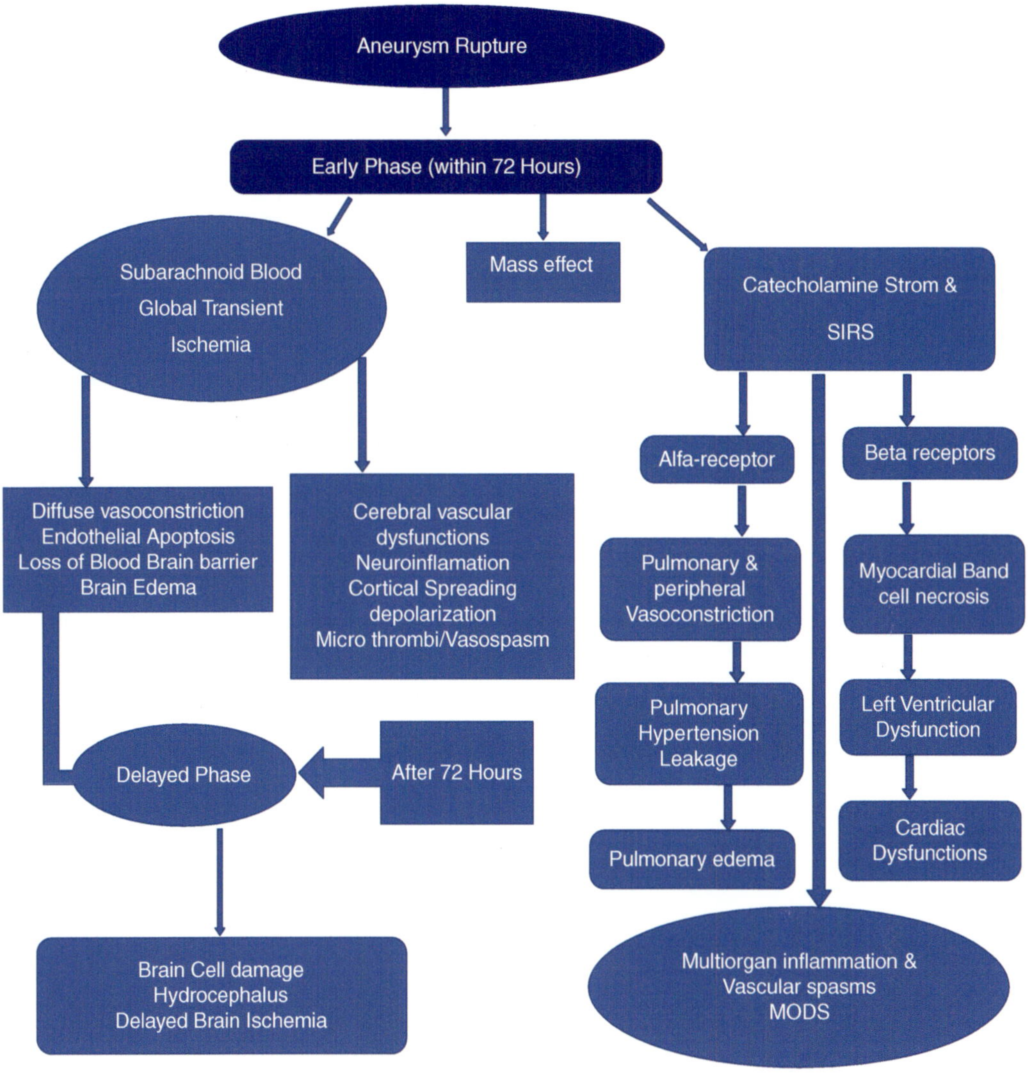

Fig. 1.5 Cerebral aneurysm rupture causing brain and distal organ injuries (Courtesy of Dr. Nissar Shaikh)

1.4 Conclusion

Although the global incidence of aSAH shows a decreasing trend, the morbidity and mortality remain high despite developments in diagnostic and therapeutic options. There are well-known risk factors that increase cerebral aneurysm formation, growth and rupture, namely recreational drug abuse, hypertension, gender, low body mass index, hypercholesterolemia, and genetic risk. Apart from these, connective tissue disorders and occupational stress can increase the risk of cerebral aneurysms formation and rupture which is commonly seen in anterior circulation. All these risks and environmental factors cause increased elastase activity in the vascular wall leading to elastin destruction, increased collagen load, collagen remodelling, decreased strength with net results in vascular weakness, and bulging out with aneurysm formation. If the increased hemodynamic stress persists or progress will lead to aneurysm rupture. The ruptured aneurysm will cause transient global ischemia, loss of blood–brain barrier, brain oedema, cerebral vascular dysregulation, neuroinflammation, microthrombi, and vasospasm. A sudden surge of catecholamine due to aSAH will cause non-neural distal organ dysfunction. The delayed ischemia occurs if the changes persist for a longer duration. Blood and its products will block the subarachnoid villi leading to the late development of normal pressure communicating hydrocephalus.

References

1. Zacharia BE, Hickman ZL, Grobelny BT, DeRosa P, Kotchetkov I, Ducruet AF, et al. Epidemiology of aneurysmal subarachnoid hemorrhage. Neurosurg Clin N Am. 2010;21(2):221–33.
2. Etminan N, Chang HS, Hackenberg K, de Rooij NK, Vergouwen MDI, Rinkel GJE, et al. Worldwide incidence of aneurysmal subarachnoid hemorrhage according to region, time period, blood pressure, and smoking prevalence in the population: a systematic review and meta-analysis. JAMA Neurol. 2019;76(5):588–97.
3. Ahmed AE, Ganaw AMT, Mohamed AO, Khair B. Aneurysmal subarachnoid hemorrhage. ICU Book, Intechopen; 2017. p. 73–99.
4. Dasenbrock HH, Rudy RF, Rosalind Lai PM, Smith TR, Frerichs KU, Gormley WB, et al. Cigarette smoking and outcomes after aneurysmal subarachnoid hemorrhage: a nationwide analysis. J Neurosurg. 2018;129(2):446–57.
5. Starke RM, Thompson JW, Ali MS, Pascale CL, Martinez Lege A, Ding D, et al. Cigarette smoke initiates oxidative stress-induced cellular phenotypic modulation leading to cerebral aneurysm pathogenesis. Arterioscler Thromb Vasc Biol. 2018;38(3):610–21.
6. Broderick JP, Viscoli CM, Brott T, Kernan WN, Brass LM, Feldmann E, et al. Major risk factors for aneurysmal subarachnoid hemorrhage in the young are modifiable. Stroke. 2003;34(6):1375–81.
7. Singh PK, Marzo A, Howard B, Rufenacht DA, Bijlenga P, Frangi AF, et al. Effects of smoking and hypertension on wall shear stress and oscillatory shear index at the site of intracranial aneurysm formation. Clin Neurol Neurosurg. 2010;112(4):306–13.
8. Bonita R. Cigarette smoking, hypertension and the risk of subarachnoid hemorrhage: a population-based case-control study. Stroke. 1986;17(5):831–5.
9. Inci S, Spetzler RF. Intracranial aneurysms and arterial hypertension: a review and hypothesis. Surg Neurol. 2000;53(6):530–40. Discussion 40–2.
10. Bau PF, Bau CH, Rosito GA, Manfroi WC, Fuchs FD. Alcohol consumption, cardiovascular health, and endothelial function markers. Alcohol. 2007;41(7):479–88.
11. Martin-Schild S, Albright KC, Hallevi H, Barreto AD, Philip M, Misra V, et al. Intracerebral hemorrhage in cocaine users. Stroke. 2010;41(4):680–4.
12. Nanda A, Vannemreddy PS, Polin RS, Willis BK. Intracranial aneurysms and cocaine abuse: analysis of prognostic indicators. Neurosurgery. 2000;46(5):1063–7. Discussion 7–9.
13. Rumalla K, Reddy AY, Mittal MK. Association of recreational marijuana use with aneurysmal subarachnoid hemorrhage. J Stroke Cerebrovasc Dis. 2016;25(2):452–60.
14. Behrouz R, Birnbaum L, Grandhi R, Johnson J, Misra V, Palacio S, et al. Cannabis use and outcomes in patients with aneurysmal subarachnoid hemorrhage. Stroke. 2016;47(5):1371–3.
15. Mohr JP, Wolf PA, Grotta JC, Moskowitz MA, Mayberg MR, von Kummer R, editors. Stroke 5th ed. Elsevier; 2011. 1520 p.
16. Tirschwell DL, Smith NL, Heckbert SR, Lemaitre RN, Longstreth WT Jr, Psaty BM. Association of cholesterol with stroke risk varies in stroke subtypes and patient subgroups. Neurology. 2004;63(10): 1868–75.
17. Lindbohm JV, Kaprio J, Korja M. Cholesterol as a risk factor for subarachnoid hemorrhage: a systematic review. PLoS One. 2016;11(4):e0152568.
18. Bolger C, Phillips J, Gilligan S, Zourob T, Farrell M, Croake D, et al. Elevated levels of lipoprotein (a) in association with cerebrovascular saccular aneurysmal disease. Neurosurgery. 1995;37(2):241–5.
19. Kosierkiewicz TA, Factor SM, Dickson DW. Immunocytochemical studies of atherosclerotic lesions of cerebral berry aneurysms. J Neuropathol Exp Neurol. 1994;53(4):399–406.
20. Yan T, Chopp M, Ning R, Zacharek A, Roberts C, Chen J. Intracranial aneurysm formation in type-one diabetes rats. PLoS One. 2013;8(7):e67949.
21. Can A, Castro VM, Yu S, Dligach D, Finan S, Gainer VS, et al. Antihyperglycemic agents are inversely associated with intracranial aneurysm rupture. Stroke. 2018;49(1):34–9.
22. Lindgren AE, Kurki MI, Riihinen A, Koivisto T, Ronkainen A, Rinne J, et al. Type 2 diabetes and risk of rupture of saccular intracranial aneurysm in eastern Finland. Diabetes Care. 2013;36(7):2020–6.
23. Kawate N, Kayaba K, Hara M, Hamaguchi T, Kotani K, Ishikawa S. Body mass index and incidence of subarachnoid hemorrhage in Japanese community residents: the jichi medical school cohort study. J Stroke Cerebrovasc Dis. 2017;26(8):1683–8.
24. Jakovljevic D, Sivenius J, Sarti C, Torppa J, Mahonen M, Immonen-Raiha P, et al. Socioeconomic inequalities in the incidence, mortality and prognosis of subarachnoid hemorrhage: the FINMONICA Stroke Register. Cerebrovasc Dis. 2001;12(1):7–13.
25. Ghods AJ, Lopes D, Chen M. Gender differences in cerebral aneurysm location. Front Neurol. 2012;3:78.
26. Imaizumi Y, Mizutani T, Shimizu K, Sato Y, Taguchi J. Detection rates and sites of unruptured intracranial aneurysms according to sex and age: an analysis of MR angiography-based brain examinations of 4070 healthy Japanese adults. J Neurosurg. 2018;130(2):573–8.
27. Onda H, Kasuya H, Yoneyama T, Takakura K, Hori T, Takeda J, et al. Genomewide-linkage and haplotype-

association studies map intracranial aneurysm to chromosome 7q11. Am J Hum Genet. 2001;69(4):804–19.
28. Jung KH. New pathophysiological considerations on cerebral aneurysms. Neurointervention. 2018;13(2):73–83.
29. Olson JM, Vongpunsawad S, Kuivaniemi H, Ronkainen A, Hernesniemi J, Ryynanen M, et al. Search for intracranial aneurysm susceptibility gene(s) using Finnish families. BMC Med Genet. 2002;3:7.
30. Lee JS, Park IS, Park KB, Kang DH, Lee CH, Hwang SH. Familial intracranial aneurysms. J Korean Neurosurg Soc. 2008;44(3):136–40.
31. Schievink WI, Torres VE, Piepgras DG, Wiebers DO. Saccular intracranial aneurysms in autosomal dominant polycystic kidney disease. J Am Soc Nephrol. 1992;3(1):88–95.
32. Chen S, Li Q, Wu H, Krafft PR, Wang Z, Zhang JH. The harmful effects of subarachnoid hemorrhage on extracerebral organs. Biomed Res Int. 2014;2014:858496.
33. Biancardi VC, Son SJ, Ahmadi S, Filosa JA, Stern JE. Circulating angiotensin II gains access to the hypothalamus and brain stem during hypertension via breakdown of the blood-brain barrier. Hypertension. 2014;63(3):572–9.
34. Dhar R, Diringer MN. The burden of the systemic inflammatory response predicts vasospasm and outcome after subarachnoid hemorrhage. Neurocrit Care. 2008;8(3):404–12.

2 Cerebral Circulation and Its Clinical Impact

M. A. Rahman, Nissar Shaikh, Adnan Khan, Shoaib Nawaz, Aisha Alkubiasi, M. M. Nainthramveetil, Adel E. Ahmed Ganaw, and Stefan Rohrig

2.1 Background

The brain circulation is movement of blood in and out of cranial cavity and brain. About 1/sixth of the cardiac output goes to the brain and it consumes 1/fifth of the total oxygen supply of the body. The continuous and uninterrupted blood supply is essential for the normal functioning of the brain. Human brain is a vital and precious organ of the body. Hence it is protected by around 10 mm thick skull bone. The brain floats in the cerebrospinal fluid and firmly covered with meningeal layers. Apart from these, another protective layer for the brain comes from blood–brain barrier (BBB). It allows dynamic interactions between cerebral blood capillaries and the neuronal cells and provides an adequate control of molecules that are transported in and out of the brain [1]. Cerebral autoregulation is another physiological process which regulates and maintains cerebral blood flow constant with a range of blood pressures [2].

We will discuss the circulation and protection in the following headings.

2.2 Blood Supply of the Brain

Blood supply to the brain is from two sets of arteries from the dorsal aorta and carotid arteries. The vertebral artery arises from the subclavian arteries, and internal carotid arteries are the branches of the common carotid arteries in the neck.

2.2.1 Internal Carotid Arteries

The common carotid artery bifurcates at the level of cervical vertebra 4–5 in the neck into the external and internal carotid arteries (ICA). The ICA proceeds through the carotid canal within the petrous part of the temporal bone and enters the cranium. ICA further passes anteriorly through the cavernous sinus and distal to the cavernous sinus it gives of its branches, the anterior cerebral artery and middle cerebral artery which forms the anterior circulation of brain as they supply to the forebrain (Fig. 2.1) [3]. Apart from these major arteries, the internal carotid arteries give out smaller branches, namely anterior choroidal, ophthalmic, and posterior communicating arter-

M. A. Rahman (✉)
Surgical Intensive Care Unit, Hamad Medical Corporation, Doha, Qatar

Department of Anesthesia/ICU and Perioperative Medicine, Hamad Medical Corporation, Doha, Qatar
e-mail: mrahman2@hamad.qa

N. Shaikh · S. Nawaz · M. M. Nainthramveetil
A. E. A. Ganaw · S. Rohrig
Surgical Intensive Care Unit, Hamad Medical Corporation, Doha, Qatar
e-mail: Smahemoob@hamad.qa; snawaz1@hamad.qa; mnainthramveetil@hamad.qa; aganaw@hamad.qa; srohrig@hamad.qa

A. Khan · A. Alkubiasi
Department of Neurosciences, Neurosurgery Section, Hamad Medical Corporation, Doha, Qatar
e-mail: akhan15@hamad.qa; aalkubaisi8@hamad.qa

A. E. A. Ganaw et al. (eds.), *Management of Subarachnoid Hemorrhage*,
https://doi.org/10.1007/978-3-030-81333-8_2

ies. The details of anterior circulation arteries are given in Table 2.1.

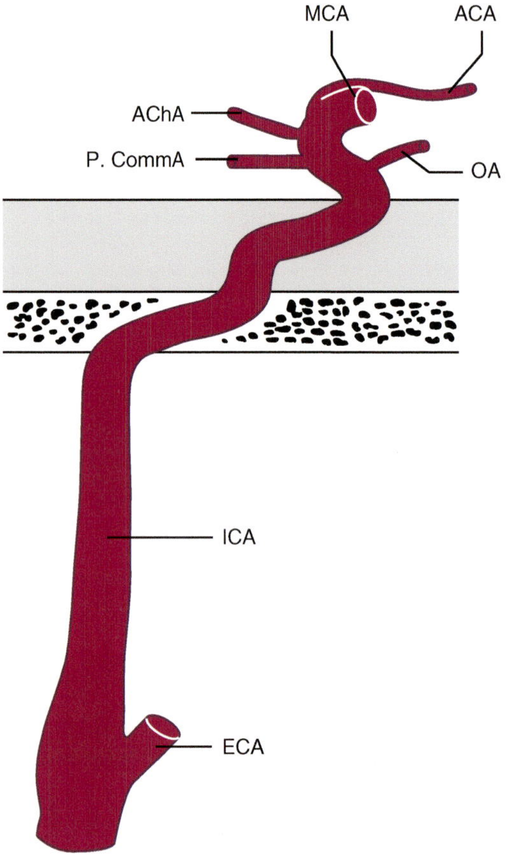

Fig. 2.1 Anterior circulation of brain [3]

Table 2.1 Anterior circulation arteries and its blood supply

Cerebral artery	Blood supply
Anterior cerebral artery (ACA)	Medial side of the frontal lobes and superior medial parietal lobes
Posterior communicating arteries	Medial thalamic surface and the walls of the third ventricle
Anterior Choroidal Arteries	Crus cerebri of the midbrain, lateral geniculate body, choroid plexus of the lateral ventricles and third ventricle, Globus pallidus, caudate nucleus, amygdala, hypothalamus, red nucleus, substantia nigra, posterior limb of the internal capsule, optic tract, hippocampus
Ophthalmic arteries	Supplies all the structure of the orbit and meninges
Middle cerebral arteries	Anterior temporal lobes, insular and lateral cerebral cortex

Table 2.2 Showing ICA segments [4]

Segment of ICA	Name
C1	Cervical
C2	Petrous
C3	Lacerum
C4	Cavernous
C5	Clinoid
C6	Ophthalmic
C7	Terminal communicating

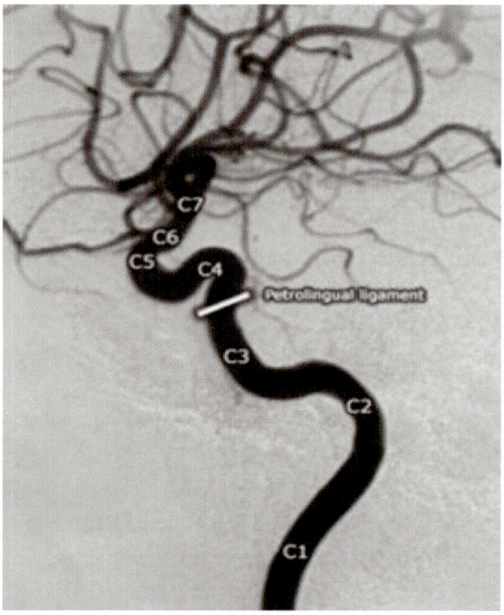

Fig. 2.2 Internal carotid artery and its segments [4]

2.2.2 The Bouthillier Classification

This classification is useful in describing the internal carotid artery (ICA) aneurysm, pathologies and divided into the seven segments as shown in Table 2.2 and Fig. 2.2.

2.3 Posterior Circulation

Both the vertebral arteries arise from the respective subclavian arteries, proceed to enter the transverse foramen of the cervical spines at the C5 level and after passing through the C1 foramen, both vertebral arteries enter through cranium and at the base of pons join to form single basilar artery thus forming the posterior circulation of brain (Fig. 2.3) [3]. Before forming the

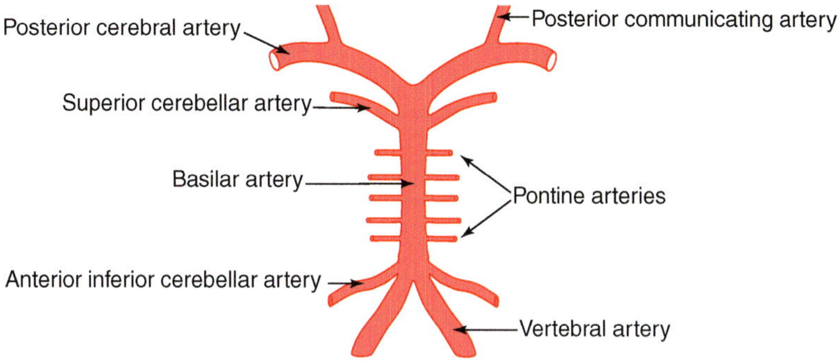

Fig. 2.3 Posterior circulation of brain [3]

Table 2.3 The branches of posterior circulation arteries and their area of blood supply [5]

Brach artery	Area supplied
Posterior inferior cerebellar artery (PICA)	It is the largest branch of the vertebral artery. It is one of the three main arteries that supplies blood to the cerebellum, a part of the brain
Anterior inferior cerebellar artery (AICA)	Pairs of arteries that supply blood to the cerebellum
Pontine branches	These are a number of small vessels which come off at right angles from either side of the basilar artery and supply the pons and adjacent parts of the brain
Superior cerebellar artery (SCA)	Arises near the termination of the basilar artery. Blood supply to the superior half of the cerebellum and the parts of the midbrain
Posterior cerebral artery (PCA)	Pair of arteries that supply oxygenated blood to the occipital lobe, part of the back of the human brain

basilar artery the vertebral artery gives rise to the posterior inferior cerebellar artery (PICA) The posterior circulation of brain is responsible for supplying the oxygenated blood to occipital lobe, cerebellum, and brain stem (Table 2.3).

2.4 Circle of Willis (COW)

Nearly 400 years back COW was described. It is a compensatory arterial circle formed by the arteries at the base of brain. COW compensates up to some extent in the case of obstruction to one of the component arteries. Typically it is important in older patients who have limited ability to compensate acute changes and thus are at a greater risk for developing ischemic stroke or brain hypoperfusion [6]. Approximately 1:3 patients have a complete COW, up to 50% of healthy patients and 80% of the patients with dysfunctional brain have at least one artery which is underdeveloped or absent. The topological anomalies of COW may be fused arteries, string-like vessels, missing communicating vessels, and presence of an extra artery [7].

The simplified anatomy of the COW is, the three major arteries going into the circle of Willis are the major anterior and posterior circulation arteries namely two internal carotids and one basilar artery. Six arteries leave the COW in pairs, anterior cerebral arteries, middle cerebral arteries and posterior communicating arteries. The three arteries completing the COW are two posterior communicating arteries and one anterior communicating artery (Fig. 2.4).

2.5 Venous Drainage from Brain

The venous drainage of brain is different the rest of the organs in the body. The brain veins are not following the arteries, lack in muscular layer and the valves [8].

The brain parenchymal venous drainage is divided into the superficial and deep veins. The superficial veins drain from the cerebral cortex, while deep veins drain the blood from deeper and internal structures of the brain, namely thalamus, hypothalamus, internal capsule, septum, corpus striates, white matter and the choroid plexuses [8]. The venous sinus is a peculiarity of venous drainage of the brain (channels of a branching complex sinus network that lies in the subarachnoid space and functions to collect venous blood).

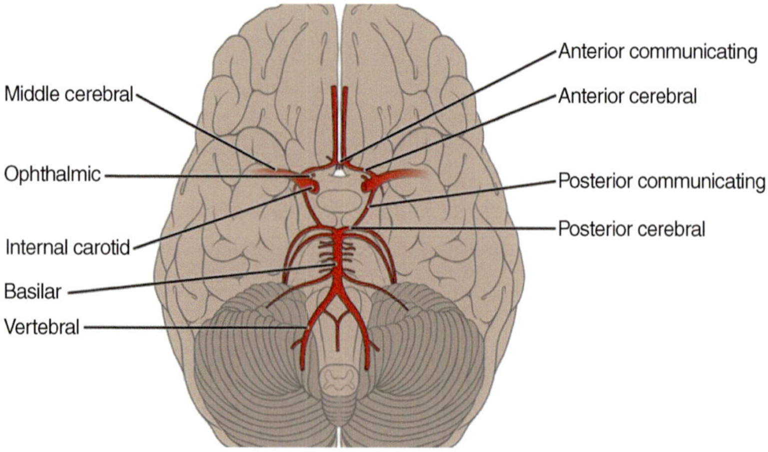

Fig. 2.4 Circle of Willis (COW) [6, 7]

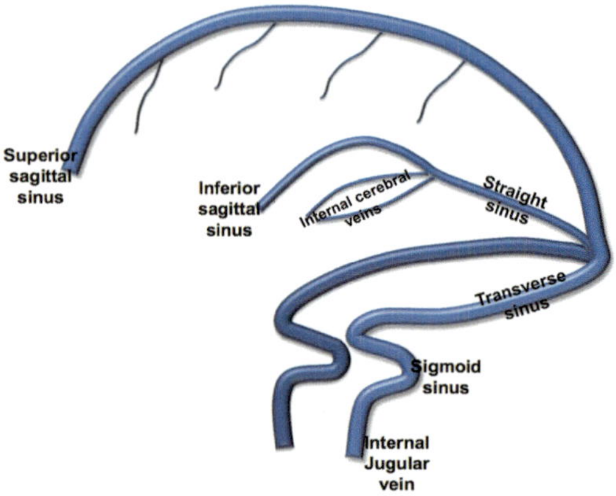

Fig. 2.5 Cerebral venous sinuses [8]

The superficial venous system drains into the sagittal sinus, whereas the deeper veins drain into transverse, straight, and the sigmoid sinuses (Fig. 2.5) [8]. As these sinuses are closely related to the venous drainage of the nasal sinuses, cerebral sinuses can get infected by retrograde bacterial transmission causing sinus thrombosis.

2.6 Cerebrospinal Fluid (CSF)

Brain floats in the cerebrospinal fluid (CSF), CSF cushions the brain in the skull bone and serves as a shock absorber for the central nervous system, it also circulates nutrients and chemicals filtered from the blood and up to some state removes waste products from the brain [9]. CSF is secreted at the rate of around 25 ml/hour and at any given time there is around 125 ml of the CSF in the brain. It is secreted by the choroid plexuses in lateral ventricles by diffusion, pinocytosis, and active transfer. Choroid plexuses are the nothing but tufts of capillaries within thin fenestrated endothelial cells. CSF circulation is helped by the pulsation in choroidal plexuses [9]. As CSF is formed from the plasma, it contains 2/3rd of the glucose level compared to the plasma and it is a protein free fluid in physiological circumstances. CSF circulation is shown in Fig. 2.6, and finally gets absorbed into the subarachnoid granulation or villi and drains into the superior sagittal sinuses. CSF pressure is maintained in range of 8–15 mm of Hg. CSF leakage will drop the intracranial pressure and obstruction to the flow of CSF will increase the intracranial pressure and lead to hydrocephalus.

2.7 Blood–Brain Barrier (BB)

Blood–brain barrier (BBB) is a carrier as well as a barrier. The carrier function of BBB is carrying nutrients to the brain and removing the products of cellular metabolism. The barrier function is by restricting the transfer of harmful substances to the brain [10].

BBB is formed by endothelial cells, which form a continuous sheet covering the surface of capillaries, and tight junctions to form a belt like structure interconnect endothelium. The endothelium is engulfed in the basal membrane called

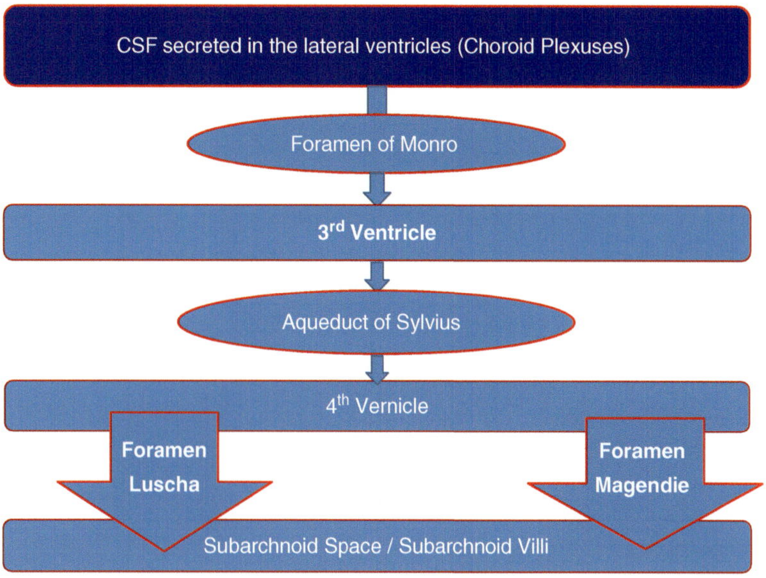

Fig. 2.6 CSF circulation

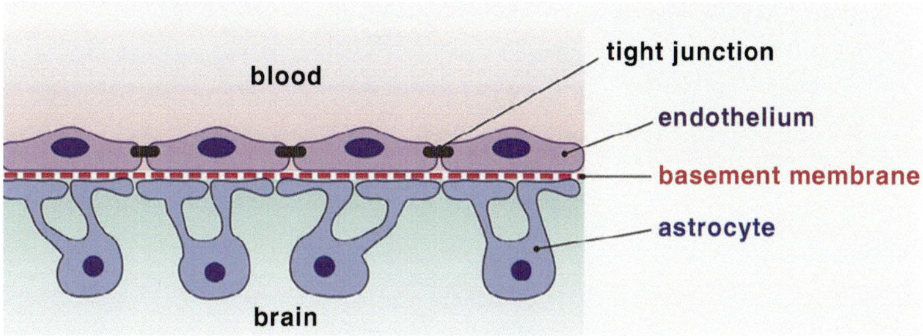

Fig. 2.7 The blood brain barrier

pericytes. Pericytes cover approximately 32% of the endothelium. Pericytes regulate proliferation, angiogenesis, and inflammatory processes. Tight junctions strengthen and maintain control on astrocytes and pericytes (Fig. 2.7). Hence the BBB stabilizes the environment for the proper brain cellular function, facilitates neurotransmission, prevents macromolecules entry into the brain, protects brain from the neurotoxic substances, and allows immune-surveillance and response with a minimal cell damage and inflammation [10].

2.8 Conclusion

Human brain is a vital organ in the body, hence well protected in the bony skull covered with meninges and floats in the cerebrospinal fluid (CSF).

The uninterrupted blood circulation is essential for normal brain function. Blood supply of the brain is unique. Anterior circulation comes from a pair of internal carotid arteries and the posterior circulation is from the basilar artery formed by joining of two vertebral arteries. Both anterior and posterior circulation arteries join and form the circle of Willis (COW) and provide blood supply to the brain. COW ensures and compensates the blood supply in case of obstruction to one the component arteries. Due to hemodynamic stress outpouching of one or multiple cerebral arteries occurs to form the cerebral aneurysms.

The venous drainage from the brain is through the superficial and deep veins of the brain. Blood from cerebrum and internal brain parts get drained into sagittal and sigmoid sinuses, respectively. Venous blood from cerebral sinuses goes to internal jugular veins and ultimately reaches to the heart and lungs.

CSF is secreted from the lateral ventricles by the choroidal plexuses and circulates through brain and spinal cords before getting absorbed by the subarachnoid villi. Any obstruction to the CSF flow will lead to increased intracranial pressure and hydrocephalus.

Blood–brain barrier protects and restricts the particles circulating in the blood reaching the brain. The BBB is formed by the specific anatomy of the astrocytes held together by tight junctions, which maintains the homeostasis in the brain.

References

1. Haddad-Tóvolli R, Dragano NRV, Ramalho AFS, Velloso LA. Development and function of the blood-brain barrier in the context of metabolic control. Front Neurosci. 2017;11:224.
2. Armstead WM. Cerebral blood flow autoregulation and dysautoregulation. Anesthesiol Clin. 2016;34(3):465–77.
3. Menshawi K, Mohr JP, Gutierrez J. A functional perspective on the embryology and anatomy of the cerebral blood supply. J Stroke. 2015;17(2):144–58.
4. Bouthillier A, van Loveren HR, Keller JT. Segments of the internal carotid artery: a new classification. Neurosurgery. 1996;38(3):425–32.
5. Akgun A, Battal B, Bozkurt Y, Oguzhan OZ, Hamcans SS, Akgun H. Normal anatomical features and variations of the vertebrobasilar circulation and its branches: an analysis with 64-detector row CT and 3T MR angiographies. Sci World J. 2013;2013:7.
6. Vrselja Z, Brkic H, Mrdenovic S, Radic R, Curic G. Function of circle of Willis. J Cereb Blood Flow Metab. 2014;34(4):578–84.
7. Alpers BJ, Berry PG, Paddison RM. Anatomical studies if circle of Willis in normal brain. AMA Arch Neur Psych. 1959;81(4):409–18.
8. Piazza G. Cerebral venous thrombosis. Circulation. 2012;125:1704–9.
9. Pollay M. The function and structure of the cerebrospinal fluid outflow system. Cerebrospinal Fluid Res. 2010;7:9.
10. Daneman R, Prat A. The blood-brain barrier. Cold Spring Harb Perspect Biol. 2015;7(1):a020412.

Central Nervous System Neurophysiology

3

Pragasan Dean Gopalan and Alexa de Castro

3.1 Introduction

The human nervous system mediates a wide range of functions essential for survival and well-being. The approximately 10^{11} neurons in the human brain offer limitless potential for the creation of complex neuronal circuits and inter-connectivity.

Neurophysiology refers to the study of neurons, and their various arrangements into nerves and nervous systems, describing their functions and the mechanisms by which they achieve these functions. When this is restricted to the brain and its various structures in the central nervous system (CNS), it may be termed central neurophysiology. A clear understanding of central neurophysiology is relevant to better appreciate the variety of pathophysiological states, including subarachnoid haemorrhage, that affect the brain.

P. D. Gopalan (✉)
Anaesthesiology and Critical Care, Nelson R Mandela School of Medicine, UKZN, Berea, South Africa
e-mail: Gopalan@ukzn.ac.za

A. de Castro
Inkosi Albert Luthuli Central Hospital, and Honorary Lecturer, Discipline, Anaesthesiology and Critical Care, Nelson R Mandela School of Medicine, UKZN, Berea, South Africa

3.2 Electrophysiology

A neuron is a specialised cell with two fundamental properties that define its functioning and importance, namely excitability and conductivity. Excitability of a neuron refers to its ability to respond to changes in or stimuli from the environment; conductivity is the ability to transmit or convey an impulse, action potential or state of excitation from one part of the cell to another. This section addresses the basic principles of neuro-electrophysiology.

3.2.1 Neuron Structure

Neuronal signals are transmitted as electrical signals by a vast network of neurons in the central and peripheral nervous system. Fibre-like processes called dendrites receive and transmit signals to the cell body, where proteins are synthesised in the basophilic granules (Nissl substances) of the rough endoplasmic reticulum. A fibre-like structure called an axon, leaves the cell body and consists of axoplasm filled with mitochondria, microtubules, neurofilaments and smooth endoplasmic reticulum. The axon ends in a nerve terminal, where neurotransmitters are released to bind with receptors on target tissue (Fig. 3.1) [2]. An axon may or may not be surrounded by a myelin sheath. Myelin sheaths consist of Schwann cells that surround the axon and slow the conduction of

A. E. A. Ganaw et al. (eds.), *Management of Subarachnoid Hemorrhage*,
https://doi.org/10.1007/978-3-030-81333-8_3

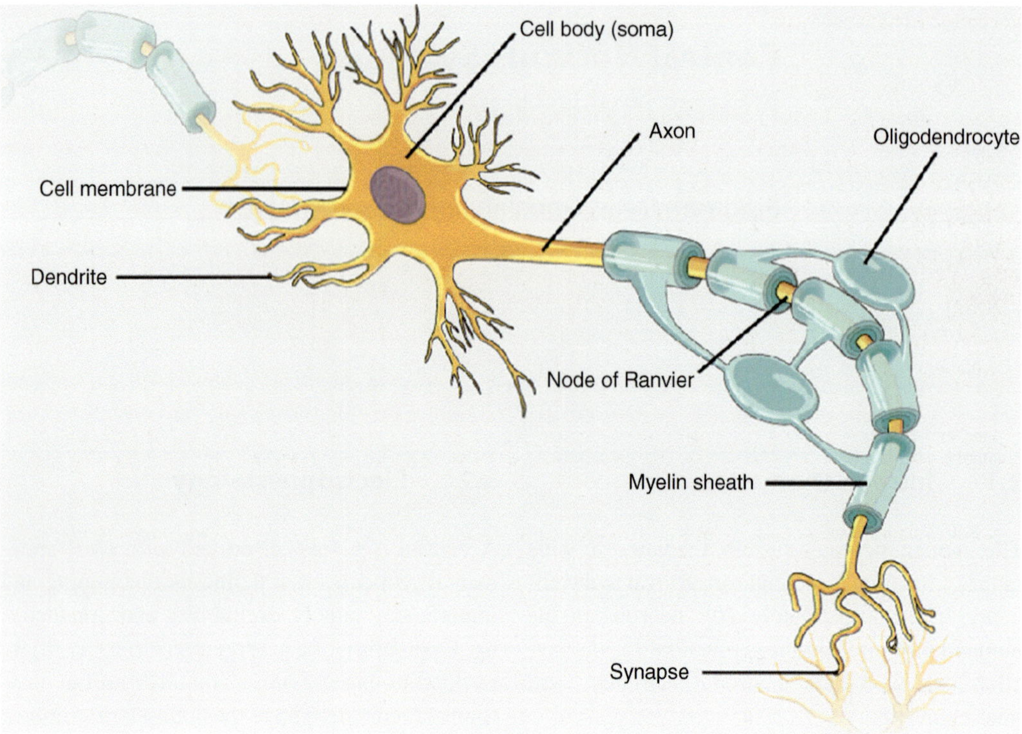

Fig. 3.1 Basic anatomy of a neuron (From OpenStax College [1]—Creative Commons Attribution 4.0 International License)

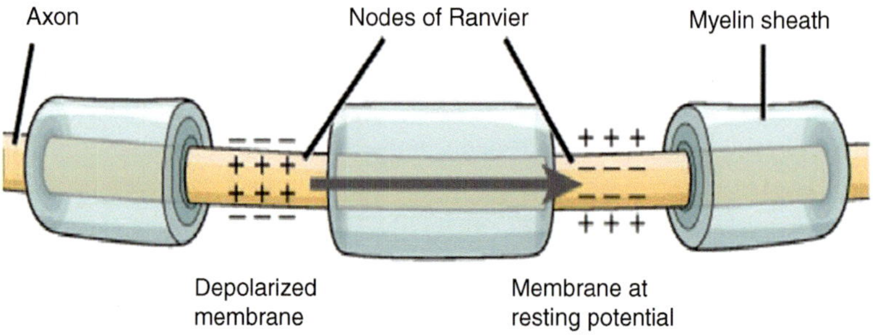

Fig. 3.2 Anatomy of a myelinated nerve fibre with nodes of Ranvier (From OpenStax College [3]—Creative Commons Attribution 4.0 International License)

electrical signals by reducing ion transfer through the axonal membrane (Fig. 3.2). The junction between two adjacent Schwann cells is interrupted by a node of Ranvier, a small uninsulated area consisting of closely packed sodium channels, allowing for fast passage of ions. Electrical action potentials are able to jump between these nodes, referred to as saltatory conduction, resulting in increased velocity of nerve signal transmission with limited energy expenditure.

3.2.2 The Resting Membrane Potential

During the resting state, the electrical difference across a selectively permeable membrane is determined by the difference in ion concentrations on either sides of the membrane. This is called the resting membrane potential and in nervous system cells is determined by the relatively higher intracellular concentration of K^+ ions

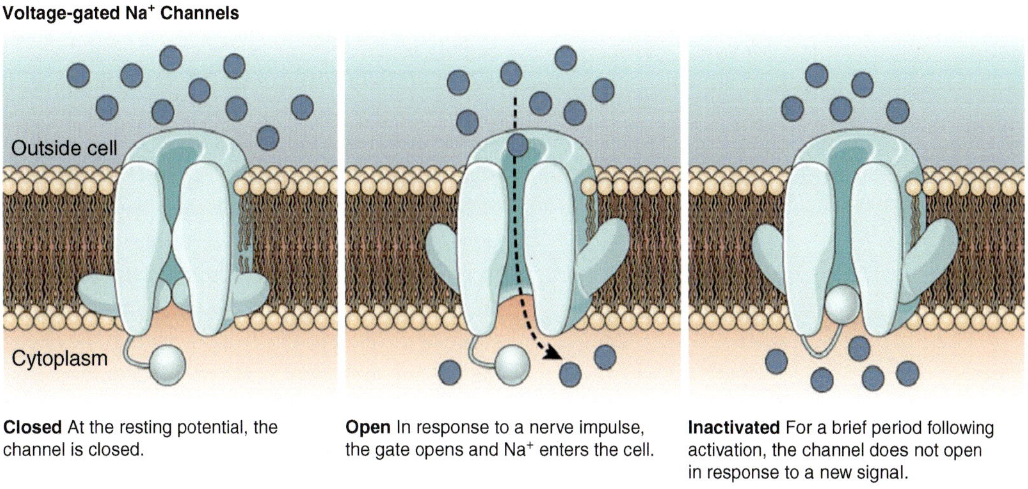

Fig. 3.3 Voltage-gated sodium channels showing successive activation and inactivation during an action potential (From OpenStax College [3]—Creative Commons Attribution 4.0 International License)

compared to the relatively higher extracellular concentration of Na^+ ions. The resting membrane potential is maintained by the active Na^+/K^+/ATPase transport mechanism that is present in all cells of the human body. A net deficit of positive ions inside the cell is maintained by the continual pumping of three sodium ions outwards in exchange for two potassium ions inward, and creates the negative resting membrane potential of about −90 mV. This sets up large concentration gradients across the resting cell membrane, ready for activation of an action potential.

3.2.3 Depolarisation

Any stimuli, including mechanical, chemical, or electrical stimuli, that can cause a rapid change in the membrane potential by influencing permeability of the sodium and potassium ion channels, can generate electrochemical impulses necessary to transmit nerve signals. Each action potential begins with depolarisation, creating a change from the negative membrane potential to a more positive potential. An action potential will only develop if a threshold potential of between −70 and −50 mV is reached, at which point a conformational change of the voltage-gated sodium channels occur, activating the voltage-gated channel to an open state. Sodium ions stream into the cell at a high rate, causing the opening of more sodium channels (Fig. 3.3). The membrane potential quickly depolarises to about +30 mV. The inactivation gate of the sodium channel is activated at the same time but the conformational change is slower, allowing the passage of sodium ions before closing (Fig. 3.4). No further passage of sodium ions is allowed and opening of the inactivation gate will not occur until the resting membrane potential is reached, thereby avoiding any further action potentials until repolarisation is complete, also called the refractory period.

3.2.4 Repolarisation

When the membrane potential increases toward 0 mV, a conformational opening of the potassium channels occur just as the sodium channels start to close. This allows the rapid movement of potassium ions out of the cell, rapidly restoring the membrane potential back to −90 mV. At this point the potassium channels return to their resting closed state. The active Na+/K+ ATPase channel is responsible for re-establishing the sodium and potassium ion gradients of the resting state, ready for the next action potential.

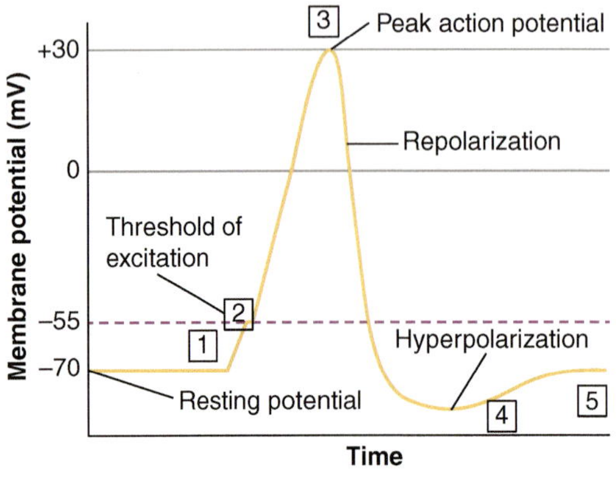

Fig. 3.4 Typical voltage changes during an action potential. The formation of an action potential can be divided into five steps: (1) A stimulus from a sensory cell or another neuron causes the target cell to depolarise toward the threshold potential. (2) If the threshold of excitation is reached, all Na^+ channels open and the membrane depolarises. (3) At the peak action potential, K^+ channels open and K^+ begins to leave the cell. At the same time, Na^+ channels close. (4) The membrane becomes hyperpolarised as K^+ ions continue to leave the cell. The hyperpolarised membrane is in a refractory period and cannot fire. (5) The K^+ channels close and the Na^+/K^+ transporter restores the resting potential. (From OpenStax College [3]—Creative Commons Attribution 4.0 International License)

3.2.5 Nerve Impulse

Propagation of the action potential occurs as the depolarisation process spreads along the nerve fibre, exciting the adjacent membrane. This occurs in one direction only, spreading along the entire length of the fibre, and is called the nerve impulse. The velocity of the nerve impulse is increased in myelinated fibres and is also accelerated in axons of larger diameter.

3.2.6 Synaptic Transmission

The connection between a nerve terminal and other nerves, muscles or glands, is called a synapse, and permits the transmission of a neural impulse from one nerve to another. Transmission in mammals occur via chemical neurotransmission. Impulses can be received from several nerves (convergence) or may be transmitted via synaptic contact with many other neurons (divergence) The action potential is propagated along the axon, reaching the nerve terminal to open voltage-gated calcium channels which release neurotransmitter from vesicles into the synaptic cleft via a process called exocytosis. Thereafter, the neurotransmitters diffuse across the cleft to bind to receptors on the post-synaptic cleft either opening ion channels or activating a second messenger system (Fig. 3.5). Neurotransmitter activity in the synaptic cleft is terminated by enzymatic breakdown, reuptake into the presynaptic membrane or diffusion away from the site. If the opening of ion channels resulted in depolarisation reaching the threshold potential, the action potential is further transmitted along the new nerve.

3.3 Cerebral Metabolism

A description of cerebral metabolism under normal conditions allows for a better understanding of metabolic responses to pathological states. This section reviews the basic principles of cerebral metabolism.

The brain is one of the most metabolically active of all organs in the body. The regulation of cellular energy metabolism and metabolic supply is essential to the highly dynamic energy consumption of the CNS that is needed for cellular function and generation of electrophysiological signals. Increased neuronal activity requires adequate delivery of oxygen and nutrients to meet the increased consumption of energy. Concurrently, compensatory metabolic and vascular mechanisms are initiated to enhance neuronal function [4]. Tight metabolic control is essential for normal brain function and survival. The relationship between metabolism and neuronal activity likely involves various complex regulatory pathways [5].

3.3.1 Oxygen

The brain is the largest consumer of energy in the body. With a mass of only 2–3% (1200–1400 g) of total body mass, the brain uses 20% of the total body oxygen consumption, 25% of total glucose consumption, and receives 15–20% of the car-

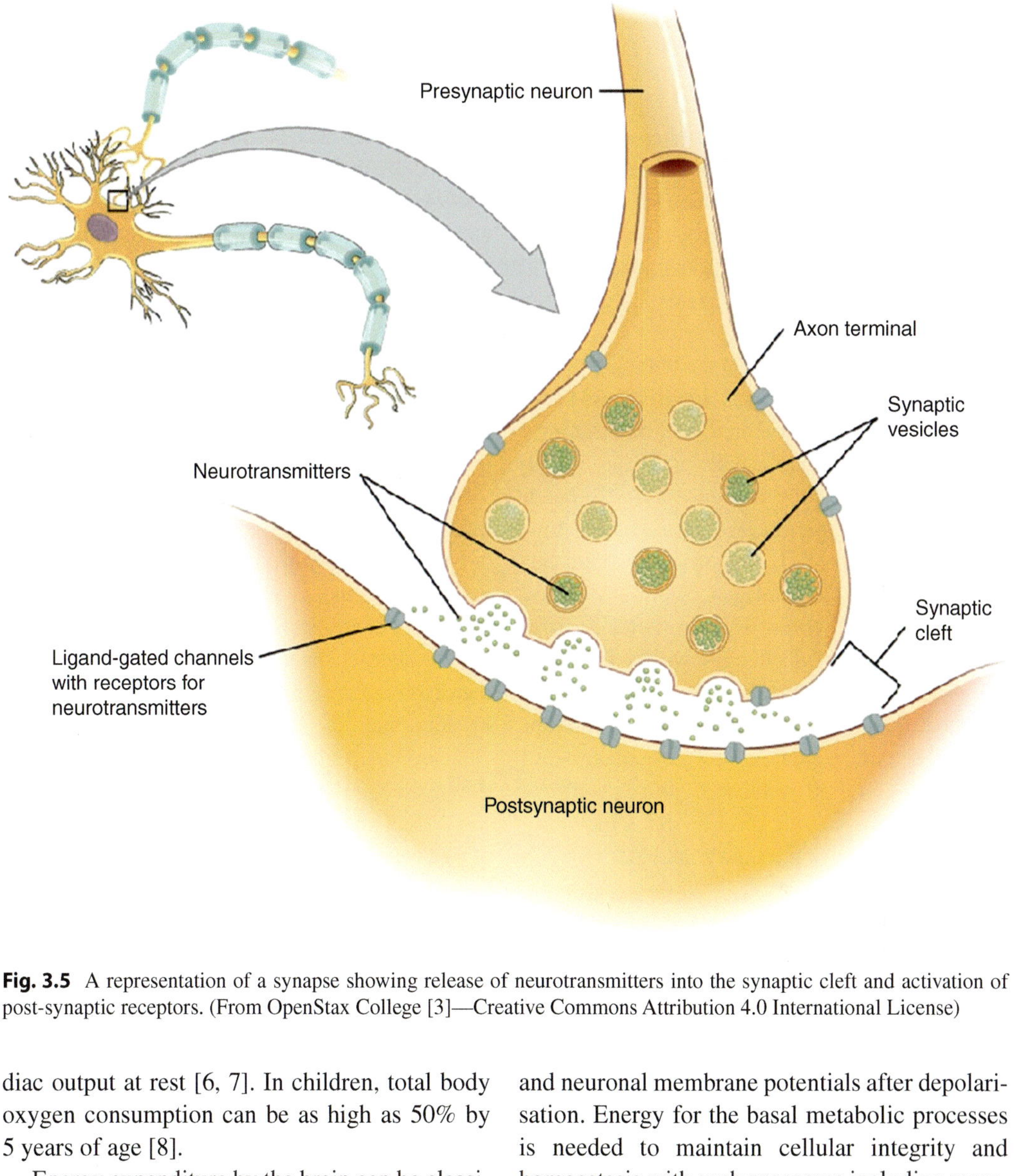

Fig. 3.5 A representation of a synapse showing release of neurotransmitters into the synaptic cleft and activation of post-synaptic receptors. (From OpenStax College [3]—Creative Commons Attribution 4.0 International License)

diac output at rest [6, 7]. In children, total body oxygen consumption can be as high as 50% by 5 years of age [8].

Energy expenditure by the brain can be classified into two broad categories: (1) "activation energy" is the energy expended by the brain in the work of generating electric signals and consumes 55% of the total cerebral energy consumption and (2) basal metabolic processes consume the remaining 45% of the brain's energy production [9]. The "activation energy" is used to generate adenosine triphosphate (ATP) and support neuronal electrical activity. This energy is primarily utilised at the synapse to drive ion pumps and sustain and restore ionic gradients and neuronal membrane potentials after depolarisation. Energy for the basal metabolic processes is needed to maintain cellular integrity and homeostasis with such processes including membrane stabilisation, ion pumping to preserve membrane ion gradients, and synthesis of structural and functional molecules [10]. Neurotransmitter synthesis, vesicle recycling, and axoplasmic transport contribute to the elevated metabolic requirements in neurons [5].

The normal human brain consumes oxygen at a rate of 156 μmol/100 g tissue/min in the conscious state. The production of CO_2 is the same, leading to a respiratory quotient of quotient of 1.0 [11]. The cerebral metabolic rate (CMR) of oxygen consumption ($CMRO_2$) in a normal, conscious, young adult is approximately 3.5 ml/100 g brain/min with a range of 3–3.8 ml/100 g/min equating to approximately 50 ml/min in adults. This energy consumption continues throughout the day and night and may be increased during rapid eye movement (REM) sleep [5, 8]. Energy requirements are not uniformly spread throughout the CNS. Requirements parallel cortical electrical activity and are greatest in the grey matter of the cerebral cortex.

The brain is absolutely dependent on an uninterrupted supply of oxygen to drive oxidative metabolism for the maintenance of structural and functional integrity. The brain has no O_2 stores itself, and unconsciousness will occur after 10 s of complete cessation of blood flow. The critical level of O_2 tension in the brain lies between 15 and 20 mmHg. Cessation of blood flow is followed within a few minutes by irreversible pathological changes within the brain [8]. Within 3–8 min all ATP stores will be depleted, leading to irreversible injury. The hippocampus and cerebellum are most sensitive to this injury. Cerebral metabolism of oxygen may be impaired in various disease states including stroke, traumatic brain injury, and Alzheimer's disease [11].

3.3.2 Energy Substrates

Most tissues in the body operate facultatively in choosing energy substrates with an ability to use such substrates interchangeably according to their availability. The brain does possess the capacity to utilise various substrates for metabolism to generate the energy requirements for its numerous needs. Such substrates include glucose, ketone bodies, lactate, glycerol, fatty acids, and amino acids. However, in vivo the brain appears inflexible in substrate choice with glucose, by far, the primary source of energy.

The rate of brain glucose utilisation is estimated as 31 μmol/100 g/min [12]. Carrier-mediated mechanisms account for the majority of glucose transport with only 4% of glucose entering via simple diffusion [9]. The transport of glucose through cell membranes of neurons is not dependent on insulin.

Cellular respiration to metabolise glucose for energy release in the form of ATP occurs in two sequential phases. Glycolysis occurs in the cytosol of cells without the influence of oxygen and results in the production of two molecules of ATP and pyruvate per molecule of glucose, the pyruvate being subsequently converted to lactate. Oxidative phosphorylation occurs on the inner mitochondrial membrane and, in the presence of oxygen, produces 36 molecules of ATP. In the resting brain, aerobic metabolism accounts for 99% of energy production and is directly related to glucose consumption [10].

Cerebral glycogen stores are limited to approximately 0.3–0.4 μmol/100 g tissue [13] providing only a 2-min supply of glucose generated from glycogen in the neurons. Glucose deprivation results in aberrations of cerebral function with mental state changes from mild sensory disturbances to coma. These clinical effects, paralleled by abnormalities in EEG patterns and the CMR [12], are independent of decreased cerebral blood flow (CBF). In special situations, the energy needs of the brain may be partly fulfilled with substrates other than glucose. During starvation and ketosis, for example, ketone bodies (acetoacetate and β-hydroxybutyrate) become the major source of energy substrates [14].

In the brain, as in other tissues, glycolysis results in pyruvate that is subsequently converted into lactate. In some situations, such as immediately after injury, there may be a relative increase in glycolysis, termed "hyperglycolysis" that leads to increased lactate production [15]. The CMR for lactate depends on the balance between production, uptake, and disposal [16]. In humans the extent of lactate production is typically overlooked because production is balanced by removal rate. However, the role of lactate may be under-appreciated. Lactate may have a significant role in normal and pathophysiological states.

3.3.3 Neurometabolic Coupling

Lactate exchange, termed "lactate shuttle", may occur among various cellular sites of production and removal [17]. It has been postulated that a similar process occurs in the brain [18]. Such exchanges among neurons and other cells depend on the metabolic rates within cells and on the extracellular environment influenced by cellular metabolism and vascular delivery and removal [19]. Cellular compartmentalisation of bioenergetics has been suggested with different phases occurring in different cell types [20]. Glucose in the cerebral circulation is thought to be primarily consumed anaerobically by astrocytes. The resultant lactate released into the extracellular space is thought to be consumed aerobically by neurons [21]. The close association of astrocytes with capillaries and neuronal synaptic clefts allow them to crucially regulate neurometabolic coupling during neuronal activity by, for example, maintaining neurotransmitter stores via the glutamine-glutamate cycle [5]. This is supported by distinct gene expression patterns and expressions of, for example, lactate transporter proteins in astrocytes and neurons. This coupling of neuronal activity to astrocytic glycolysis suggests a far more complex cerebral bioenergetic process than previously considered.

3.4 Cerebral Blood Flow (CBF)

Total CBF in adults is approximately 50 ml/100 g tissue/min with a range of 50–60 ml/100 g/min [22]. Levels are usually higher in children and adolescents and decreases with age [23]. The flow varies to the different tissues with grey matter receiving 80 ml/100 g/min and white matter 20 ml/100 g/min. Total CBF is thus approximately 750 ml/min (range 750–900) in an adult which constitutes 15–20% of the cardiac output. The brain does not tolerate any major drop in perfusion. A CBF of less than 20–25 ml/100 g/min can lead to cerebral impairment. Flows of 15–20 ml/100 g/min cause a flat EEG, and anything less than 10 ml/100 g/min will cause irreversible brain damage.

The CBF depends on the arterial blood pressure, the intracranial pressure (ICP), or back pressure in the cerebral venous system, and the resistance of the small cerebral vessels. Cerebral vessels rapidly adapt to the chemical environment of the brain, neuronal signals and to pressures within the vessels themselves. Maintenance of optimal CBF relies on the relationship between cardiovascular, respiratory, and neurological physiology [22].

3.4.1 Cerebral Metabolic Rate of Oxygen Consumption

The lack of significant brain storage capacity necessitates tight coupling of cerebral metabolism, CBF, and oxygen extraction. Fick's equation best describes this relationship:

$$CMRO_2 = CBF \times AVDO_2$$

($CMRO_2$ = cerebral metabolic rate of oxygen; CBF = cerebral blood flow; $AVDO_2$ = arterio-venous difference of oxygen)

The CBF thus varies with brain metabolic activity (Fig. 3.6). Neurovascular and neurometabolic coupling mechanisms enhance blood flow and utilisation of metabolism to compensate for varying energy demands throughout the brain [5]. Regional CBF is directly related to metabolic activity in that area, e.g. moving an arm. Regional blood flow ranges from 10 to 300 ml/100 g/min. This flow-metabolism coupling or "functional hyperaemia" may be the most relevant of the CBF regulation mechanisms, as cerebral tissue is among the least tolerant of ischemia [25].

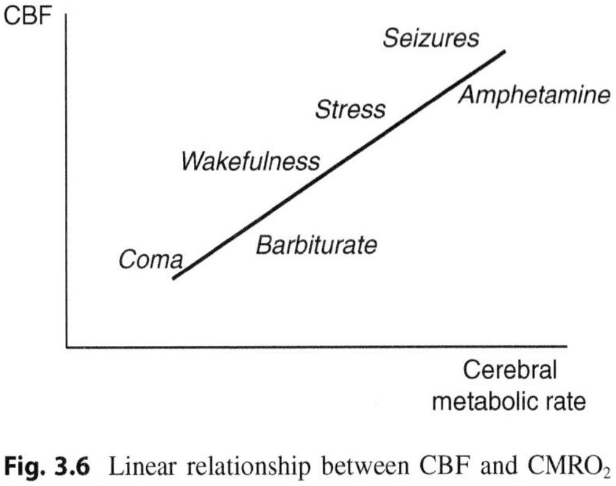

Fig. 3.6 Linear relationship between CBF and $CMRO_2$ (From Nordstrom et al. [24]—Creative Commons Attribution 4.0 International License)

3.4.2 Cerebral Perfusion Pressure

The pressure that supplies the cerebral vessels is dependent on arterial blood pressure, which in turn is dependent on factors outside the brain, namely cardiac output and the peripheral vascular resistance. Any physiological or pathological event affecting these factors has the potential to affect CBF. The CBF is also impaired by conditions that increase ICP or impede cerebral venous outflow. Cerebral perfusion pressure (CPP) is therefore related to both the mean arterial pressure and the back pressure, i.e. the higher of either ICP or CVP (central venous pressure):

$$\text{CPP} = \text{MAP} - \text{ICP} \ (\text{or CVP if higher})$$

The normal CPP is approximately 80–100 mmHg. Levels of ICP >30 mmHg compromise CPP and CBF. Levels of CPP <50 mmHg demonstrate slowing on EEG, 25–40 mmHg produce a flat EEG, and <25 mmHg cause irreversible brain damage.

3.4.3 Autoregulation

Cerebral autoregulation is the homeostatic phenomenon under normal conditions whereby cerebral vessel caliber is changed in response to changes in cerebral metabolism and/or CPP in order to regulate and maintain a constant CBF across a range of blood pressures. Cerebral vascularity has the ability to rapidly adapt to changes within 10–60 s. A decreased CPP will cause cerebral vasodilation, whereas an increased CPP will lead to vasoconstriction.

The CBF is maintained at a constant level between mean arterial pressures (MAP) of 60–160 mmHg. For MAPs outside these limits, CBF becomes pressure dependent (Fig. 3.7). Levels of MAP >150–160 mmHg can disrupt the blood–brain barrier (BBB) and may cause cerebral oedema or haemorrhage. In chronic hypertensive patients, this curve is shifted to the right to offer protection to the higher arterial pressures.

The major site of active regulation is thought to be at the level of the arterioles because of the thick smooth muscle layer and the ability to rapidly constrict and dilate. Conversely cerebral veins and venules have a low density of smooth muscle cells and react to increases in pressure with increasing volume. In healthy individuals, this is most evident during neuronal activity which elicits a significant increase in CBF through vessel dilation. However, during ischaemic stroke or vasospasm, cerebral arteries constrict, causing a local increase in cerebral vascular

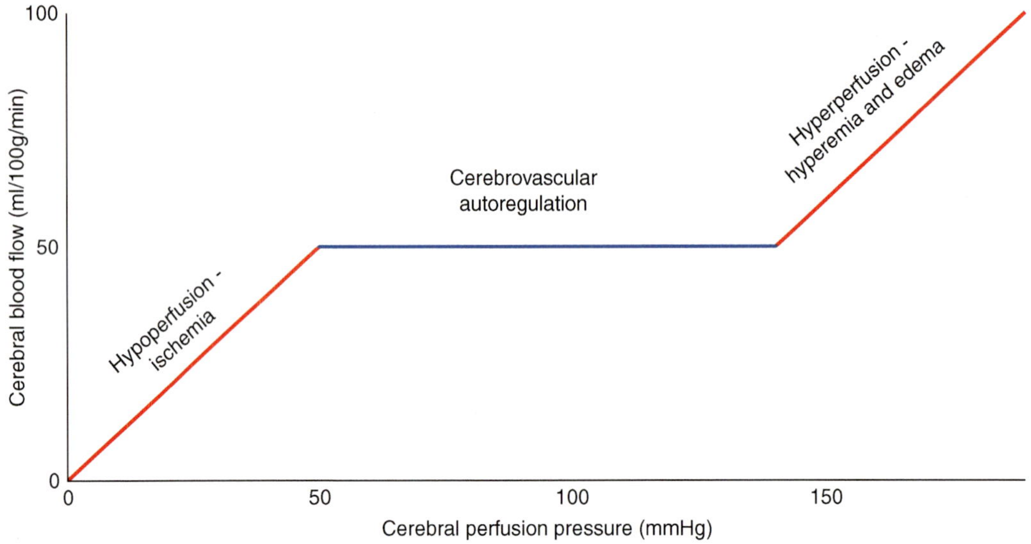

Fig. 3.7 Relationship between CBF and MAP (From Harary et al. [26]—Creative Commons Attribution 4.0 International License)

resistance and, by extension, a decrease in CBF [22].

Various mechanisms have been proposed to account for the changes in vascular tone of cerebral vessels. The myogenic mechanism proposes a response of vascular smooth muscle to transmural pressure changes that occurs through arterial membrane depolarisation, with a resultant change in the concentration of Ca^{2+} in the arterial wall [27]. The metabolic mechanism proposes that altered concentrations of vasoactive metabolites (such as adenosine) resulting from initial blood pressure-induced changes in blood flow accounts for changes in vascular calibre [28]. In the neurogenic mechanism, perivascular neurons are proposed to have autoregulatory effects on cerebral arterioles via an extensive arborisation of perivascular nerves [29].

Neurovascular coupling, first described by Roy and Sherrington, refers to the relationship between local neural activity and subsequent changes in CBF [4]. The exact mechanism for this activity-coupled increases in local CBF remains unclear. Glutamate release following synaptic transmission may be a key stimulus for neurovascular coupling through production of vasoactive metabolites which include arachidonic acid derivatives, adenosine, lactate and nitric oxide. These substances produce changes in intracellular calcium concentration in the smooth muscle fibres of the arterioles or capillaries, altering the degree of vessel constriction [22]. Of these metabolites, nitric oxide (•NO) may play a key role [30]. Astrocytes are also thought to play a key role in regulating blood flow. The processes from these cells ensheath brain capillaries. During neuronal activation, Ca^{2+} release triggered at astrocytic end feet induces pathways downstream that regulate vasodilation [31].

3.4.4 Extrinsic Regulatory Mechanisms

3.4.4.1 Respiratory Gas Tensions

Blood and CSF tension of respiratory gases affect cerebral blood flow (Fig. 3.8). Cerebral vasculature is extremely sensitive to changes in $PaCO_2$ and levels between 20 and 60 mmHg are directly related to CBF. A decrease in $PaCO_2$ constricts cerebral resistance vessels, while an increase leads to dilation. The CBF increases by 1–2 ml/100 g/min per mmHg change in $PaCO_2$. A 70% increase in $PaCO_2$ doubles CBF. Extracellular H+ concentration resulting from diffusion of $PaCO_2$ probably plays an important role. Changes in CBF secondary to fluctuations in the pH of CSF and brain tissue occur immediately. $PaCO_2$ of <20 mmHg shifts the oxyhaemoglobin dissociation curve to the left and may cause cerebral impairment. The PaO_2 only influences CBF if

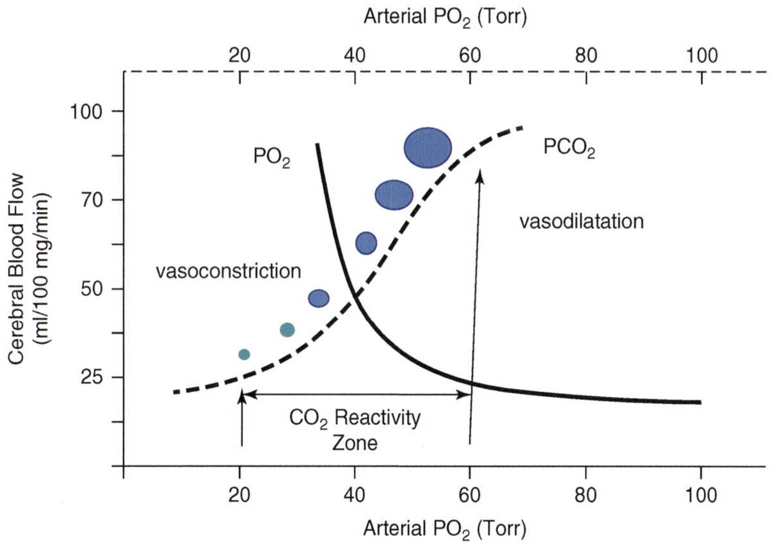

Fig. 3.8 Relationship between CBF and respiratory gas tensions. The autoregulatory curve depicting CBF according to shifting $PaCO_2$ resembles a sigmoid function with a CO_2 reactivity zone between 20 and 60 mmHg. (1 Torr = 1 mmHg). (From Godoy et al. [32]—Creative Commons Attribution 4.0 International License)

marked changes occur. Hyperoxia causes a minimal decrease of approximately 10% in CBF, whereas $PaO_2 < 50$ mmHg greatly increases CBF.

3.4.4.2 Temperature

The CBF changes by 5–7% per 1 °C change in temperature. Hypothermia decreases CMR and CBF. Conversely, hyperthermia increases CMR and CBF. Between 17 and 37 °C, for every 10 °C drop in temperature, CBF halves. At 20 °C the EEG is isoelectric and with temperatures >42 °C neuronal cell injury can occur.

3.4.4.3 Viscosity

A decrease in haematocrit decreases the viscosity of blood, causing an increase in CBF but also decreasing the O_2 carrying capacity. Conversely, an increase in haematocrit will cause a decrease in CBF. The ideal haematocrit still remains controversial but is thought to be about 30% (30–34%).

3.4.4.4 Autonomic Influences

Intracranial vessels are innervated by both sympathetic and parasympathetic fibres. Sympathetic activity causes vasoconstriction and leads to a decrease in CBF. Conversely, parasympathetic activation causes vasodilation and increases CBF. This may play an important role in vasospasm after brain injury or stroke. Sympathetic innervation arises from the superior cervical sympathetic ganglia in the neck and travels into the brain along with the cerebral arteries. Mild to moderate stimulation or transection will have little effect. Blood flow autoregulation mechanisms can override the nervous system effects. Increased MAP caused by the sympathetic nervous system constricts large- and medium-sized arteries to prevent pressure reaching the smaller vessels. This can be preventative of vascular haemorrhage or "cerebral stroke".

3.5 Blood–Brain Barrier

The preservation of normal brain activity requires a narrow and stable homeostatic environment. For this to occur, dynamic ion balance is needed, effective nutrient transport must occur and there must be a functional barrier to harmful molecules, toxic substances, and infective agents at the interface of the CNS and circulatory system [33]. Key in achieving this is the BBB.

3.5.1 Structure and Function

The BBB is a tightly regulated boundary between the CNS and the peripheral circulation that consists of three barrier layers: (1) a highly specialised endothelial cell layer separating blood and brain interstitial fluid, (2) the choroid plexus epithelium forming the blood-cerebrospinal fluid (CSF) barrier, and (3) the arachnoid epithelium that separates blood from the subarachnoid CSF [34]. Loss of function of this barrier is a major pathophysiological mechanism in many neurological diseases.

Capillaries in the CNS consist of a single, non-fenestrated, continuous layer of specialised endothelial cells with each cell encircling the microcapillary. The endothelial cells are highly polarised with distinct apical and basolateral compartments [35]. This polarity is demonstrated in the vital barrier properties that maintain the functioning and integrity of the BBB [36]. Substances from the microcapillary to the brain must travel either via the paracellular or the transcellular route [37]. The endothelial cells are nearly fused with tight junctions that form a barrier to ions and small hydrophilic molecules [38]. Tight junctions are composed of tight junction proteins such as occludin and claudin, adhesion junction proteins such as cadherin, junctional adhesion molecules and adaptor proteins such as zona occludens. CNS endothelial cells have limited vesicle-mediated transcellular movement (transcytosis) [39]. CNS endothelial cells use polarised cellular transporters for nutrient influx (e.g. glucose transporter 1) and efflux of toxins and metabolic wastes via ATP-binding cassette transporters [40]. CNS endothelial cells lack leukocyte adhesion molecules that prevent immune cell entry making the healthy brain immune-privileged [41].

The endothelium is further surrounded by pericytes and astroglial foot processes forming an additional continuous stratum [34]. There is some distance between the endothelial cells and brain tissue around the penetrating vessels. These form the Virchow–Robin space in which perivascular macrophages are found. The intimate contact and functional interactions and signalling between neurons, microglia, pericytes, astrocytes, and blood vessels form a dynamic functional unit, the neurovascular unit that is capable of rapid response to stressors (Fig. 3.9) [34, 37]. The basement membrane, a 30–40 nm thick lamina encloses pericytes and endothelial cells and is closely adjacent to the astrocyte end feet surrounding the cerebral capillaries. Astrocytes play a key role in maintenance of the BBB and homeostasis of extracellular transmitters, ions, metabolites, and water [34].

Areas of the brain such as the area postrema, pineal gland, and median eminence do not possess a BBB and are collectively termed the circumventricular organs. The barrier properties of such areas are significantly reduced so as to allow for easy transfer of molecules to and from the bloodstream [43].

The three BBB layers provide a physical and functional barrier affecting transport, metabolic, and immunological functions in a dynamic manner. Factors determining transport across the BBB include the size, charge, lipid solubility, and degree of protein binding of sub-

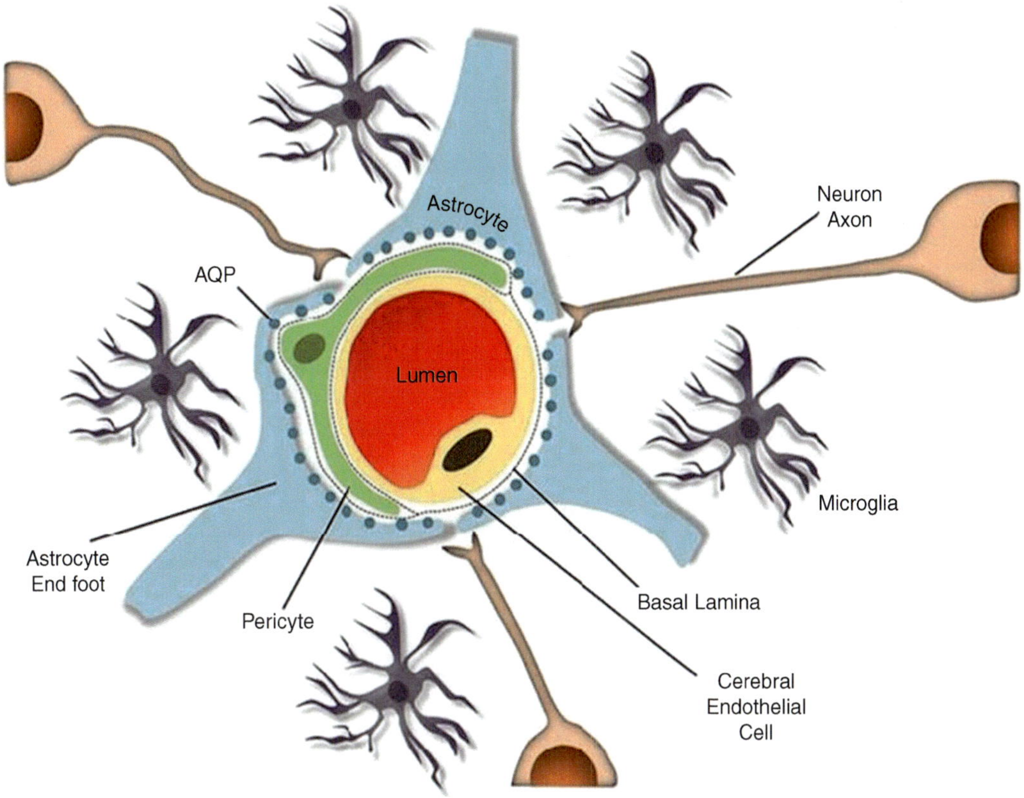

Fig. 3.9 Schematic representation of the neurovascular unit at the capillary level. The blood–brain barrier is composed of several cell types and extracellular matrix molecules in close association. Highly specialised and polarised endothelial cells, basal lamina, pericytes, and astrocyte end feet, which by wrapping the micro-vessel walls, establish communication with neurons in the neurovascular unit. The neurovascular unit is important to maintain optimal brain function. Pericytes and astrocytes are important in barrier induction and maintenance. Microglia are CNS-resident immune cells. AQP—aquaporins; (Diagram by de Spohr, TCLS. Adapted from Abbott, 2013). (From Dubois et al. [42]—Creative Commons Attribution 4.0 International License)

stances. Lipid-soluble substances pass through via diffusion. The BBB is permeable to O_2, CO_2, and other gases such as helium, xenon, nitrogen, and anaesthetic agents. The BBB is also permeable to water. Ionised and large molecules enter the brain in a restricted and regulated manner through the BBB. The BBB plays a role in CNS immunity by regulating the recruitment of leukocytes and innate immune elements. Loss of integrity of the BBB leaves the brain vulnerable to potentially harmful concentrations of substances. This may have a detrimental effect on brain homeostasis and neuronal signalling [37].

3.5.2 Transport of Glucose and Amino Acids

Essential polar molecules such as glucose, amino acids, and nucleosides cannot diffuse through the cell membrane and therefore enter via passive or secondarily active carrier-mediated influx. A family of glucose transporters (GLUT) is expressed by different cells. Endothelial cells of the microvasculature, astrocytes, and the choroid plexus express the insulin independent glucose transporter GLUT1 [34]. GLUT1 expression is upregulated by hypoglycaemia. The GLUT 4 transporter is also expressed in the BBB. GLUT3, expressed in neurons, likely provides glucose uptake into neurons. This uptake bypasses the glucose lactate shuffle through astrocytes that provides lactate as an energy substrate [34]. A sustainable supply of essential amino acids across the BBB is dependent on specific solute carriers expressed in the endothelium. As part of brain protection, the BBB is largely impermeable to neuroactive substances, e.g. aspartate and glutamate.

3.5.3 Transport of Ions

Specific ion channels and transporters act to preserve an optimal environment for synaptic and neural functioning. The BBB is largely impermeable to most ions thereby defending neural cells against significant variations in ion concentrations that may affect neuronal activity. Neuronal firing and synaptic transmission are associated with the influx of Na^+ and Ca^{2+} and an increase in the concentrations of K^+ and neurotransmitters extracellularly. However, regulated ionic movement maintains potassium concentration in the CSF and brain interstitial fluid at ~2.5–2.9 mM despite higher plasma concentration of potassium. The BBB is largely impermeable to ions such as Ca^{2+} and Mg^{2+}. Astrocytes have an important role in maintaining brain extracellular environment despite continuous neuronal activity [34]. Water moves freely with bulk flow but depends on the presence of aquaporins.

3.5.4 Transport of Macromolecules

The presence of certain proteins and peptide macromolecules in the brain can initiate cascades that may lead to seizure activity, synaptic plasticity, and cell damage. Regulated movement of such molecules across the BBB is thus vital. Endocytic vesicles provide the main delivery of large molecular weight proteins and peptide molecules across the BBB by the process of transcytosis. Internalisation into the endothelial cell cytoplasm and exocytosis to the opposite pole accounts for transport of these molecules. This process may be receptor-mediated, for example, with insulin or adsorptive-mediated, for example, with cationised albumin [34].

Figure 3.10 summarises the movement of various substances across the BBB. The BBB can be disrupted by a multitude of factors including severe hypertension, tumours, stroke, trauma, infection, CO_2, O_2, and sustained seizure activity. In these situations, movement of the various substances becomes affected. Fluid movement, for example, becomes dependent on hydrostatic pressures more than osmotic gradients.

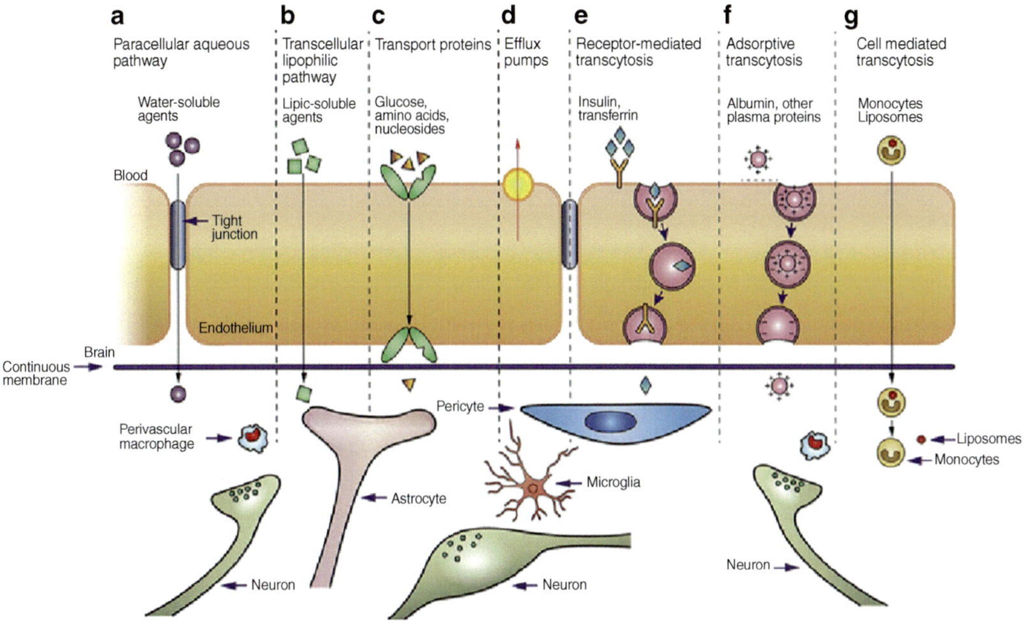

Fig. 3.10 Potential routes for infiltration and transport across the endothelial cells forming the blood–brain barrier. (From Vidu et al. [44]—Creative Commons Attribution 3.0 Unported License)

3.6 Cerebrospinal Fluid

Within the rigid bony structure of the cranium, the brain is vulnerable to mechanical trauma. To protect the brain and spinal cord, it is suspended in a specialised extracellular fluid that fills the ventricular and subarachnoid spaces. This CSF serves many roles to preserve optimal nervous system functioning. The CSF has a protective purpose by preventing deformation and damage caused by acceleration and deceleration during head movement. The buoyancy effect of CSF is thought to reduce the effective weight of the brain to about 25 g. This allows the brain to maintain its density without compression of its blood supply. It also has a key role in maintaining homeostasis by regulating fluid and electrolyte composition, transporting essential molecules, removal of substances, and is proposed to be involved in brain development and health [45]. The CSF represents an alternate point of entrance and exit for some substances that are not able to cross the BBB.

3.6.1 Production and Secretion

The production of CSF mainly occurs within the choroid plexuses in the lateral, third and fourth ventricles. Some production also occurs in the ventricular ependymal cell linings. The choroid plexus, comprised of microvilli and granular meningeal protrusions that extend into the ventricles, has a vast capillary network and filters plasma passively down a pressure gradient through the fenestrated capillary endothelium into the choroidal interstitial space. The epithelial cells of the choroid plexus are joined to the arachnoid membrane cells by tight junctions, limiting passive flow of water and are referred to as the blood–CSF barrier.

Active transport is required for the ultrafiltrate of plasma from the choroidal interstitial spaces, across the choroidal epithelium into the ventricular space, a process regulated by carbonic anhydrase and other membrane ion carrier proteins. Facilitated by aquaporin I in the apical membrane, water follows the osmotic gradient created by ATP-dependent ion pumps transporting Na^+, Cl^-, K^+, and $HCO3^-$ into the ventricles. CSF volume and composition is closely regulated by the bidirectional flow of ions facilitated by $Na/K_2/Cl$ co-transporters in the choroidal membrane. Fluid leaking from interstitial and perivascular spaces at extrachoroidal sites probably contribute minimally to production of CSF.

The gap junctions found in the pial and ependymal linings allow free diffusion between CSF and the extracellular space of the brain (ECSB). The CSF-ECSB may thus be considered a collective compartment with CSF playing an important part in homeostasis of the ECSB and brain tissue [46]. The variable distance of different cerebral tissues to the ECSB makes equilibration slow and transient differences may occur.

In a young, healthy adult, CSF is produced at a rate of about 400–600 ml/day which equates to approximately 21 ml/h. With a turnover rate of 4–5 times/day, the total amount of CSF around the brain at any given time is about 150 ml, with one-sixth of this volume filling the ventricles and the rest suspended in the subarachnoid space around the brain and spinal cord.

The volume and composition of CSF is finely regulated by multiple factors that influence the production and secretion of CSF. Autonomic innervation of the choroidal cells increases CSF secretion via cholinergic stimulation and conversely decreases secretion by sympathetic stimulation. Raised ICP has a minimal influence on the rate of CSF production as long as the CPP is above 70 mmHg. The decrease of the pressure gradient will minimally decrease filtration and secretion of CSF to act as compensation for rising intraventricular pressure, but this capacity to adapt is limited and rapidly exhausted. However, when CPP drops to below levels of 70 mmHg, CSF secretion decreases because of reduced cerebral and choroid plexus blood flow. Monoamine and neuropeptides play a role in CSF secretion. Both atrial natriuretic peptide and arginine vasopressin have been shown to decrease secretion. Aquaporins, enzymes, and membrane carrier proteins involved with CSF are influenced by humoral regulation and acid base disorders. The activity of carbonic anhydrase is also influenced by acid base disorders and carbonic anhydrase inhibitors. The production of CSF is decreased by several other pharmacological agents including corticosteroids, spironolactone, furosemide, isoflurane, and vasopressors [45].

3.6.2 Composition

CSF is mainly composed of water. The osmotic pressure of CSF approximates that of plasma. The hydrostatic pressure of CSF is 5–15 mmHg with a pH of 7.32. The composition of CSF differs greatly from plasma. Although CSF concentration of Na^+ ions is similar to plasma, Cl^- and Mg^{2+} concentrations are higher, whereas K^+ and Ca^{2+} concentrations are lower. The osmolality of CSF is maintained by bulk flow of H_2O molecules. Small amounts of plasma proteins, mostly albumin enter the CSF either via passing through epithelial cell junctions or via vesicular transport across the epithelial cells at the choroid plexus. A minimal amount of protein can enter via extrachoroidal sites or via bulk flow from the extracellular space of the brain. CSF therefore has a protein concentration that is much lower than that of plasma (0.025 g/100 ml versus 7 g/100 ml) [47]. The ratio of glucose levels in CSF to plasma is about 0.6 and the cell count is usually less than 5 cells/ml. Microglial cells constantly remove unwanted or damaged tissue into the extracellular cerebral space and CSF, thus also contributing to CSF composition. The presence of certain immunological tissues or leukocytes in the CSF indicates possible neural damage and/or inflammation.

The CSF contains other substances and micronutrients including growth factor, vitamins B1, B12, and C, folate, B2-microglobulin, arginine vasopressin, nitric oxide (NO), peptides, proteins, and other ions that are thought to contribute to tissue repair, giving merit to the proposed idea of CSF being a "nourishing liquor" [47]. This is true for many ions and some organic molecules found in CSF but not for macronutrients which are not able to pass into CSF. The transfer of drugs via the CSF is finely regulated and depends mainly on size, charge, lipid solubility, and plasma protein binding of the drug.

3.6.3 Circulation

CSF circulates continually around the brain and spinal cord to maintain homeostasis. It flows to the beat of the systolic pulse wave but is also affected to a lesser extent by respiratory waves, posture, and physical effort, and is assisted by beating ciliated ependymal cells.

The CSF flows from the lateral ventricles toward the cisterna magna. Through the intraventricular foramen of Monro, CSF enters the third ventricle and exits via the aqueduct of Sylvia to the fourth ventricle. From here it passes to the cerebellomedullary cisterns via the lateral foramen of Luschka and the midline foramen of Magendie. Even though flow was previously thought to be unidirectional, oscillatory bidirectional flow through the aqueduct of Sylvia, propagated by the arterial pulse, respiration, and posture is now thought to occur [48]. These gentle ebbs and flows create mixing of CSF. However, the net flow of about 0.4 ml/min still remains from the ventricles toward the basal subarachnoid spaces. Multidirectional flow in the subarachnoid space circulates CSF around the brain and spinal cord.

3.6.4 Absorption

Absorption of CSF into the bloodstream occurs mainly via the arachnoid villi, and to a lesser degree, through the lymphatic system. Arachnoid granulations are responsible for the absorption of CSF via a dynamic pressure gradient dependent process. Finger-like villi are present over the cerebral hemispheres and in the spinal nerve roots. These are endothelium lined protrusions that facilitate translocation of CSF through vesicular passages into large venous sinuses that drain into the internal jugular system. Approximately 85–90% of CSF absorption occurs in the cerebral villi, and the rest in the spinal arachnoid villi. Free flow of large particles and proteins including red and white blood cells occur along a pressure gradient, provided this gradient remains greater than about 3–5 mmHg [47]. In the event of raised CSF pressure above 7 mmHg, absorption of CSF increases. This is accomplished by the development of more arachnoid villi increasing the surface area for absorption. Increased pinocytosis and opening of intercellular spaces also contribute to the increased absorption rate. As ICP increases, so does the absorption rate of CSF in a linear fashion up to an ICP of 30 cm H_2O, at which point no further increase in absorption rate is possible. Conversely, increased venous pressure caused by obstruction, either of the internal jugular venous system or obstruction of villi in diseased states, decrease the pressure gradient, thereby decreasing absorption of CSF. Posture is also thought to influence absorption rate to a minimal degree.

To a lesser extent, CSF is also absorbed through the nasal cribriform plate and along the nerve root sleeves of cranial and spinal nerves providing a direct route to the extracranial lymphatics. Experimental data suggest a possible alternate pathway involving the Virchow–Robin perivascular spaces found around penetrating arteries and veins which lead directly to the cervical lymphatics [49]. As the brain and spinal cord lacks any lymphatic tissue, this process acts to return perivascular and interstitial protein to the blood.

3.6.5 Pathophysiology Related to Cerebrospinal Fluid

Inflammation and bleeding into the subarachnoid space can interfere with normal physiology and disruption of CSF homeostasis, resulting in altered secretion or absorption of CSF. Subarachnoid haemorrhage (SAH) and intraventricular bleeding caused by the disruption of a vessel into the subarachnoid space may cause obstruction of CSF flow in the ventricles. Inflammation leads to scarring, and further obstruction of arachnoid granulations occur. The resulting hydrocephalus and raised ICP explain the classic symptoms of headache, nausea and vomiting, seizures, vision disturbances, and loss of consciousness or death associated with SAH. Analysis of CSF will demonstrate erythrocytes or visible xanthochromia.

3.7 Intracranial Pressure

Intracranial pressure (ICP) refers to the pressure of the contents within the cranial vault. The ICP is a key determinant of the CPP. In many CNS disease states the contributing pathophysiology that results in brain death is as a result of cerebral oedema and intracranial hypertension. Understanding the changes in ICP in pathologies such as head trauma, subarachnoid haemorrhage, and intracranial tumours helps to better manage these conditions in the quest for better outcomes.

3.7.1 Volume/Pressure Relationship

The cranial vault is a rigid compartment with a fixed total volume consisting of the brain (80%), blood (12%), and CSF (8%). The Monro–Kellie hypothesis states if an increase occurs in the volume of one component, the volume of one or more other components must decrease, or ICP will be elevated. Physiological values of ICP range between 3 and 4 mmHg before the age of 1 year, and between 10 and 15 mmHg in supine adults. Respiration and the cardiac cycle lead to cyclical variations in ICP. The ICP also varies with body position and clinical conditions. Coughing, sneezing, and straining may transiently increase ICP to 30–50 mmHg.

The capacity of the intracranial contents to adapt to volume changes is defined as brain compliance (Fig. 3.11). Changes in the CSF and blood components are the initial buffer mechanisms to defend the ICP. Compensatory CSF pressure changes are regulated at all levels including CSF displacement from cranial to spinal space, decreased CSF secretion and circulation, and increased CSF absorption. An increased intraventricular pressure decreases the pressure gradient across the blood–CSF barrier at the choroidal plexus. Neuropeptides such as atrial natriuretic

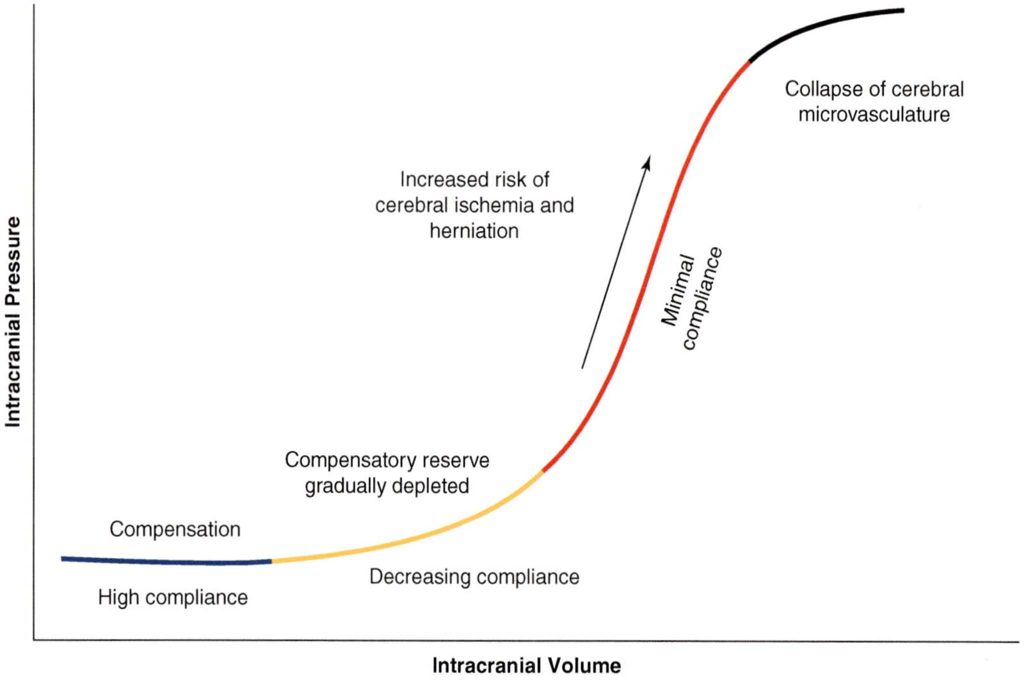

Fig. 3.11 Pressure–volume curve for ICP. Four "zones" may be delineated: (1) baseline intracranial volume with good compensatory reserve and high compliance (blue); (2) gradual depletion of compensatory reserve as intracranial volume increases (yellow); (3) poor compensatory reserve and increased risk of cerebral ischemia and herniation (red); and (4) critically high ICP causing collapse of cerebral microvasculature and disturbed cerebrovascular reactivity (grey) (Harary et al. [26]—Creative Commons Attribution 4.0 International License)

peptide and arginine vasopressin decrease choroidal secretion of CSF and cause pial artery dilation. Compensatory changes in the blood component are from a decrease in the total cerebral blood volume with the venous component primarily affected. Other CBF regulatory mechanisms are covered in the preceding section on CBF.

3.7.2 ICP Waves

As the brain floats in the CSF, cardiac and respiratory pulse waves are transmitted intracranially to reflect a characteristic ICP waveform. The mean ICP is a reflection of the time average (Fig. 3.12a). Three components of the waveform are described: i) respiratory waveforms (0.1–0.3 Hz) associated with the respiratory cycle, (2) pulse pressure waveforms that are equal to the heart rate, and (3) slow vasogenic waveforms (e.g., "Lundberg A and B waves"). The pulse pressure waveform generated by the arterial pulse shows three distinct components (Fig. 3.12b). The percussion wave (P1) correlates with the arterial pulsation that is transmitted through the choroid plexus into the CSF. The P2 wave, also called the tidal wave, indirectly represents cerebral compliance as it is thought to be the arterial pulse wave reflecting off the brain parenchyma. The dicrotic wave (P3) reflects the pressure transmitted as a result of the aortic valve closure. All these waves are

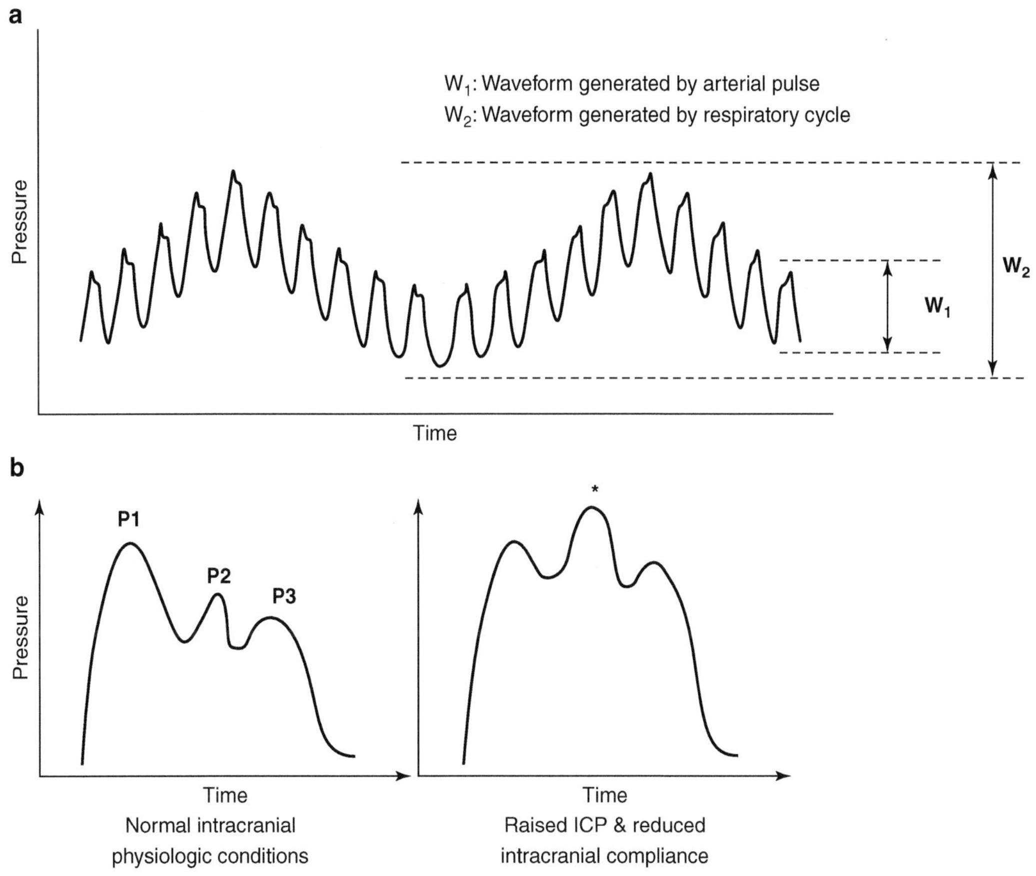

Fig. 3.12 ICP pressure waves. (**a**) ICP fluctuations in response to the respiratory cycle (W2) and the arterial cycle (W1); (**b**) close-up of ICP waveform due to the systemic arterial cycle. Components are P1 (Percussion wave = representative of arterial pulsation), P2 (Tidal wave = a proxy for intracranial compliance), and P3 (Dicrotic wave = pressure transmission of aortic valve closure). A raised P2 wave is an indicator of raised ICP and reduced intracranial compliance (*). (Harary et al. [26]—Creative Commons Attribution 4.0 International License)

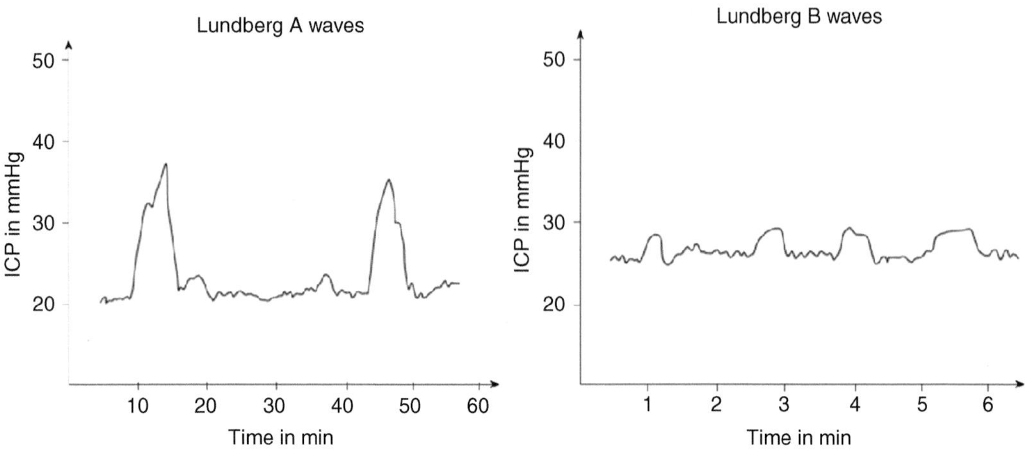

Fig. 3.13 Lundberg waves. (From Nag et al. [51]—Creative Commons Attribution-Non-commercial License)

rarely more than 4 mmHg in amplitude, or 10–30% of the mean ICP. The ICP wave is usually in synchronisation with the QRS complex on the ECG or the arterial waveform on an invasive arterial line.

The ICP waveform changes with any compromise of intracranial compliance. Lundberg first described the change in morphology in the global ICP waveform, observing three patterns [50]. (Fig. 3.13)

- Lundberg "A" or plateau waves: periodic steep ramp, large amplitude (up to 50–100 mmHg) increases in ICP that persist for 5–20 min before returning to baseline. These waves can be observed in healthy asymptomatic individuals, but their long-term presence may be indicative of decreased CPP and poor prognosis.
- Lundberg "B" waves: periodic, self-limited ICP increases of 20 to 50 mmHg lasting 1–2 min. These waves are related to changes in physiological or pathological CBF and may be due to cerebral vasospasm. They can progress to "A" waves.
- Lundberg "C" waves: periodic, self-limited ICP increases of 20 mmHg occurring with a frequency of 4–8 per minute. They may result from the transmission of arterial pressure waves and have no pathological significance [52].

Data from ICP recordings usually provide a global view of intracranial status. Such data need to be interpreted in conjunction with other general patient data and cerebral oxygenation and metabolic status from healthy and pathological territories of the CNS.

3.7.3 Increased ICP

The two main mechanisms of injury from increased ICP are cerebral ischemia and brain herniation. A level of ICP persistently raised above 15 mmHg is considered intracranial hypertension. Such a level decreases the CPP, and if prolonged, leads to focal and global ischaemia. High ICP (HICP) can cause secondary brain injury and death. HICP, traditionally defined as ICP > 20 mmHg, has been redefined as 22 mmHg [53]. However, a single threshold is controversial. Time spent above a threshold and its intensity ("ICP dose") may be more important than the single threshold value [54]. Prolonged exposure to ICP values below the threshold may also be associated with poor outcomes [55]. If CPP is critically low, for example, as a result of a very low MAP, the utility of ICP for outcome prediction becomes limited.

Severe and sustained increases in ICP may lead to herniation of brain matter with resultant syndromes related to the sites of herniation, for example, transtentorial herniation of the uncus of the temporal lobe downwards through the tentorium, subfalcine herniation of the cingulate gyrus beneath the free edge of the falx cerebri and the potentially fatal tonsillar herniation of the cerebellar tonsils through the foramen magnum.

3.7.4 Intracranial Pressure Monitors

Various methods are available to measure intracranial pressure. Such methods may be broadly considered as invasive and non-invasive. Although non-invasive techniques minimise the risk of complications, invasive methods are still considered to be superior in accuracy [51].

3.7.4.1 Invasive Techniques

Invasive techniques measure intracranial pressure through fluid-filled systems or transducer-tipped catheters and can be used in a variety of anatomical locations including intraventricular, intraparenchymal, subarachnoid, subdural or epidural spaces (Fig. 3.14).

External Ventricular Drainage (EVD)

Fluid-filled systems include the widely used and generally accepted gold standard technique of external ventricular drainage (EVD) [56]. The inexpensive catheter device placed through a burr hole into a ventricle has the added benefit of allowing drainage of CSF and can be recalibrated in vivo. It carries a risk of bleeding and infection. Trauma can be caused during insertion and these devices are prone to leaking and blockage [57].

Implantable Microtransducer ICP Monitoring Devices

Transducer-tipped catheters are directly placed in the intraventricular, intraparenchymal, subarachnoid or epidural space [56]. The most commonly used compartment is the parenchymal space. These devices are simpler to insert and not affected by blockage as with EVD systems. Bleeding and infection remain concerns. These devices are considered to be as accurate as EVDs, however, a significant disadvantage is that they have a higher cost and no recalibration is possible after placement [56]. Strain gauge, fibre-optic, microchip, and pneumatic sensor microtransducer devices are available. Fibre-optic devices transmit pressure dependent light through a fiberoptic cable to a movable mirror. The degree of movement of the flexible mirror changes the properties of the reflected light which is then translated into an ICP value [58]. Strain gauge devices calculate the change in resistance in the transducer in response to intracranial pressure [58]. Newer implantable devices are capable of telemetric ICP measurement wirelessly. These can be left in for several months with limited drift and may monitor ICP under normal daily living conditions in outpatient settings. The clinical use of such devices remains to be established.

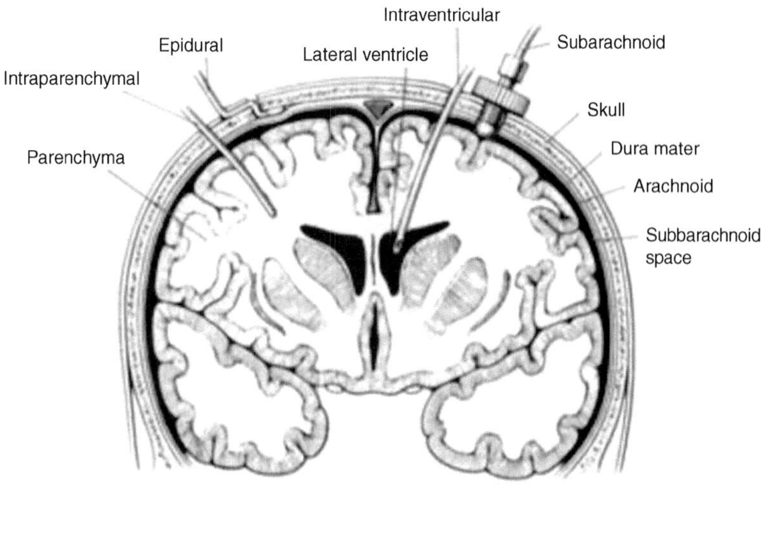

Fig. 3.14 Potential sites for invasive monitoring of intracranial pressure. (Harary et al. [26]—Creative Commons Attribution 4.0 International License)

Other Devices
Subarachnoid screws, bolts or catheters employ fluid-filled systems placed directly in the subarachnoid compartment. These devices are less prone to trauma and infection but tend to underestimate ICP [58]. Epidural and subdural devices are easier to insert and carry a lower risk of infection than EVDs. They, however, have low accuracy with sensor drift and cannot be calibrated in vivo. These devices are seldom used currently.

3.7.4.2 Non-Invasive Techniques

Non-invasive techniques in general measure physiological variables that indirectly correlate with ICP. Such techniques have less complications but are not as accurate as invasive techniques and are therefore not advocated for routine use.

Various non-invasive monitoring methods have been described [51, 56]. *Transcranial Doppler Ultrasonography* (TCD) measures the blood flow velocity in the middle cerebral artery. This technique requires training and experience and has significant intra- and inter-observer variability. *Tympanic Membrane Displacement* (TMD) measures the movement of the tympanic membrane caused by stimulation of the stapedial reflex. *Optic Nerve Sheath Diameter* (ONSD) is an affordable and efficient method but also requires training and is subject to intra-and inter-observer variability. *Fundoscopy* and observation of papilloedema is a subjective assessment. As papilloedema takes some time to develop it is not applicable in the acute setting and other causes of papilloedema should also be considered [56].

The choice of ICP monitor should be made on a case-by-case basis. Specific consideration should be given to the specific pathology and risk of bleeding of the patient as well as the accuracy and cost of the chosen technique and the possible mechanical problems of specific devices.

3.8 Conclusion

A clear and detailed understanding of central neurophysiology is essential to better appreciate the pathophysiology of subarachnoid haemorrhage. The complex components of the nervous system and their intricate interactions form the cornerstones of such an understanding. The essential electrophysiology, the balance of cerebral metabolism and blood flow, the importance of the blood–brain barrier, the complexity of cerebrospinal fluid, and the impact of intracranial pressure all serve to form a firm foundation in the study of brain pathologies.

References

1. OpenStax College, Biology. OpenStax College. 30 May 2013. https://cnx.org/contents/GFy_h8cu@9.87:c9j4p0aj@3/Neurons-and-Glial-Cells. Accessed 13 Apr 2020.
2. Guyton AC, Hall JE. Textbook of medical physiology. 11th ed. Philadelphia: Elsevier Saunders; 2006. p. 57–71.
3. OpenStax College, Biology. OpenStax College. 30 May 2013. https://cnx.org/contents/GFy_h8cu@9.87:cs_Pb-GW@5/How-Neurons-Communicate Accessed 13 Apr 2020.
4. Roy CS, Sherrington CS. On the regulation of the blood-supply of the brain. J Physiol. 1890;11(1-2):85–108. https://doi.org/10.1113/jphysiol.1890.sp000321.
5. Watts ME, Pocock R, Claudianos C. Brain energy and oxygen metabolism: emerging role in normal function and disease. Front Mol Neurosci. 2018;11:216. https://doi.org/10.3389/fnmol.2018.00216.
6. Wade OL, Bishop JM. Cardiac output and regional blood flow. Oxford: Blackwell Scientific Publications; 1962.
7. Go KG. The cerebral blood supply. Energy metabolism of the brain. In: Go KG, editor. Cerebral pathophysiology. Amsterdam: Elsevier; 1991. p. 66–172.
8. Clarke DD, Sokoloff L. Circulation and energy metabolism of the brain. In: Siegel GJ, Agranoff BW, Albers RW, et al., editors. Basic neurochemistry: molecular, cellular and medical aspects. 6th ed. Philadelphia: Lippincott-Raven; 1999. p. 637–69.
9. Briones-Galang M, Robertson C. Cerebral metabolism: implications for Neurocritically ill patients. In: Suarez JI, editor. Critical care neurology and neurosurgery. Current Clinical Neurology. Totowa, NJ: Humana Press; 2004. p. 37–46. https://doi.org/10.1007/978-1-59259-660-7_4.
10. Astrup J. Energy requiring cell functions in the ischemic brain: their critical supply and possible inhibition in protective therapy. J Neurosurg. 1982;56(4):482–97. https://doi.org/10.3171/jns.1982.56.4.0482.
11. Chong SP, Merkle CW, Leahy C, Srinivasan VJ. Cerebral metabolic rate of oxygen ($CMRO_2$) assessed by combined Doppler and spectroscopic OCT. Biomed Opt Express. 2015;6(10):3941–51. https://doi.org/10.1364/BOE.6.003941.

12. Sokoloff L. The metabolism of the central nervous system in vivo. In: Field J, Magoun HW, Hall VE, editors. Handbook of physiology—neurophysiology, vol. 3. Washington, DC: American Physiological Society; 1960. p. 1843–64.
13. Oz G, Seaquist ER, Kumar A, Criego AB, Benedict LE, Rao JP, et al. Human brain glycogen content and metabolism: implications on its role in brain energy metabolism. Am J Physiol Endocrinol Metab. 2007;292(3):E946–51. https://doi.org/10.1152/ajpendo.00424.2006.
14. Hasselbalch SG, Knudsen GM, Jakobsen J, Hageman LP, Holm S, Paulsen OB. Brain metabolism during short-term starvation in humans. J Cereb Blood Flow Metab. 1994;14(1):125–31. https://doi.org/10.1038/jcbfm.1994.17.
15. Bergsneider M, Hovda DA, Shalmon E, Kelly DF, Vespa PM, Martin NA, et al. Cerebral hyperglycolysis following severe traumatic brain injury in humans: a positron emission tomography study. J Neurosurg. 1997;86(2):241–51. https://doi.org/10.3171/jns.1997.86.2.0241.
16. Glenn TC, Martin NA, Horning MA, McArthur DL, Hovda DA, Vespa P, et al. Lactate: brain fuel following traumatic brain injury: a comparison with normal healthy control subjects. J Neurotrauma. 2015;32(11):820–32. https://doi.org/10.1089/neu.2014.3483.
17. Brooks GA. Lactate: glycolytic end product and oxidative substrate during sustained exercise in mammals—the "lactate shuttle". In: Gilles R, editor. Circulation, respiration, and metabolism. Proceedings in life sciences. Berlin, Heidelberg: Springer; 1985. p. 208–18. https://doi.org/10.1007/978-3-642-70610-3_15.
18. Pellerin L, Magistretti PJ. Glutamate uptake into astrocytes stimulates aerobic glycolysis: a mechanism coupling neuronal activity to glucose utilization. Proc Natl Acad Sci U S A. 1994;91(22):10625–9. https://doi.org/10.1073/pnas.91.22.10625.
19. Brooks GA, Martin NA. Cerebral metabolism following traumatic brain injury: new discoveries with implications for treatment. Front Neurosci. 2015;8(408):1–13. https://doi.org/10.3389/fnins.2014.00408.
20. Tsacopoulos M, Magiestretti PJ. Metabolic coupling between glia and neurons. J Neurosci. 1996;16(3):877–85. https://doi.org/10.1523/JNEUROSCI.16-03-00877.1996.
21. Kasischke KA, Vishwasrao HD, Fisher PJ, Zipfel WR, Webb WW. Neural activity triggers neuronal oxidative metabolism followed by astrocytic glycolysis. Science. 2004;305(5680):99–103. https://doi.org/10.1126/science.1096485.
22. Donnely J, Budohoski KP, Smielewski P, Czosnyka M. Regulation of the cerebral circulation: bedside assessment and clinical implications. Crit Care. 2016;20(1):129. https://doi.org/10.1186/s13054-016-1293-6.
23. Melamed E, Lavy S, Bentin S, Cooper G, Rinot Y. Reduction in regional cerebral blood flow during normal aging in man. Stroke. 1980;11(1):31–5. https://doi.org/10.1161/01.str.11.1.31.
24. Nordstrom CH, Koskinen LO, Olivecrona M. Aspects on the physiological and biochemical foundations of neurocritical care. Front Neurol. 2017;8:274. https://doi.org/10.3389/fneur.2017.00274.
25. Peterson EC, Wang Z, Britz G. Regulation of cerebral blood flow. Int J Vasc Med. 2011. 2011823525. https://doi.org/10.1155/2011/823525.
26. Harary M, Dolmans RGF, Gormley WB. Intracranial pressure monitoring – review and avenues for development. Sensors. 2018;18(2):465. https://doi.org/10.3390/s18020465.
27. Knot HJ, Nelson MT. Regulation of arterial diameter and wall [Ca2+] in cerebral arteries of rat by membrane potential and intravascular pressure. J Physiol. 1998;508(1):199–209. https://doi.org/10.1111/j.1469-7793.1998.199br.x.
28. Kontos HA. Regulation of the cerebral circulation. Annu Rev Physiol. 1981;43:397–407. https://doi.org/10.1146/annurev.ph.43.030181.002145.
29. Iadecola C. Neurovascular regulation in the normal brain and in Alzheimer's disease. Nat Rev Neurosci. 2004;5(5):347–60. https://doi.org/10.1038/nrn1387.
30. Archer SL, Huang JM, Hampl V, Nelson DP, Shultz PJ, Weir EK. Nitric oxide and cGMP cause vasorelaxation by activation of a charybdotoxin-sensitive K^+ channel by cGMP-dependent protein kinase. Proc Natl Acad Sci U S A. 1994;91(16):7583–7. https://doi.org/10.1073/pnas.91.16.7583.
31. Takano T, Tian GF, Peng W, Lou N, Libionka W, Han X, et al. Astrocyte-mediated control of cerebral blood flow. Nat Neurosci. 2006;9(2):260–7. https://doi.org/10.1038/nn1623.
32. Godoy DA, Seifi A, Garza D, et al. Hyperventilation therapy for control of posttraumatic intracranial hypertension. Front Neurol. 2017;8:250. https://doi.org/10.3389/fneur.2017.00250.
33. Gupta S, Dhanda S, Sandhir R. Anatomy and physiology of blood-brain barrier. In: Gao H, Gao X, editors. Brain targeted drug delivery systems: a focus on nanotechnology and nanoparticulates. Academic Press Elsevier; 2019. p. 7–31. https://doi.org/10.1016/B978-0-12-814001-7.00002-0.
34. Serlin Y, Shelef I, Knyazer B, Friedman A. Anatomy and physiology of the blood-brain barrier. Semin Cell Dev Biol. 2015;38:2–6. https://doi.org/10.1016/j.semcdb.2015.01.002.
35. Betz AL, Goldstein GW. Polarity of the blood-brain barrier: neutral amino acid transport into isolated brain capillaries. Science. 1978;202(4364):225–7. https://doi.org/10.1126/science.211586.
36. Daneman R, Prat A. The blood-brain barrier. Cold Spring Harb Perspect Biol. 2015;7(1):a020412. https://doi.org/10.1101/cshperspect.a020412.
37. McCaffrey G, Davis TP. Physiology and pathophysiology of the blood brain barrier: P-glycoprotein and occludin trafficking as therapeutic targets to optimize central nervous system drug delivery. J Investig

Med. 2012;60(8):1131–40. https://doi.org/10.2310/JIM.0b013e318276de79.
38. Brightman MW, Reese TS. Junctions between intimately apposed cell membranes in the vertebrate brain. J Cell Biol. 1969;40(3):648–77. https://doi.org/10.1083/jcb.40.3.648.
39. Tuma PL, Hubbard AL. Transcytosis: crossing cellular barriers. Physiol Rev. 2003;83(3):871–932. https://doi.org/10.1152/physrev.00001.2003.
40. Chow BW, Gu C. The molecular constituents of the blood-brain barrier. Trends Neurosci. 2015;38(10):598–608. https://doi.org/10.1016/j.tins.2015.08.003.
41. Engelhardt B, Ransohoff RM. Capture, crawl, cross: the T cell code to breach the blood-brain barriers. Trends Immunol. 2012;33(12):579–89. https://doi.org/10.1016/j.it.2012.07.004.
42. Dubois LG, Campanati L, Righy C, et al. Gliomas and the vascular fragility of the blood brain barrier. Front Cell Neurosci. 2014;8:418. https://doi.org/10.3389/fncel.2014.00418.
43. Kaur C, Ling EA. The circumventricular organs. Histol Histopathol. 2017;32(9):879–92. https://doi.org/10.14670/HH-11-881.
44. Vidu R, Rahman M, Mahmoudi M, et al. Nanostructures: a platform for brain repair and augmentation. Front Neurol. 2014;9:91. https://doi.org/10.3389/fnsys.2014.00091.
45. Sakka L, Coll G, Chazal J. Anatomy and physiology of cerebrospinal fluid. Eur Ann Otorhinolaryngol Head Neck Dis. 2011;128(6):309–16. https://doi.org/10.1016/j.anorl.2011.03.002.
46. Whish S, Dziegielewska KM, Møllgård K, Noor NM, Liddelow SA, Habgood MD, et al. The inner csf brain barrier: developmentally controlled access to the brain via intercellular junctions. Front Neurosci. 2015;9:16. https://doi.org/10.3389/fnins.2015.00016.
47. Spector R, Robert Snodgrass S, Johanson CE. A balanced view of the cerebrospinal fluid composition and functions: focus on adult humans. Exp Neurol. 2015;273:57–68. https://doi.org/10.1016/j.expneurol.2015.07.027.
48. Dreha-Kulaczewski S, Joseph AA, Merboldt KD, Ludwig HC, Gärtner J, Frahm J. Inspiration is the major regulator of human CSF flow. J Neurosci. 2015;35(6):2485–91. https://doi.org/10.1523/JNEUROSCI.3246-14.2015.
49. Khasawneh AH, Garling RJ, Harris CA. Cerebrospinal fluid circulation: what do we know and how do we know it? Brain Circ. 2018;4(1):14–8. https://doi.org/10.4103/bc.bc_3_18.
50. Lundberg N. Continuous recording and control of ventricular fluid pressure in neurosurgical practice. Acta Psychiatr Scand Suppl. 1960;36(149):1–193. https://doi.org/10.1111/j.1600-0447.1961.tb06112.x.
51. Nag DS, Sahu S, Swain A, et al. Intracranial pressure monitoring: gold standard and recent innovations. World J Clin Cases. 2019;7(13):1535–53. https://doi.org/10.12998/wjcc.v7.i13.1535.
52. Rodríguez-Boto G, Rivero-Garvía M, Gutiérrez-González R, Márquez-Rivas J. Conceptos básicos sobre lafisiopatología cerebral y la monitorización de la presión intracraneal. Neurologia. 2015;30(1):16–22. https://doi.org/10.1016/j.nrl.2012.09.002.
53. Carney N, Totten AM, O'Reilly C, Ullman JS, Hawryluk GW, Bell MJ, et al. Guidelines for the management of severe traumatic brain injury, fourth edition. Neurosurgery. 2017;80(1):6–15. https://doi.org/10.1227/NEU.0000000000001432.
54. Vik A, Nag T, Fredriksli OA, Skandsen T, Moen KG, Schirmer-Mikalsen K, et al. Relationship of "dose" of intracranial hypertension to outcome in severe traumatic brain injury. J Neurosurg. 2008;109(4):678–84. https://doi.org/10.3171/JNS/2008/109/10/0678.
55. Güiza F, Depreitere B, Piper I, Citerio G, Chambers I, Jones PA, et al. Visualizing the pressure and time burden of intracranial hypertension in adult and paediatric traumatic brain injury. Intensive Care Med. 2015;41(6):1067–76. https://doi.org/10.1007/s00134-015-3806-1.
56. Ravoel PH, Bartek J, Andresen M, Bellander BM, Romner B. Intracranial pressure monitoring: invasive versus non-invasive methods – a review. Crit Care Res Prac. 2012;2012:950393. https://doi.org/10.1155/2012/950393.
57. Le Roux P. Intracranial pressure monitoring and management. In: Laskowitz D, Grant G, editors. Translational research in traumatic brain injury. Boca Raton, FL: CRC Press/Taylor and Francis Group; 2016. Chapter 15. Available from: https://www.ncbi.nlm.nih.gov/books/NBK326713/.
58. Kawoos U, McCarron RM, Auker CR, Chavko M. Advances in intracranial pressure monitoring and its significance in managing traumatic brain injury. Int J Mol Sci. 2015;16:28979–97.

Neuroprotection in Subarachnoid Hemorrhage

4

Arunabha Karmakar, Yasir M. Abdelwahid, and Gustav Strandvik

4.1 Introduction

Neuroprotection is a term used to describe interventions and strategies that are used to slow the progression of neuronal injury. The aim is to disrupt the metabolic and biochemical events that lead to neuroinflammation and nerve cell death. As the primary insult occurs almost instantaneously, neuroprotective measures mitigate *secondary injury* by modifying the cellular response to ischemia and energy deprivation; thereby leading to an improved neurological outcome. The pathological processes leading to secondary brain injury that need to be targeted include neuroinflammation, microthrombosis, generation of reactive oxygen species, mitochondrial dysfunction, and excitotoxicity. These lead to cell injury and death by apoptosis and cytoskeletal proteolysis [1].

A. Karmakar · Y. M. Abdelwahid
Department of Anesthesia, Perioperative Medicine and Critical Care, Hamad Medical Corporation, Doha, Qatar
e-mail: AKarmakar@Hamad.qa; YAlhajali@Hamad.qa

G. Strandvik (✉)
Department of Trauma Intensive Care Unit, Hamad Medical Corporation, Doha, Qatar

Weill Cornell Medical School, Ar-Rayyan, Qatar

College of Medicine at Qatar University, Doha, Qatar
e-mail: GStrandvik@Hamad.qa

4.2 Primary and Secondary Brain Injury

Causes of subarachnoid hemorrhage vary from spontaneous rupture of cerebral aneurysm and bleeding from an arteriovenous malformation to trauma-induced hemorrhage. In all cases this can lead to an increase in intracranial pressure secondary to the mass effect of blood or secondary to the development of acute hydrocephalus. This increase in intracranial pressure leads to a reduction in cerebral perfusion pressure, with consequent ischemic neuronal damage. Primary brain injury occurs at disease onset and usually outside the hospital, and thus cannot be prevented.

A cascade of secondary pathophysiologic events follows (Fig. 4.1), including:

1. Disruption of the blood–brain barrier.
2. Neuroinflammation.
3. Oxidative cascades.

Various mediators of these processes have been studied and are targets for the prevention of secondary brain injury.

The distinction between primary and secondary insults as described for tramatic brain injury (TBI), is not as clearly appreciated in subarachnoid hemorrhage; the initial is closely associated with subsequent injury. The sequence of events that occur before the onset of delayed vasospasm is collectively referred

A. E. A. Ganaw et al. (eds.), *Management of Subarachnoid Hemorrhage*,
https://doi.org/10.1007/978-3-030-81333-8_4

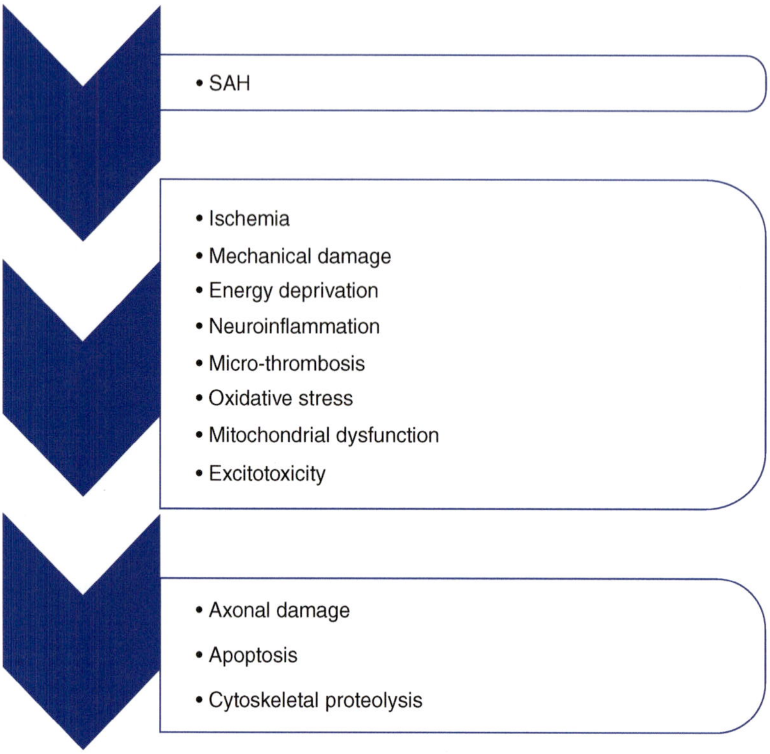

Fig. 4.1 Possible pathophysiological mechanisms of secondary brain injury after subarachnoid hemorrhage. (Courtesy of Dr. Yasir)

to as early brain injury; delayed brain injury occurs after the onset of cerebral vasospasm (delayed cerebral ischemia (DCI)). Recent research has led to the understanding that reversing vasospasm alone does not lead to better outcomes and thus many neuroprotective strategies are designed to treat early brain injury in addition to preventing or treating delayed cerebral ischemia [2].

4.3 Neuroprotective Strategies

Despite advancements in neuroscience in recent years, evidence supporting currently used neuroprotective strategies is still lacking, and many proposed strategies have conflicting evidence behind them. Many of these strategies show some benefit in experimental trials (mainly animal studies) but not in human studies [3]. The main difficulty appears to be related identifying appropriate therapeutic targets, as the process leading to the injury is complex and yet not fully understood.

4.3.1 General Measures

4.3.1.1 Cerebral Perfusion

Effective cerebral perfusion (flow) relies on the balance between the pressure of blood entering the cranial cavity, and the pressure within that cavity. The mean arterial pressure (MAP) as a function of both systolic and diastolic pressure dynamics is counteracted by the intracranial pressure (ICP). The product is the cerebral perfusion pressure (CPP).

$$CPP = MAP - ICP$$

In health, the brain can autoregulates the cerebral blood flow by mitigating or augmenting transmission of the MAP to the brain. This is predominantly a vascular tone phenomenon, mediated by local myogenic factors in cerebral blood vessels, produced in response to cerebral flow needs. Other factors affect the vasomotor tone of cerebral blood vessels; in particular, carbon dioxide levels have a powerful influence on vasoconstriction and vasodilatation of cerebral blood vessels. In disease states of the brain, including aneurysmal SAH, the ability of the brain to adjust the volume of blood entering the brain is often lost, and the CPP becomes directly proportional to cerebral flow (CBF) [4]. For more details please refer to Chap. 3 (central nervous system neurophysiology). For the purposes of neuroprotection, it is evident that, in the presence of a continuously bleeding blood vessel, the cerebral flow should be minimized. Thus, we divide neuroprotection into two phases: pre- and post-securing of the aneurysm.

Pre-securing of the aneurysm, it is important to provide adequate cerebral perfusion while avoiding the risk of excess blood loss or re-bleeding from the aneurysm. The bleeding is usually arrested after the initial event due to local coagulation dynamics, but high pressures transmitted to the brain can cause re-bleeding from the damaged blood vessel. This usually occurs from 2 to 10 h after the sentinel event. Although it would thus seem sensible to reduce the systemic blood pressure, there is evidence that hypotension in aneurysmal SAH may worsen outcomes [5] Evidence for a specific target systolic blood pressure to reduce the re-bleeding risk is limited. Based on the existing literature, it is standard practice to limit the systolic blood pressure to less than 160 mmHg in an un-secured aneurysmal SAH [6, 7].

Post-securing of the aneurysm, systolic blood pressure targets may be relaxed. The primary concern in the 10–14 days following the sentinel event is delayed cerebral ischemia due to cerebral vasospasm. The patient needs to be monitored closely for evidence of delayed cerebral ischemia (DCI). In good grade aSAH, the best monitor is clinical examination; a drop of GCS of two points or more is considered significant, although more subtle signs may be present [7]. In poorer grades, bedside tools such as regular measurement of middle cerebral artery velocities with transcranial Doppler (TCD) may be employed, although evidence for their effectiveness is lacking [8] There is currently little evidence for empirically augmenting the mean arterial pressure to provide any given cerebral perfusion pressure to prevent cerebral vasospasm and delayed cerebral ischemia. Maintaining a "normal" cerebral perfusion pressure of 60–70 mm Hg is cited as a reasonable target [9] In patients without an intracranial pressure monitor in situ, a mean arterial pressure target of 80–90 mmHg should ensure an adequate CPP. However, there is evidence that, should DCI develop, a target CPP of 80-120 mmHg may be effective at reversing the vasospasm [2]. Targets should be individualized depending on resolution of symptoms of DCI.

4.3.1.2 Normoxia and Normocapnia

Despite it's relatively small size (around 2% of the total body weight), the brain has a very high, accounting for only around 2% of the total body weight, its well known that the brain has a very high basal metabolic rate (approximately 3.5 ml/100 g brain/min) [10]. This is better understood when compared to the total body oxygen consumption. The total oxygen consumption by the entire brain (an average weight of 1400 grams) is around 50 ml/min which accounts for 20% or *one fifth* of the total body oxygen consumption (250 ml/min) [11]. There is no doubt that maintaining tissue oxygenation is vital for normal cellular function and that hypoxia is harmful and could be fatal; therefore, providing supplementary oxygen plays a major role in the management of critically ill patients in whom hypoxia is more likely to cause detrimental effects. On the other hand, it should not be assumed that providing extra oxygen (hyperoxia) is beneficial or that the injured tissues will be able to utilize this extra oxygen; and the side effects of having such high oxygen levels should not be overlooked. Having high levels of oxygen can actually cause direct tissue injury by producing reactive oxygen species (ROS) and stimulating the inflammatory response leading to cellular death by apoptosis. A retrospective cohort study by Davis et al. in 2009 which included 3420 patients with moderate to severe traumatic brain injury showed that maintaining a partial pressure of oxygen (PaO_2) value of 110–487 mmHg is optimal and a higher PaO_2 value was associated with a decreased survival rate, Fig. 4.2 [13]. Another retrospective study (Brenner et al. in 2012) included 1547 patients with severe TBI and found that both hypoxia and hyperoxia were associated with an increased mortality rate; but patients with hyperoxia had a higher in-hospital

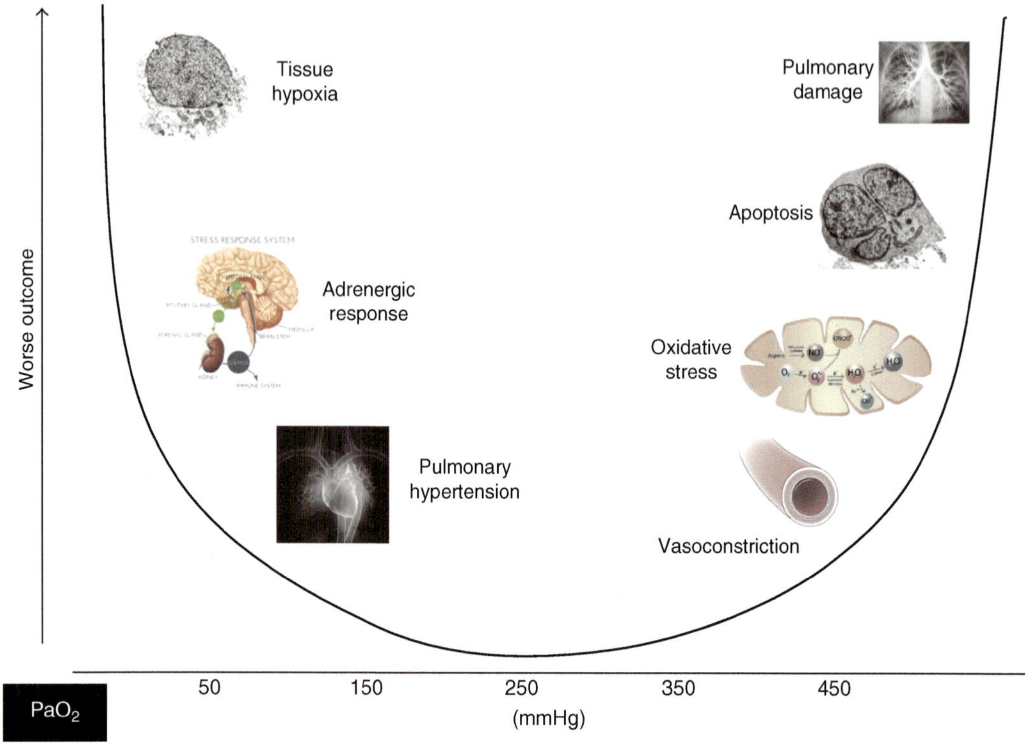

Fig. 4.2 Schematic showing U-shaped association of PaO_2 and outcome. (Reproduced under the Creative Commons Attribution License from reference [12])

mortality and lower Glasgow coma scales on discharge [14]. A more recent observational retrospective study conducted by Jeon et al. in 2014 included 252 patients with subarachnoid hemorrhage, and linked hyperoxia to a higher incidence of delayed cerebral ischemia. Hyperoxia was also associated with a worse neurological outcome at 3 months after the SAH [15]. Thus, while the optimal level of PaO_2 remains unclear, it should be remembered that maintaining levels higher than the physiological range has been associated with poor outcome.

As noted in previous chapters, the effect of CO_2 levels on vascular reactivity in the brain can be profound. Manipulation of the $PaCO_2$ is commonly utilized in the setting of raised intracranial pressure; changes in CO_2 levels have real-time effects on cerebral blood flow [16]. For more details please refer to Chap. 3.

4.3.1.3 Therapeutic Hypothermia

It is well established that mild therapeutic hypothermia improves neurological outcome after cardiac arrest due to ventricular fibrillation [17]. However, there are very few human studies examining the effect of therapeutic hypothermia in patients with subarachnoid hemorrhage. Kuramatsu et al. found that early (<48 h after ictus), mild (35 °C) and prolonged (7 ± 1 days) therapeutic hypothermia was associated with a reduced degree of macrovascular vasospasm and significantly decreased occurrence of DCI (87.5% in non-therapeutic hypothermia vs 50% in therapeutic hypothermia group). Additionally, favorable functional outcomes at 6 months (modified Rankin scale score of 0–2) were twice as likely in the therapeutic hypothermia group (66.7%) versus the non-therapeutic hypothermia group (33.3%) [18]. Choi et al. studied the safety and feasibility of mild therapeutic hypothermia (core body temperature <36 °C for >95% of a 48-h treatment period) in poor grade (Hunt and Hess Scale 4,5 and modified Fisher Scale 3,4) subarachnoid hemorrhage patients following successful aneurysm control. They reported that fewer patients in the therapeutic hypothermia group suffered symptomatic vasospasm and DCI, although these differences were not statistically significant. They reported good-to-moderate functional outcomes (0–3 modified Rankin Scale) at 3 months post study in 54.5% of the therapeutic hypothermia group compared with 9% in the control group [19]. Both studies agree that larger studies are required to provide conclusive evidence for the support of routine therapeutic hypothermia in the management of subarachnoid hemorrhage.

4.3.1.4 Prevention of Fever

Core temperatures of ≥38.3 °C (101 °F) occur in up to 72% of patients with aneurysmal SAH, have been linked to negative outcomes [20]. Andrews et al. published a consensus opinion regarding Targeted Temperature Management (TTM) for subarachnoid hemorrhage, intracerebral hemorrhage (ICH), and acute ischemic stroke (AIS) patients. They opined that fever and shivering should both be controlled by TTM. They proposed that the target temperature for patients who develop neurogenic fever is 37.0 ± 0.5 °C. TTM should be maintained for as long as there is potential for secondary brain damage, and there should be advanced TTM methods to enable precise temperature control [21]. Most evidence on fever prevention in patients in critical care is observational in nature and the exact role that fever plays in causing secondary brain injury is unclear. Results from The Impact of Fever Prevention in Brain Injured Patients Study (NCT02996266) are awaited.

4.3.1.5 Glycemic Management

Multiple studies have shown that patients with hyperglycemia on admission for SAH develop DCI and cerebral infarction more often than patients with normal blood glucose levels. Furthermore, aneurysmal SAH patients with pre-existent diabetes mellitus are at an increased risk of DCI compared with aneurysmal SAH patients without pre-existent diabetes mellitus [22]. Fontera et al. as part of an SAH outcomes project prospectively studied the glucose burden (GB) in 580 patients admitted with spontaneous SAH. They found that GB was associated with increased intensive care unit length of stay, congestive heart failure, respiratory failure, pneumonia, and brain stem compression from herniation. After adjusting for Hunt–Hess grade, aneurysm size and age, GB was an independent predictor of death or severe disability [23]. The Neurocritical Care Society's Multidisciplinary Consensus Conference panel agreed that extreme systemic hyperglycemia is a marker of severity of SAH as well as a risk factor for infection. They also expressed concern that patients being treated with insulin infusions may have inappropriately low cerebral glucose concentrations, which could go undetected due to the limited availability and use of cerebral microdialysis catheters (to measure cerebral glucose and other cerebral metabolic crisis) in clinical management. They recommended that hypoglycemia (serum glucose <80 mg/dl) should be avoided, that serum glucose should be maintained below 200 mg/dl, and that (if available) microdialysis-guided serum glucose adjustment may avoid low cerebral glucose [24].

4.3.1.6 Dysnatremia and Sodium Management

Low serum sodium (hyponatremia) is seen in almost 56.6% of SAH patients, and is more common post aneurysmal rather than non-aneurysmal SAH. The etiopathology includes syndrome of inappropriate ADH secretion (SIADH), cerebral salt wasting syndrome, and glucocorticoid deficiency [25]. Hyponatremia may be an independent risk factor for poor outcome. Hyponatremia and associated hypotonicity result in a shift of water from the extracellular to intracellular space, thereby worsening cerebral edema and intracranial hypertension, increasing risk of seizures and neurological injury. Natriuresis and volume contraction may exacerbate vasospasm and DCI [26]. Determination of the cause of hyponatremia includes clinical examination and biochemical hormone measurement. Comprehensive electrolyte and fluid balance monitoring on a daily basis may ensure early detection and efficient management. The Neurocritical Care Society expert panel [24] recommends vigilant fluid balance management as the foundation for monitoring intravascular volume status. There is no particular recommendation for the type of monitoring technology to be used. They advised that central venous lines should not be placed solely to obtain CVP measurements and that fluid management based solely on CVP measurements is not recommended. Routine use of pulmonary artery catheters is also not recommended. There was a broad agreement that hypovolemia was to be avoided following SAH. Studies have, however, showed no benefit with prophylactic hypervolemia, which has been associated with an increased risk of cardiopulmonary complications. They recommend that intravascular volume management should target euvolemia and that prophylactic hypervolemia should be avoided. Isotonic crystalloid is the preferred agent for volume replacement. In patients with persistent negative fluid balance, the use of [24] fludrocortisone or hydrocortisone may be considered. Prospective randomized controlled trials on the use of fludrocortisone and hydrocortisone to prevent hyponatremia in SAH suggest that their use may reduce the amount of fluid required to maintain euvolemia [24].

While there exists support for the use of fludrocortisone and hydrocortisone in patients with excessive diuresis, there is a concern about the impact of high dose hydrocortisone on glucose management. Overall both corticosteroids are consistently effective in limiting natriuresis and hyponatremia when started early after the onset of SAH. Use of corticosteroids is associated with an increased incidence of hyperglycemia and hypokalemia, both of which were treatable. Vasopressin receptor antagonists such as conivaptan are effective for the treatment of hyponatremia associated with euvolemic or hypervolemic conditions, and in hyponatremic SAH patients. They can, however, produce a significant rise in urine output raising a concern about intravascular volume contraction, especially in the setting of DCI [24]. Generally, the trigger used for treatment of hyponatremia is serum sodium concentration <135 mEq/l or if neurological deterioration is attributed to falling sodium concentration. Fluid restriction should not be used to treat hyponatremia. Mild hypertonic saline solutions can be used for correction. Free water intake via intravenous and enteral routes should be limited [24].

4.3.1.7 Seizure Prophylaxis

Clinical seizures are often due to aneurysm rerupture in patients with un-secured aneurysm rather than the initial aneurysm rupture. Risk factors include surgical aneurysm repair in patients >65 years of age of age more than 65 years, thick subarachnoid clot and possible intraparenchymal hematoma or infarction. While prophylactic anticonvulsant use was common, studies have shown worsened long-term outcomes. However, most of these studies used phenytoin and outcome with another anti-convulsant use is not clear [24]. The Neurocritical Care Society expert panel stated that the routine use of prophylactic anticonvulsant prophylaxis with phenytoin is not recommended while the use of other anti-convulsant agents may be considered. If used, short duration (3–7 days) is recommended. In patients who suffer a seizure after presentation, anti-convulsant should be continued for a duration defined by local practice (no evidence base supporting the duration). Continuous EEG monitoring should be considered in patients with poor-grade SAH who fail to improve or who have neurological deterioration of undetermined etiology; non-convulsive status epilepticus should be excluded [24].

4.3.1.8 Anemia

Anemia is common after subarachnoid hemorrhage. A secondary analysis of 413 SAH patients in the CONSCIOUS-1 study (Clazosentan to Overcome Neurological Ischemia and Infarction After Subarachnoid Hemorrhage) found that Hemoglobin <10 g/dl was present in 5% of patients at presentation, 29% of patients after aneurysm securing (days 1–3) and in 32% of patients during the peak delayed cerebral ischemia risk period (days 5–9). Anemia after aneurysm securing and during the delayed cerebral ischemia window was independently associated with poor neurological outcomes; anemia post-aneurysm securing but not during the delayed cerebral ischemia window was associated with death. The same study (using propensity score-matched cohorts) found that transfusion of anemic patients did not improve long-term outcome or mortality rates. However, transfusion of patients with Hemoglobin <10 g/dl was associated with improved neurological outcomes with no differences in mortality [27]. A retrospective review of 421 consecutive patients with SAH, admitted to a neurocritical care unit after surgical occlusion of their ruptured aneurysm, concluded that blood transfusions are associated with unfavorable outcome after SAH, particularly when DCI is absent. However, when DCI is present, red blood cell transfusion may help improve outcome [28]. The results of the Aneurysmal Subarachnoid Hemorrhage-Red Blood Cell Transfusion and Outcome (SAHaRA) (NCT02483351)—A pilot Randomized Controlled trial is awaited.

4.3.1.9 Nutrition

Resolution of inflammation in SAH can be a potential therapeutic target to prevent secondary injury. Omega 3 fatty acids such as Eicosapentaenoic acid (EPA) and Docosahexaenoic acid (DHA) are precursors of key mediators involved in resolution of inflammation and endogenous neuroprotection. EPA is also involved in microvascular function. DHA is widely distributed in membrane phospholipids and is abundant in brain and retinal tissue. It is an essential component of neuronal membrane architecture, composition and promotes selective accumulation of Phosphatidyl serine which is involved in intracellular signal events. DHA is also a precursor for Docosanoids and other important bioactive compounds needed for normal neuronal function, tissue homeostasis, and neuronal survival.

There are increased levels of free DHA in CSF after SAH which is likely because DHA was cleaved from membrane phospholipids by either direct structural damage or an increase in phospholipase A2 activity in response to neuroinflammation. Increased consumption of DHA by the brain may occur following SAH due to increased generation of neuroprotective derivatives [29]. A small pilot trial examining the impact of long chain omega 3 fatty acids in aneurysmal SAH suggested that the intervention group did not suffer from increased post-operative intracranial bleeding complications and did not suffer unexpected harm. Larger trials would be required to show any outcome changes in SAH patients who are given omega 3 fatty acids [30].

4.4 Specific Pharmacological Measures

4.4.1 Corticosteroids

The neurocritical care society expert panel [24] recommends that early treatment with hydrocortisone or fludrocortisone may be used in acute SAH to limit natriuresis and hyponatremia. However, no clear evidence exists in terms of outcome improvement. Hypothalamic dysfunction appears to occur acutely in a minority of patients with SAH. The diagnosis should be considered in patients who are unresponsive to vasopressors. Administration of stress dose steroids for patients with vasospasm and un-responsiveness to induced hypertension may be considered. Steroids (mostly dexamethasone) have been studied for their potential studied for its potential anti-inflammatory role in SAH patients. The mechanisms are poorly understood and though to be related to general interruption of inflammatory processes. Multiple studies showed mixed results and sample sizes are too small to draw firm conclusions. Although some evidence does exist for potential improvement in long-term functional outcomes, the studies are small [31], a Cochrane review concluded that no clear evidence existed for benefit or harm of steroid use in the acute management of SAH patients [32]. Thus, administration of high dose corticosteroids is not recommended in acute SAH as use of high dose steroids in patients with neurocritical illness can cause serious adverse effects, increased mortality and no benefit.

4.4.2 Calcium Channel Antagonists

Studies have shown that calcium channel antagonists may prevent or reverse vasospasm, and have neuroprotective properties. A Cochrane review found that calcium channel antagonists reduce the risk of poor outcome and secondary ischemia after aneurysmal SAH. The results for poor outcome depend largely on a single large trial of oral Nimodipine. The evidence for other calcium antagonists is inconclusive. Given the potential benefits and modest risk of treatment, oral Nimodipine is currently indicated in patients with aneurysmal SAH. Intravenous administration of calcium channel antagonists cannot be recommended for routine practice based on present evidence [33].

4.4.3 Statins

Statins inhibit 3 hydroxy-3 methylglutaryl coenzyme A reductase and block the formation of mevalonate which is an important precursor for both cholesterol and other non-sterol products. Statins have a good safety record and have several potential beneficial effects after SAH, including cerebral blood flow enhancement, raised cerebral endothelial nitric oxide synthase expression, improved endothelial function, and protection against ischemia. Some studies have reported reduced vasospasm, delayed ischemic neurological deficit and mortality [34]. A 2008 meta-analysis by Sillberg et al. supported these conclusions, but a 2009 meta-analysis by Vergouwen and colleagues did not find any evidence to support the beneficial effects of statins in SAH.

In view of contrasting evidence, a multicenter randomized controlled trial—the STASH (Simvastatin in Aneurysmal Subarachnoid Hemorrhage) trial recruited 803 patients 18–65 years of age with confirmatory evidence of aneurysmal SAH. Patients presenting less than 96 h from ictus were recruited and randomized to receive either simvastatin 40 mg or placebo once a day for up to 21 days. The primary outcome of the trial was distribution of modified Rankin Scale (mRS) score at 6 months. The STASH trial did not detect any benefit in the use of simvastatin for long-term or short-term outcome in patients with aneurysmal subarachnoid hemorrhage. The authors of the trial concluded that patients with subarachnoid hemorrhage should not be routinely treated with simvastatin during the acute stages [35].

4.4.4 Magnesium

Magnesium is a non-competitive calcium antagonist with potential neuroprotective effects. It promotes vasodilation by blocking voltage-dependent calcium channels, decreasing glutamate release. Magnesium can attenuate the effect of potent vasoconstrictors including endothelin 1, and also blocks the including endothelin 1, and blocks the formation of reactive oxygen species [24]. However, the MASH-2 trial (magnesium for aneurysmal subarachnoid hemorrhage), a randomized placebo controlled trial that studied 1203 patients, found that intravenous magnesium sulfate did not improve clinical outcome after aneurysmal SAH and therefore routine administration of magnesium cannot be recommended [36].

4.4.5 Erythropoietin (EPO)

It is believed that EPO may exert beneficial neuroprotective effects via inhibition of apoptosis in tissues adjacent to a lesion, modulate nitric oxide synthesis in the vascular endothelium, promote neurotransmitter release, and reduce blood brain barrier dysfunction [37]. A small randomized controlled trial of 80 patients randomized participants to receive 30,000 units of erythropoietin beta every other day for 3 doses within 72 h after subarachnoid hemorrhage. The study showed no difference in overall incidence of vasospasm but reduced incidence of severe vasospasm and delayed neurological deficit. However, most authors agree that larger trials are needed before making a conclusive decision on the benefit of erythropoietin for subarachnoid hemorrhage management [38].

4.4.6 Anti-platelet Therapy

Platelet aggregation may play a role in secondary ischemia and experimental studies have suggested that anti-platelet therapy might offer benefit to reduce secondary ischemia. A Cochrane review from 2007 showed a trend towards better outcome in patients with SAH treated with antiplatelet agents. However, the results were not statistically significant and thus no definite conclusions could be drawn [39]. Ven Den Berg et al. as part of the MASH (Magnesium and Acetylsalicylic acid in subarachnoid Hemorrhage) study examined whether acetylsalicylic acid reduced the risk of delayed ischemic neurological deficit (DIND) in patients with subarachnoid hemorrhage. Patients in whom aneurysm treatment was started 4 days after subarachnoid hemorrhage were included. Fourteen daily suppositories with 100 mg Acetylsalicylic acid or placebo was started within 12 h after the aneurysm was occluded. The study was stopped at 161 of 200 planned patients because by then the chances of a positive effect were negligible. It was concluded that acetylsalicylic acid given after aneurysm treatment does not appreciably reduce the occurrence of delayed ischemic neurological deficit [40]. Risk of re-bleeding is very high in the first 24 h. Making the administration of anti-platelet agents very risky in un-secured aneurysm.

Another benefit that anti-platelets may give is the prevention of thromboembolic complications during endovascular treatment of aneurysms. Van Den Bergh conducted a questionnaire study to the participating centers of The International Subarachnoid Aneurysm Trial (ISAT) Collaborative Group. The questionnaire study involved 19 of the 43 participating centers, which involved 1422 of the 2143 ISAT patients. The questionnaire asked whether the centers never, sometimes or always prescribed anti-platelets during or after coiling of aneurysmal subarachnoid hemorrhage. Based on the individual patient data, the relative risks of coiling versus clipping were calculated separately for patients treated in hospitals with standard prescription during or after coiling versus patients treated in hospitals with no standard prescription of anti-platelets. The results of the study did not support anti-platelets during or after endovascular coiling in terms of improved outcomes in patients with SAH [41].

4.4.7 Endothelin A Antagonist

Endothelin has been implicated as a possible cause of delayed ischemic neurological deficit by causing blood vessel constriction. A Cochrane review of four trials involving 2024 patients showed that endothelin receptor antagonists reduced the risk of delayed ischemic neurologic deficit and angiographic vasospasm but did not improve clinical outcomes, with potentially serious side effects such as low blood pressure and chest infection. The authors stated that there is not enough evidence to conclude that endothelin A receptor antagonists are beneficial in subarachnoid hemorrhage patients [42].

4.4.8 Beta Blockers/ Dexmedetomidine

Many of the adverse outcomes of subarachnoid hemorrhage can be linked to the sympathetic surge which might cause neurologic complications (re-bleeding, vasospasm) and cardiovascular complications (myocardial stunning, stress induced cardiomyopathy, troponin elevation, ECG changes, regional wall motion abnormalities). It is believed that beta blocker therapy might help to prevent this sympathetic surge. A retrospective analysis of 218 patients admitted to the surgical intensive care unit for management of ruptured subarachnoid hemorrhage was done by Chang et al. They identified three classes of patients: No/No were patients who did not have any beta blocker, No/Yes were patients who received post admission beta blockade, and Yes/Yes were patients who were on home beta blockade and continued. They found that when compared to No/No patients, No/Yes patients had significantly increased vasospasm. However, these patients had significantly fewer deaths and need for long-term care with decreased tendency for infarcts. When compared to No/No patients, Yes/Yes patients had increased trend towards vasospasm that led to infarction but with decreased mortality or need for long-term care [43]. Another study looked at the association between dexmedetomidine use and neurological outcomes in aneurysmal subarachnoid hemorrhages. They found that low dose dexmedetomidine during the first 24 h after admission was associated with favorable neurological outcomes [44].

4.4.9 Heparin

Heparin was found to have neuroprotective interactions, possible by decreasing the transcription of Endothelin-1 (ET-1) and the ET-1 promoter, and also decreased expression of the erythroid transcription factor family binding capacity which is essential for ET-1 function in the endothelial cells. Heparin and its low molecular weight derivatives are also potent inhibitors of the adhesion molecules P- and L-selectin which cause leucocyte rolling (one of the initial steps responsible for inflammation). The anticoagulation effect of heparin may also prevent microthromboembolism, which is a possible contributor to delayed neurological deficits [45]. A retrospective analysis as conducted of 86 consecutive patients with Fisher Grade 3 aneurysmal subarachnoid hemorrhage due to rupture of a supratentorial aneurysm, who presented within 36 h and were treated by surgical clipping within 48 h of their ictus. Forty-three of 86 patients were managed postoperatively with a low dose intravenous heparin infusion (Heparin group) while the remaining 43 received conventional subcutaneous heparin twice daily as deep vein thrombosis prophylaxis (control group). The control group had higher incidence of clinical vasospasm (20 of 43 patients, i.e. 47%) requiring rescue therapy (induced hypertension, selective intra-arterial verapamil, and angioplasty) and 21% of patients experienced a delayed infarct on CT scan. In the heparin group, the incidence of clinical vasospasm requiring rescue therapy was 9% and no patient suffered a delayed infarct [46]. Heparin infusions appear safe as long as vigilance for bleeding complications is maintained. Evidence for its benefit in preventing delayed neurological injury is inconclusive. A major hurdle continues to be concerns about bleeding. Larger randomized controlled studies are required to promote its large-scale implementation [47].

4.4.10 Hydrogen Rich Saline

Hong Y et al. did a rat study involving injection of hydrogen rich saline intraperitoneally into rats with experimental SAH models (cisterna magna blood injection) and found that hydrogen rich saline significantly improved neurological outcomes and attenuated morphological vasospasm of the basilar artery after subarachnoid hemorrhage. They also found that the beneficial effects of hydrogen rich saline on cerebral vasospasm were associated with decreased levels of lipid peroxidation, increased activity of anti-oxidant enzymes, and reduced levels of pro-inflammatory cytokines in the basilar artery [48]. Zong Zhuang et al. showed that intra-peritoneal hydrogen rich saline could alleviate oxidative stress and brain edema after subarachnoid hemorrhage in rabbit models. Clinical studies in humans are awaited [49].

4.4.11 Ghrelin

Xiao-ke Hao et al. showed that ghrelin significantly improved neurological function and reduced neuronal apoptosis and brain edema at 24 h after subarachnoid hemorrhage in rat models. They found that levels of p-Akt expressed in many neurons were markedly up-regulated. Additionally, the level of Caspase-3 was decreased. They proposed that Ghrelin may be useful to reduce early brain injury after subarachnoid hemorrhage and that these beneficial effects may be due to a mechanism involving the PI3K/Akt signaling pathway [50].

4.4.12 ADAMTS13

ADAMTS13 (A disintegrin and Metalloprotease with Thrombospondin repeats −12) deficiency can lead to higher concentrations of large von Willebrand factor multimers resulting in microthrombosis. Vergouwen et al. in a study of 31 patients after aneurysmal subarachnoid hemorrhage found that 11 of the 31 patients (35%) patients who developed delayed cerebral ischemia were found to also have a decrease in ADAMST13 activity and a more profound increase in Von Willebrand Factor antigen, Von Willebrand factor pro-peptide, and Von Willebrand factor activity in the first few days after hemorrhage. The authors concluded that their results suggest that micro-thrombosis may have a role in the pathogenesis of delayed cerebral ischemia [51].

4.4.13 Fasudil

FasudilHCl(Hexahydro-1-5-isoquinolinesulfonyl)-1H-1.4-diazepine HCl) is a Rho-kinase inhibitor, which has been shown by experimental studies in dogs to dilate spastic arteries without causing systemic hypotension. This effect was also shown in human studies. It is routinely used in Japan for patients with subarachnoid hemorrhage. It has been shown that Rho-kinase is observed not only in spastic arteries but also in ischemic brain tissue. Fasudil specifically increased regional cerebral blood flow in areas with vasospasm. Fasudil may also improve cerebral blood flow by limiting vascular endothelial and also by minimizing the inflammatory response implicated in cerebral vasospasm development [52]. A retrospective cohort study by Funakoshi H et al. looked at 24068 patients who were older than 18 years and underwent surgical clipping or endovascular coil embolization within 72 h from admission with subarachnoid hemorrhage. Patients with unknown modified Rankin scale (mRS) or coma (Japan coma scale 100 or higher) at the time of visit and those who died within 3 days after intervention were excluded. The study found that prophylactic administration of Fasudil Hydrochloride for cerebral vasospasm prevention to patient with subarachnoid hemorrhage did not reduce the 30-day mortality.

However, Fasudil Hydrochloride significantly reduced poor neurological outcome (modified Rankin scale >2) upon discharge [53] of eight studies by Liu et al., found that Fasudil greatly reduces the occurrence of cerebral vasospasm and cerebral infarction in subarachnoid hemorrhage patients and significantly improves the clinical outcomes of the patients (as assessed by the Glasgow Outcome Scale). Due to the limited number of trials and samples available for analysis, these results need to be validated with results from large randomized, controlled trials [54].

4.4.14 Deferoxamine

Lee JY et al. investigated hemoglobin and iron handling after subarachnoid hemorrhage, to investigate the relationship between iron and neuroglial cell changes, and whether deferoxamine reduced subarachnoid hemorrhage-induced injury. In rats induced with subarachnoid hemorrhage using an endovascular perforation technique, there was marked heme oxygenase-1 (HO-1) up-regulation at day 3, and accompanied by elevated non-heme iron, transferrin, Tf receptor, and ferritin levels. Deferoxamine treatment reduced subarachnoid hemorrhage-induced mortality, brain non-heme iron concentration, iron handling, protein expression, oxidative stress, and neuronal cell death at day 3 after subarachnoid hemorrhage. The results suggest that iron overload in the acute phase of subarachnoid hemorrhage leads to oxidative injury leading to neuronal cell death. Since Deferoxamine effectively reduces oxidative stress and neuronal cell death, it may be a potential therapeutic agent for subarachnoid hemorrhage [55].

4.5 Conclusions

Principles of neuroprotection have been developed from multiple sources within and outside the specific domain of aneurysmal subarachnoid hemorrhage. Some of these principles are inductive; they rely on applying the understanding of physiology and pathophysiology to a dynamic process that cannot at this time be directly visualized. The concept of "normal" is a reasonable starting point. If one provides what the brain needs in terms of pressure, oxygen, substrate and an optimized metabolic state, the development of secondary injury may be minimized. The one well-established therapy, Nimodipine, is itself based on robust, but relatively limited, evidence. None of these techniques have yet been found in isolation to fully protect the brain. Many investigative techniques for neuroprotection in SAH exist, and ongoing efforts need to be made to prevent the scourge of secondary brain injury. In time, a composite set of measures may help patients achieve optimal outcomes.

References

1. Park E, Bell JD, Baker AJ. Traumatic brain injury: can the consequences be stopped? Can Med Assoc J. 2008;178(9):1163–70.
2. Francoeur CL, Mayer SA. Management of delayed cerebral ischemia after subarachnoid hemorrhage. Crit Care. 2016;20(1):277.
3. Mrara B. Neuroprotection: fact and fantasy. South African J Anaesth Analg. 2015;21(1):64–6.
4. Conzen C, Becker K, Albanna W, Weiss M, Bach A, Lushina N, et al. The acute phase of experimental subarachnoid hemorrhage: intracranial pressure dynamics and their effect on cerebral blood flow and autoregulation. Transl Stroke Res. 2019;10(5):566–82.
5. Ascanio LC, Enriquez-Marulanda A, Maragkos GA, Salem MM, Alturki AY, Ravindran K, et al. Effect of blood pressure variability during the acute period of subarachnoid hemorrhage on functional outcomes. Neurosurgery. 2020;87(4):779–87.
6. Der-Nigoghossian C, Levasseur-Franklin K, Makii J. Acute blood pressure management in neurocritically ill patients. Pharmacotherapy. 2019;39(3):335–45.
7. Djilvesi D, Horvat I, Jelaca B, Golubovic J, Pajicic F, Vulekovic P. Comparison of radiological versus clinical cerebral vasospasm after aneurysmal subarachnoid hemorrhage: is vasospasm always present? Neurol Res. 2020:1–7.
8. Wartenberg KE. Critical care of poor-grade subarachnoid hemorrhage. Curr Opin Crit Care. 2011;17(2):85–93.
9. Cai J, Fang W, Chen F, Lin Z, Lin Y, Yu L, et al. Cerebral perfusion pressure threshold to prevent delayed cerebral ischemia after aneurysmal subarachnoid hemorrhage. J Clin Neurosci. 2018;54:29–32.
10. Diringer MN. Hyperoxia: good or bad for the injured brain? Curr Opin Crit Care. 2008;14(2):167–71.
11. Kennedy C, Sokoloff L. An adaptation of the nitrous oxide method to the study of the cerebral circulation in children; normal values for cerebral blood flow and cerebral metabolic rate in childhood. J Clin Invest. 1957;36(7):1130–7.
12. Vincent J-L, Taccone FS, He X. Harmful effects of hyperoxia in postcardiac arrest, sepsis, traumatic brain injury, or stroke: the importance of individualized oxygen therapy in critically ill patients. Can Respir J. 2017;2017:2834956.
13. Davis DP, Meade W, Sise MJ, Kennedy F, Simon F, Tominaga G, et al. Both hypoxemia and extreme hyperoxemia may be detrimental in patients with severe traumatic brain injury. J Neurotrauma. 2009;26(12):2217–23.
14. Brenner M, Stein D, Hu P, Kufera J, Wooford M, Scalea T. Association between early hyperoxia and worse outcomes after traumatic brain injury. Arch Surg. 2012;147(11):1042–6.
15. Jeon SB, Choi HA, Badjatia N, Schmidt JM, Lantigua H, Claassen J, et al. Hyperoxia may be related to delayed cerebral ischemia and poor outcome after subarachnoid haemorrhage. J Neurol Neurosurg Psychiatry. 2014;85(12):1301–7.
16. Cipolla MJ. Control of cerebral blood flow. In: The cerebral circulation. Morgan & Claypool Life Sciences; 2009.
17. Hypothermia after Cardiac Arrest Study Group. Mild therapeutic hypothermia to improve the neurologic outcome after cardiac arrest. N Engl J Med. 2002;346(8):549–56.
18. Kuramatsu JB, Kollmar R, Gerner ST, Madžar D, Pisarčíková A, Staykov D, et al. Is hypothermia helpful in severe subarachnoid hemorrhage? An exploratory study on macro vascular spasm, delayed cerebral infarction and functional outcome after prolonged hypothermia. Cerebrovasc Dis. 2015;40(5–6):228–35.
19. Choi W, Kwon SC, Lee WJ, Weon YC, Choi B, Lee H, et al. Feasibility and safety of mild therapeutic hypothermia in poor-grade subarachnoid hemorrhage: prospective pilot study. J Korean Med Sci. 2017;32(8):1337–44.
20. Scaravilli V, Tinchero G, Citerio G. Fever management in SAH. Neurocrit Care. 2011;15(2):287.
21. Andrews P, Verma V, Healy M, Lavinio A, Curtis C, Reddy U, et al. Targeted temperature management in patients with intracerebral haemorrhage, subarachnoid haemorrhage, or acute ischaemic stroke: consensus recommendations. Br J Anaesth. 2018;121(4):768–75.
22. Kruyt ND, Biessels GJ, DeVries JH, Luitse MJ, Vermeulen M, Rinkel GJ, et al. Hyperglycemia in aneurysmal subarachnoid hemorrhage: a potentially modifiable risk factor for poor outcome. J Cereb Blood Flow Metab. 2010;30(9):1577–87.
23. Frontera JA, Fernandez A, Claassen J, Schmidt M, Schumacher HC, Wartenberg K, et al. Hyperglycemia after SAH: predictors, associated complications, and impact on outcome. Stroke. 2006;37(1):199–203.
24. Diringer MN, Bleck TP, Claude Hemphill J 3rd, Menon D, Shutter L, Vespa P, et al. Critical care management of patients following aneurysmal subarachnoid hemorrhage: recommendations from the Neurocritical Care Society's Multidisciplinary Consensus Conference. Neurocrit Care. 2011;15(2):211–40.
25. Okazaki T, Kuroda Y. Aneurysmal subarachnoid hemorrhage: intensive care for improving neurological outcome. J Intensive Care. 2018;6:28.

26. Marupudi NI, Mittal S. Diagnosis and management of hyponatremia in patients with aneurysmal subarachnoid hemorrhage. J Clin Med. 2015;4(4): 756–67.
27. Ayling OGS, Ibrahim GM, Alotaibi NM, Gooderham PA, Macdonald RL. Anemia after aneurysmal subarachnoid hemorrhage is associated with poor outcome and death. Stroke. 2018;49(8):1859–65.
28. Kumar MA, Levine J, Faerber J, Elliott JP, Winn HR, Doerfler S, et al. The effects of red blood cell transfusion on functional outcome after aneurysmal subarachnoid hemorrhage. World Neurosurg. 2017;108:807–16.
29. Saito G, Zapata R. Aneurysmal subarachnoid hemorrhage and resolution of inflammation. Intracranial Aneurysms: IntechOpen; 2019.
30. Saito G, Zapata R, Rivera R, Zambrano H, Rojas D, Acevedo H, et al. Long-chain omega-3 fatty acids in aneurysmal subarachnoid hemorrhage: a randomized pilot trial of pharmaconutrition. Surg Neurol Int. 2017;8:304.
31. Mohney N, Williamson CA, Rothman E, Ball R, Sheehan KM, Pandey AS, et al. A propensity score analysis of the impact of dexamethasone use on delayed cerebral ischemia and poor functional outcomes after subarachnoid hemorrhage. World Neurosurg. 2018;109:e655–e61.
32. Feigin VL, Anderson N, Rinkel GJE, Algra A, van Gijn J, Bennett DA. Corticosteroids for aneurysmal subarachnoid haemorrhage and primary intracerebral haemorrhage. Cochrane Database Syst Rev. 2005;(3):CD004583.
33. Dorhout Mees SM, Rinkel GJ, Feigin VL, Algra A, van den Bergh WM, Vermeulen M, et al. Calcium antagonists for aneurysmal subarachnoid haemorrhage. The Cochrane database of systematic reviews. 2007(3):Cd000277.
34. Su S-H, Xu W, Hai J, Wu Y-F, Yu F. Effects of statins-use for patients with aneurysmal subarachnoid hemorrhage: a meta-analysis of randomized controlled trials. Sci Rep. 2014;4(1):4573.
35. Kirkpatrick PJ, Turner CL, Smith C, Hutchinson PJ, Murray GD. Simvastatin in aneurysmal subarachnoid haemorrhage (STASH): a multicentre randomised phase 3 trial. Lancet Neurol. 2014;13(7):666–75.
36. Mees SMD, Algra A, Vandertop WP, van Kooten F, Kuijsten HAJM, Boiten J, et al. Magnesium for aneurysmal subarachnoid haemorrhage (MASH-2): a randomised placebo-controlled trial. Lancet. 2012;380(9836):44–9.
37. Grasso G, Tomasello G, Noto M, Alafaci C, Cappello F. Erythropoietin for the treatment of subarachnoid hemorrhage: a feasible ingredient for a successful medical recipe. Mol Med. 2015;21(1):979–87.
38. Tseng MY, Hutchinson PJ, Richards HK, Czosnyka M, Pickard JD, Erber WN, et al. Acute systemic erythropoietin therapy to reduce delayed ischemic deficits following aneurysmal subarachnoid hemorrhage: a phase II randomized, double-blind, placebo-controlled trial. Clin Art J Neurosurg. 2009;111(1):171–80.
39. Dorhout Mees S, van den Bergh WM, Algra A, Rinkel GJE. Antiplatelet therapy for aneurysmal subarachnoid haemorrhage. Cochrane Database Syst Rev. 2007;(4):CD006184.
40. van den Bergh WM, et al. Randomized controlled trial of acetylsalicylic acid in aneurysmal subarachnoid hemorrhage. Stroke. 2006;37(9):2326–30.
41. van den Bergh WM, Kerr RSC, Algra A, Rinkel GJE, Molyneux AJ. Effect of antiplatelet therapy for endovascular coiling in aneurysmal subarachnoid hemorrhage. Stroke. 2009;40(6):1969–72.
42. Guo J, Shi Z, Yang K, Tian JH, Jiang L. Endothelin receptor antagonists for subarachnoid hemorrhage. Cochrane Database Syst Rev. 2012;(9):CD008354.
43. Chang MM, Raval RN, Southerland JJ, Adewumi DA, Bahjri KA, Samuel RK, et al. Beta blockade and clinical outcomes in aneurysmal subarachnoid hemorrhage. Open Neurol J. 2016;10:155–63.
44. Okazaki T, Hifumi T, Kawakita K, Shishido H, Ogawa D, Okauchi M, et al. Association between dexmedetomidine use and neurological outcomes in aneurysmal subarachnoid hemorrhage patients: a retrospective observational study. J Crit Care. 2018;44:111–6.
45. Khattar NK, James RF. Heparin: the silver bullet of aneurysmal subarachnoid hemorrhage? Front Neurol. 2018;9:97.
46. Simard JM, Aldrich EF, Schreibman D, James RF, Polifka A, Beaty N. Low-dose intravenous heparin infusion in patients with aneurysmal subarachnoid hemorrhage: a preliminary assessment. J Neurosurg. 2013;119(6):1611–9.
47. Khattar NK, Bak E, White AC, James RF. Heparin treatment in aneurysmal subarachnoid hemorrhage: a review of human studies. In: Martin RD, Boling W, Chen G, Zhang JH, editors. Subarachnoid hemorrhage: neurological care and protection. Cham: Springer; 2020. p. 15–9.
48. Hong Y, Guo S, Chen S, Sun C, Zhang J, Sun X. Beneficial effect of hydrogen-rich saline on cerebral vasospasm after experimental subarachnoid hemorrhage in rats. J Neurosci Res. 2012;90(8): 1670–80.
49. Zhuang Z, Zhou M-l, You W-c, Zhu L, Ma C-y, Sun X-j, et al. Hydrogen-rich saline alleviates early brain injury via reducing oxidative stress and brain edema following experimental subarachnoid hemorrhage in rabbits. BMC Neurosci. 2012;13(1):47.
50. Hao X-K, Wu W, Wang C-X, Xie G, Li T, Wu H-m, et al. Ghrelin alleviates early brain injury after subarachnoid hemorrhage via the PI3K/Akt signaling pathway. Brain Res. 2014;1587:15–22.
51. Vergouwen MD, Bakhtiari K, van Geloven N, Vermeulen M, Roos YB, Meijers JC. Reduced ADAMTS13 activity in delayed cerebral ischemia after aneurysmal subarachnoid hemorrhage. J Cereb Blood Flow Metab. 2009;29(10):1734–41.

52. Shibuya M, Meda K, Ikeda A. Fasudil (a rho kinase inhibitor) specifically increases cerebral blood flow in area of vasospasm after subarachnoid hemorrhage. Adv Preclin Study Ischem Stroke. 2012;409–18.
53. Funakoshi H, Sugawara S, Nakashima Y, Homma Y, Mizobe M, Takahashi J, et al. 268 the effectiveness of fasudil hydrochloride administration to prevent cerebral vasospasm after intervention for subarachnoid hemorrhage. Ann Emerg Med. 2017;70(4):S106.
54. Liu GJ, Wang ZJ, Wang YF, Xu LL, Wang XL, Liu Y, et al. Systematic assessment and meta-analysis of the efficacy and safety of fasudil in the treatment of cerebral vasospasm in patients with subarachnoid hemorrhage. Eur J Clin Pharmacol. 2012;68(2):131–9.
55. Lee JY, Keep RF, He Y, Sagher O, Hua Y, Xi G. Hemoglobin and iron handling in brain after subarachnoid hemorrhage and the effect of deferoxamine on early brain injury. J Cereb Blood Flow Metab. 2010;30(11):1793–803.

5 Systematic Approach for Diagnosis of Aneurysmal Subarachnoid Hemorrhage

Adel E. Ahmed Ganaw, Moad Ehfeda, Nissar Shaikh, Marcus Lance, Abdussalam Abugrara, Ali O. Mohamed Bel Khair, and Sirajeddin Belkhair

5.1 Introduction

Aneurysmal subarachnoid hemorrhage (aSAH) is considered one of the most devastating neurosurgical emergencies which is affects 10 per 100,000 with mortality rate of almost 60% in the first 6 months, it is generally affecting otherwise healthy individuals in the most productive stage of their life and less than 16% of patients will return to their premorbid status. Furthermore, persistent cognitive deficits are present in many patients who would otherwise have a good outcome.

A. E. A. Ganaw (✉) · M. Ehfeda · N. Shaikh
M. Lance · A. O. M. Bel Khair
Anesthesia, Perioperative Medicine and Critical Care Department, Hamad General Hospital, Hamad Medical Corporation, Doha, Qatar
e-mail: aganaw@hamad.qa; MEhfeda@hamad.qa; Smaheboob@hamad.qa; MLance@hamad.qa; Akhair2@hamad.qa

A. Abugrara
Radiology Department, Hamad General Hospital, Hamad Medical Corporation, Doha, Qatar
e-mail: ASaid3@hamad.qa

S. Belkhair
Neurosurgery Department, Hamad General Hospital, Hamad Medical Corporation, Doha, Qatar

Neurosurgery Department, Weill Cornell Medical College, Doha, Qatar

Neurosurgery Department, Michigan State University, East Lansing, MI, USA
e-mail: SBelkhair@hamad.qa

The prognosis of aSAH is influenced by several non-modifiable factors as well as factors that can be manipulated by prompt interventions and proper management. Early diagnosis may prevent devastating neurological and non-neurological complications of aSAH. Patients with SAH usually present with headache, photophobia, and meningism. These complaints are not specific and can be confused with meningitis and migraine headache. Therefore, almost 12% of patients who present with aSAH are misdiagnosed at initial presentation.

High index of suspicion for SAH during initial assessment increases the chance for early recognition and timely intervention. Moreover, detailed history, careful examination, full work up, and know limitations of all investigations are very important to avoid late and misdiagnosis of aSAH, which may in addition to worsening the outcome for the patient may lead to medico-legal consequences for the treating physician [1–3].

5.2 History

History of unusual severe headache is the clinical hallmark of aneurysmal subarachnoid hemorrhage (aSAH). Most of the patients (70%) who were diagnosed with aSAH present to emergency department with headache alone without

A. E. A. Ganaw et al. (eds.), *Management of Subarachnoid Hemorrhage*,
https://doi.org/10.1007/978-3-030-81333-8_5

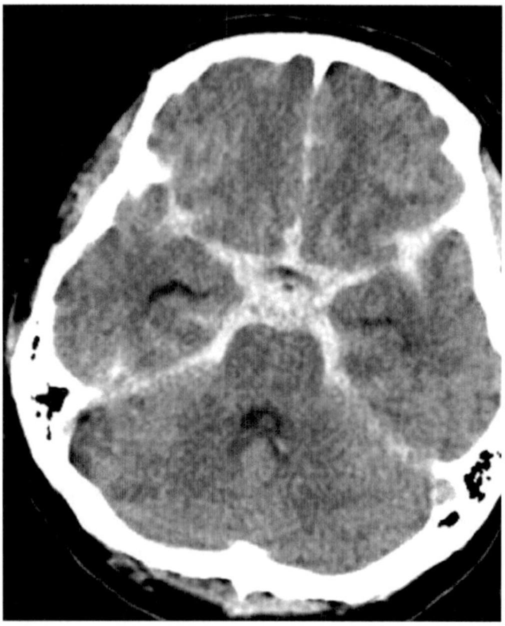

Fig. 5.2 Non contrast CT scan shows SAH in the basal cistern, both sylvian fissures, and interhemispheric fissure. This is an Open Access article distributed under the terms of the Creative Commons Attribution Non-Commercial License (http://creativecommons.org/licenses/by-nc/3.0) [13]

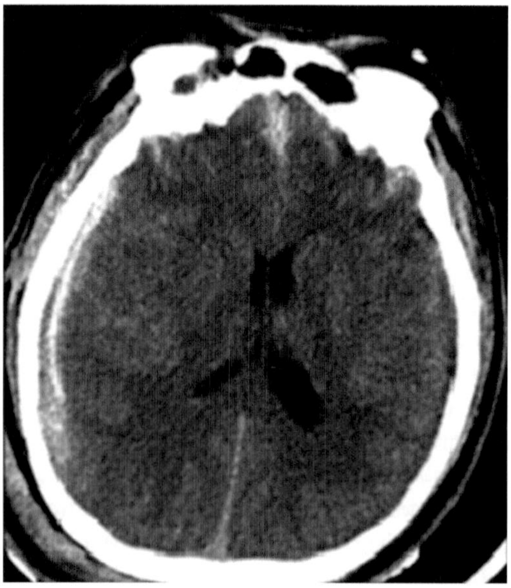

Fig. 5.3 Non-contrast brain CT scan reveals diffuse traumatic SAH and traumatic subdural hematoma on the right cerebral hemisphere [14]

abnormalities such as intraventricular, subdural hematoma, hydrocephalus, and brain edema.

Table 5.2 Limitation of Non-contrast CT [1, 5, 13]

Limitation	Comment
Timing of brain CT scan	Sensitivity of brain CT scan declines as time from symptom beginning increases.
Blood volume	CT scan may not detect small volume bleeds.
Technical challenges	Advanced scanners with thinner cuts and no motion artifacts amplify the chance of SAH diagnosis.
Anemia	Hematocrit less than 30% increase chance of false negative results.

The clinician must be aware of CT limitations in the diagnosis of the SAH (Table 5.2). The CT scan technique is very important to improve sensitivity of brain CT scan, very thin cuts (3 mm in thickness) through the base of the brain are highly recommended to avoid missing small collections of the blood. The plane of scanning need to be parallel to the hard palate. Blood and neighboring bone, which both appear white, can be hard to differentiate from one another, particularly in small hemorrhages. Furthermore, because the augmented density of blood on CT is due to hemoglobin concentration, therefore blood with a hemoglobin concentration less than 10 g/dl may appear iso-dense. Moreover, artifacts of motion during scanning of agitated patients may interfere with quality of the CT scan and obscure the diagnosis.

5.4.2 Lumbar Puncture (LP)

Given the devastating nature of aSAH and limited sensitivity of non contrast brain CT scan, especially with late presentation (more than 5 days), LP is generally recommended to augment the sensitivity of the diagnostic process. Moreover, LP may help clinicians to differentiate other pathologies that cannot be diagnosed by non-contrast brain CT scan for instance benign high ICP and meningitis [5, 12]. Nevertheless, many studies reported that emergency physicians performed LP for less than half of the patients who presented with worst-of-life headache and negative non-contrast brain CT scan [15]. In reality LP may be postponed for many reasons such as difficulty in getting patient consent, patient nervousness, phobia from complications, the patient looks normal and time limits. LP is particularly beneficial in early diagnosis of SAH in alert, neurologically normal patients who present with sudden onset, severe headache. These group of patients have high chance to have negative CT scan [16]. Perry and co-workers reported that 10% of SAH patients were diagnosed based on the positive CSF reports after normal CT results [17]. Numerous retrospective studies have reported that 2–7% of SAH is undetected by non-contrast brain CT scan, diagnosed by LP and hereafter confirmed by cerebral angiography [18]. The American Heart Association (AHA) guidelines (2012) recommend performing a LP after negative non-contrast brain CT scan for suspected patients (Table 5.3) [8]. In addition, the American college of emergency physicians (ACEP) clinical policy 2008 states that the diagnosis of SAH can be excluded if both CT and LP are negative [12].

There are number of limitations to the LP which may interfere with interpretation of CSF results (Table 5.4). First of all, traumatic tab is quite common which occurs in 15% of patients [5]. Therefore, analysis of blood-stained CSF reports can be extremely difficult. Treating physicians should be able to differentiate between true SAH and traumatic tap. The CSF is usually collected in four serial tubes, the persistence of constant numbers of red blood cells from tube one to tube four is abnormal and may be suggestive of aSAH. Furthermore, a traumatic tap is considered when there is no red blood cells in the fourth tube irrespective of the number of red blood cells in the first three tubes [5, 19]. The absolute number of red blood cells (RBCs) that confirms the diagnosis of SAH has never been established. Despite an aSAH has been reported with few hundred RBCs, although this is very rare. Therefore, if the progressive clearing of CSF is incomplete, additional diagnostic investigations such as computed tomographic angiography (CTA), magnetic resonance angiography (MRA), or conventional cerebral angiography should be considered. Moreover, timing of LP is vital in the interpretation of CSF reports, circulating CSF may dilute may dilute RBCs count, so absolute number of RBCs decreases with time from symp-

Table 5.3 AHA 2012 recommendations [8]

AHA recommendations 2012	Level of evidence
1 aSAH is a medical emergency that is frequently misdiagnosed. A high level of suspicion for aSAH should exist in patients with acute onset of severe headache	Class I; level of evidence B
2 acute diagnostic workup should include non-contrast head CT, which, if nondiagnostic, should be followed by lumbar puncture	Class I; level of evidence B
3 CTA may be considered in the workup of aSAH. If an aneurysm is detected by CTA, this study may help guide the decision for type of aneurysm repair, but if CTA is inconclusive, DSA is still recommended (except possibly in the instance of classic peri mesencephalic aSAH)	Class IIb; level of evidence C
4 magnetic resonance imaging (fluid-attenuated inversion recovery, proton density, diffusion-weighted imaging, and gradient echo sequences) may be reasonable for the diagnosis of aSAH in patients with a nondiagnostic CT scan, although a negative result does not obviate the need for cerebrospinal fluid analysis.	Class IIb; level of evidence C
5 DSA with 3-dimensional rotational angiography is indicated for detection of aneurysm in patients with aSAH (except when the aneurysm was previously diagnosed by a non-invasive angiogram) and for planning treatment (to determine whether an aneurysm is amenable to coiling or to expedite microsurgery).	Class I; level of evidence B

Table 5.4 Limitations of LP [5]

Limitations	Comments
Invasive procedure	Difficult to perform in agitated patients, may lead to serious complications and contraindicated in coagulopathic patients.
Timing of LP	Very early LP may falsely give negative reports (xanthochromia may be absent if LP performed before 12 h or after 2 weeks). Circulating CSF may dilute RBCs count.
Traumatic tap	Sometimes differentiation between traumatic tap and real SAH is challenging.
Number of RBCs	No guideline determines absolute number of RBCs to confirm diagnosis of SAH.
Diagnosis of Xanthochromia	Precise diagnosis of xanthochromia can be challenging.

toms onset. Occasionally, CSF is completely cleared from RBCs within 48 h post-ictus [5].

When suspected patients undergo LP, CSF opening pressure (OP) should be reported. For precise measurement of OP, the patient should be in the lateral recumbent position and patient's legs should be straightened while measurement of OP. Once the initial CSF confirming the location returns from the spinal needle, connect it to the manometer through a stopcock, and record the height of the fluid in the monometer (Fig. 5.4). High OP suggests aSAH. It is higher than 20 cm H_2O in almost 60% of aSAH patients. However, OP can be high due to other causes such as cerebral venous thrombosis and idiopathic high ICP [20].

Xanthochromia is another sign of SAH. Xanthochromia is yellow discoloration of CSF that results from the enzymatic degradation of hemoglobin in the CSF into oxyhemoglobin, methemoglobin, and bilirubin. It develops within 6–12 h of SAH; hence it is unlikely caused by traumatic tap. It persists at least for 2 weeks.

Xanthochromia can be assessed either by spectrophotometry or by visual inspection. Some researchers recommend using spectrophotometry for CSF analysis. Although studies reported that both methods are very reliable in the detection of xanthochromia. The ideal method of visual inspection of xanthochromia involves fast centrifuging the fourth CSF tube and matching it with an identical tube filled with an equal volume of water against a white background (Fig. 5.5). The absence of xanthochromia by either visual or spectrophotometric analysis has a high negative predictive value for SAH, with one estimate of 99%.

False positive xanthochromia may occur in certain cases such as jaundice (total bilirubin >10-15 mg/dl), use of rifampin, excessive dietary of carotenoids and increased CSF protein (>150 mg/dl) [5].

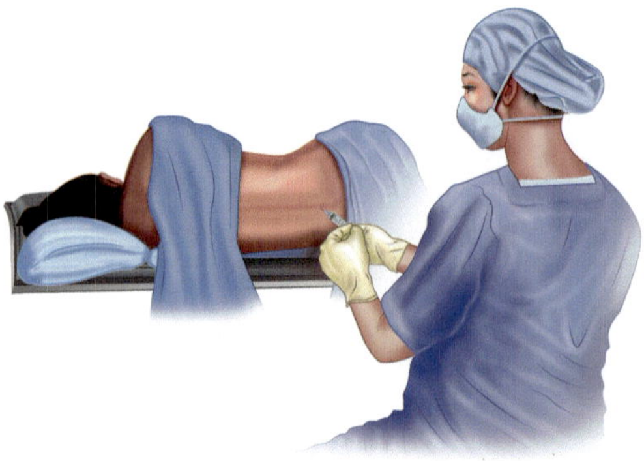

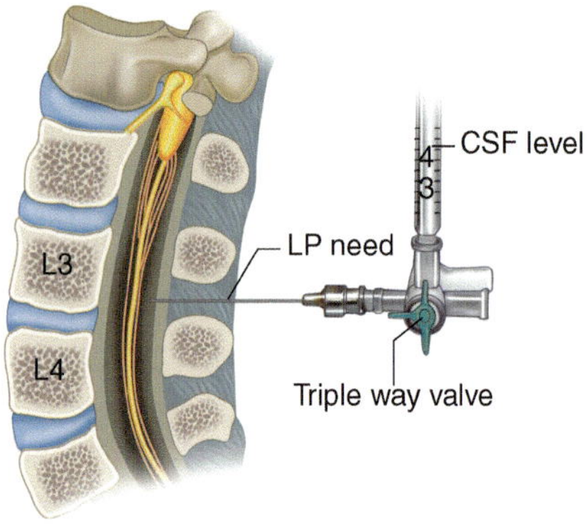

Fig. 5.4 Measurement of CSF opening pressure

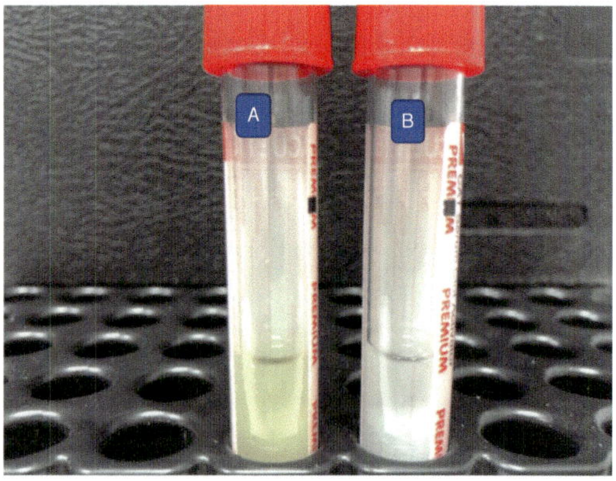

Fig. 5.5 Visual analysis of CSF: (A) Xanthochromia compared normal CSF (B)

5.4.3 Computed Tomography Angiography (CTA)

Over last 10 years, computed tomography angiography (CTA) is increasingly used for detection and characterize cerebral aneurysm in SAH patients. It can be achieved immediately after the diagnosis of SAH by non-contrast brain CT scan when the patient is still in scanner. It is non-invasive, immediately accessible with sensitivity of 98% and specificity of 100%. However, the CTA sensitivity drops significantly (92.3%) with small-sized aneurysms (<4 mm). (Fig. 5.6) [4, 21].

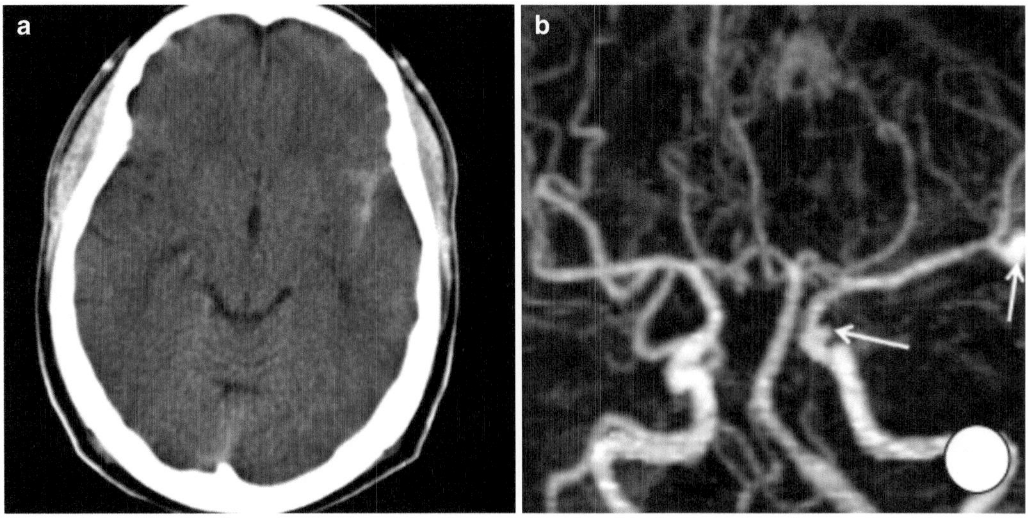

Fig. 5.6 (a) No-contrast CT scan reveals SAH limited to the left Sylvia fissure. Figure 5.6b CTA reveals aneurysms (arrows) at the left bifurcation of MCA and left ICA. distributed under the terms of the Creative Commons Attribution Non- Commercial License (http://creativecommons.org/li- censes/by-nc/3.0) [24]

There are suggestions to substitute LP with CTA after negative non-contrast brain CT scan [22]. However, with prevalence of cerebral aneurysm among general population (2–5%), incidental discovery of cerebral aneurysm may mislead treating physicians and delay diagnosis of the actual cause of headache or neurological manifestation. Therefore, further LP is still required to differentiate between incidental and symptomatic cerebral aneurysm [4, 23]. Moreover, according to the best existing data, if both non-contrast brain CT scan and CTA are negative, the possibility of SAH is less than 1% which is less than most clinicians test threshold (probability of disease below which no additional workup is need). Nonetheless, the sensitivity of CTA drops markedly with small-sized aneurysms (< 4 mm), and ruptured of small aneurysm may lead to significant morbidity and mortality [4, 21, 22]. The AHA 2012 guidelines recommend that CTA may be considered in the workup of aSAH. If an aneurysm is detected by CTA, this study may help guide the decision for type of treatment modality to secure the aneurysm, but if CTA is inconclusive, DSA is still recommended (except possibly in the instance of classic perimesencephalic" (Table 5.3) [8].

The CT-CTA approach may be considered with acknowledgment of its limits if there is any contraindication to perform LP or in acute setting, rapidly declining patient who needs emergent craniotomy for hematoma evacuation.

5.4.4 Magnetic Resonance Imaging (MRI) and Magnetic Resonance Angiography (MRA)

Magnetic resonance imaging and angiography are another radiological investigation that might be considered to investigate SAH. MRI is superior to non- contrast CT in the detection of subacute and chronic SAH, particularly with fluid attenuated- inversion recovery (Flair) T2-weighted imaging accomplished 4–14 days post ictus when sensitivity of non-contrast brain CT scan drops significantly [8].

In the first 5 days post-ictus, the sensitivity of the FLAIR sequence is 100%, while T2-weighted gradient echo has 100% sensitivity for SAH in the 6–30-day range Fig. 5.7 [25].

MRI is also useful in determination other causes of SAH when both CTA and DSA are negative. It is useful in detection cavernous angioma of brain or spinal cord as well as cerebral venous sinus thrombosis.

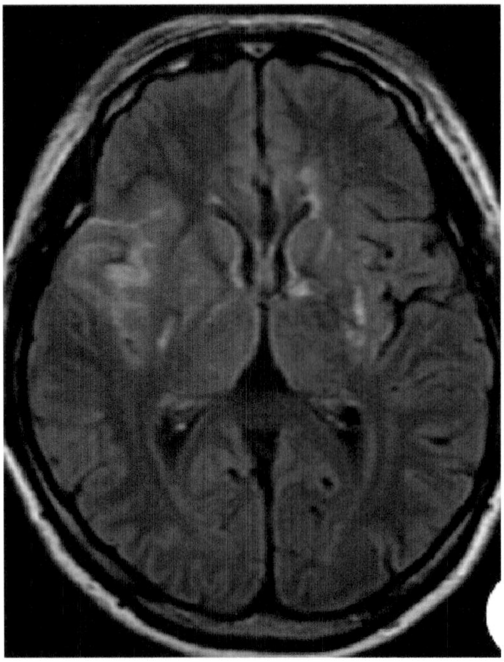

Fig. 5.7 FLAIR sequence shows SAH in right sylvian fissure [13]

There is insufficient evidence to recommend MRI as part of the routine investigation for acute diagnosis of SAH. The AHA (2012) guidelines recommend using MRI in SAH suspected cases with negative non-contrast brain CT scan; nevertheless, LP is still required if MRI is negative [5].

There are certain limitations of MRI in assessment of acute SAH, it is difficult to detect acute SAH with conventional T1-weighted and T2-weighted MRI sequences. Mixing blood with high oxygen tension CSF delays the generation of the paramagnetic deoxyhemoglobin that is better imaged with MRI. The variability in the appearance of SAH after 2 days most likely due to hemoglobin degradation, which may also interfere with the intensity of MRI signals [4, 21].

Furthermore, limited availability of MRI in emergency departments, study interpretation is difficult and requires expertise, expensive in comparison to non-contrast brain CT scan, predisposing to motion artifact and scanning of acutely ill patients who is poorly compliant to commands without sedation is extremely difficult [4].

Magnetic resonance angiography (MRA) has limited role in diagnosis SAH because of limited routine availability, time consuming, very expensive, as well as difficulty in scanning acutely sick patient who is poorly compliant to commands. It is generally used in monitoring of already diagnosed aneurysm as well as secured aneurysm with either surgical clipping or endovascular embolization. The sensitivity of MRA is directly associated with size of the aneurysm. It is comparable with CTA in medium- and large-sized aneurysm but it is inferior to CTA in aneurysms less than 5 mm. It is about 94% if the aneurysm is larger than 3 mm and drop to 38% in smaller aneurysm. The sensitivity may increase by using gadolinium-enhanced MRA. MRA may be considered in stable patients with acute aSAH who cannot receive iodinated contrast [26].

5.4.5 Digital Subtraction Angiography (DSA)

Digital subtraction angiography (DSA) is considered the gold-standard radiological investigation for detection cerebral aneurysm, determine size and location of cerebral aneurysm, study anatomical features of cerebral blood vessels as well as to determine the intervention of choice to secure the aneurysm. If SAH is confirmed and source of bleeding cannot be determined with CTA, DSA should be considered unless the blood pattern on non-contrast brain CT scan is suggesting typical peri mesencephalic SAH (extravasated blood around the midbrain with normal angiogram Figs. 5.8 and 5.9) [5, 27].

DSA is minimally invasive procedure associated with very low risk of neurological and non-neurological complications. Kaufmann et al. in retrospective study of 19,826 patients reported that the jeopardy of neurological complications ranged between 0.4% and 2.6%, the majority of these complications are transit. The most common neurological complications were transient ischemic attack (TIA) [28].

Non-neurological complications were very rare which include groin hematoma, nausea, vomiting, chest pain, arrhythmia, transient hypotension, acute kidney injury, and anaphylaxis reactions.

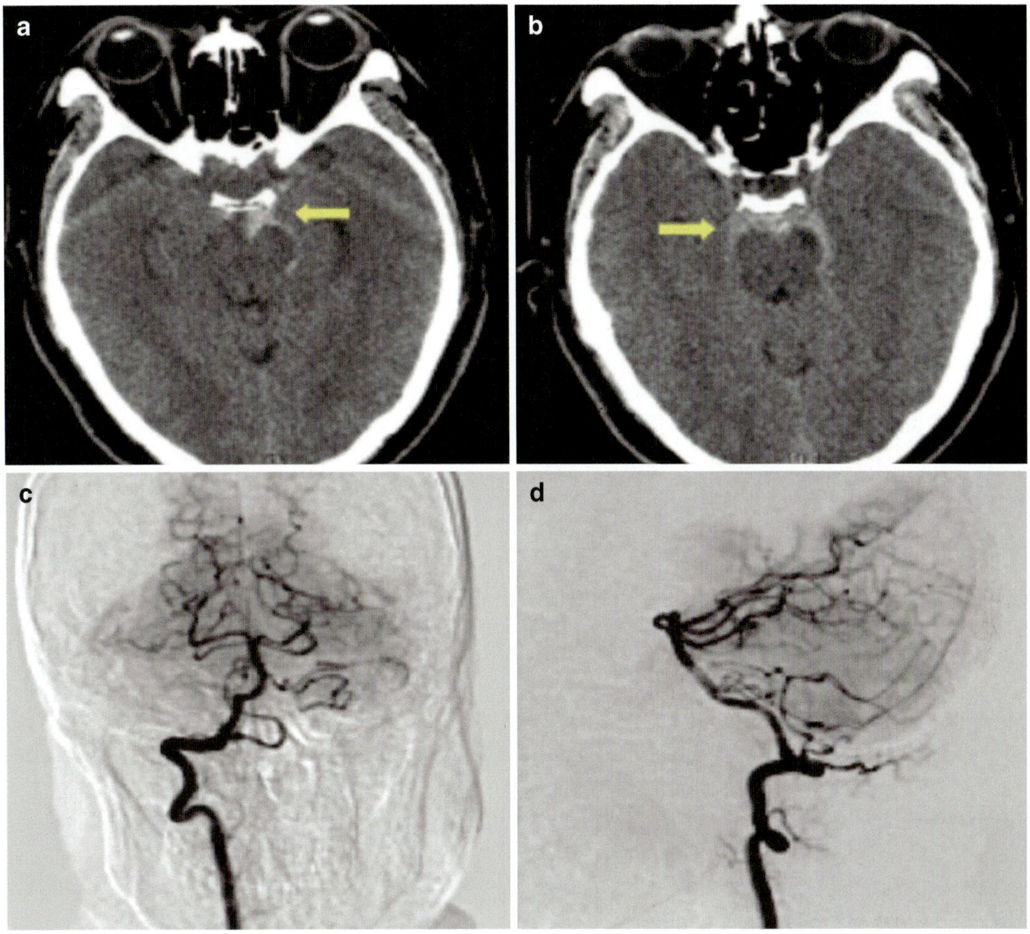

Fig. 5.8 A and B reveal (yellow arrow) localized hemorrhage in left perimesencephalic cistern in prepontine cistern (B), suggesting perimesencephalic subarachnoid hemorrhage. Figure 5.8 C and D reveal DSA on the second day after admission showed no evidence of an intracranial aneurysm or underlying vascular malformation in vertebrobasilar artery system. [30]

Most common non-neurological complication was groin hematoma, reported in 4.2% of patients. However, the incidence of groin hematomas that required surgical intervention was very low (0.03%) [28].

Although the risk associated with DSA is minimal, it has been the incentive for further assessment the efficacy of three-dimensional (3D)-CTA in comparison with DSA for diagnosis and evaluation of cerebral aneurysm after SAH. The sensitivity, specificity, and accuracy of 3D-CTA were comparable with DSA in medium- and large-sized aneurysms (> 3 mm). Nevertheless, DSA (90.9% sensitivity) was superior to 3D-CTA (81.8% sensitivity) in detection small-sized aneurysms (<3 mm) [29].

DSA-negative SAH has been observed in 10–20% of patients and the exact cause of SAH in this group is only identified in small proportion (2–21%) of patients. The most common causes of DSA-negative SAH are thrombosed aneurysm, venous perimesencephalic hemorrhage, venous sinus thrombosis, pre-eclampsia, vascular lesion of the spine, spinal neoplasm, bleeding diathesis and drugs such as anticoagulation, antiplatelet and sympathomimetics. Failure to determine the exact cause of SAH may place these group of patients at jeopardy of recurrent hemorrhage.

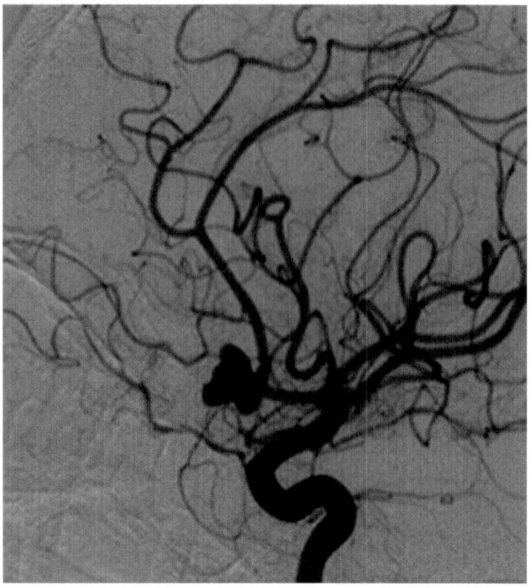

Fig. 5.9 DSA reveals AcomA aneurysm, The figure under creative common. License: CC BY-NC-SA 4.0 [31]

Thus, DSA should be repeated one to two weeks post-ictus in order to identify missed vascular lesions such as thrombosed cerebral aneurysm, micro-arteriovenous malformation, and dural or pial arteriovenous fistula. Moreover, further work up should be considered to rule out other causes of DSA negative SAH such as intracranial neoplasms, vascular cavernous malformations, drugs, Pre-eclampsia, coagulopathies and vasculitis [2, 5].

5.5 Conclusion

Aneurysmal subarachnoid hemorrhage (aSAH) is considered as one of the most devastating neurosurgical emergencies with mortality rate of almost 60% in the first 6 months and less than 16% of patients return to their premorbid status. Early diagnosis and immediate intervention are extremely important to prevent catastrophic complications and improve outcome. Unfortunately, early diagnosis of aSAH is very challenging and high index of suspicion during initial assessment increases the chance for early diagnosis. Treating physician should consider full workup and consult neurosurgeons for all suspected cases. Knowing the limitations of all radiological investigations as well as lumbar punctures is of critical importance to avoid misdiagnosis which may lead to medicolegal consequence to treating physician.

Acknowledgements Thanks are extended to Dr.Nezar Alsharef O Shlaka.

References

1. Steiner T, Juvela S, Unterberg A, Jung C, Forsting M, Rinkel G, et al. European stroke organization guidelines for the management of intracranial aneurysms and subarachnoid haemorrhage. Cerebrovasc Dis. 2013;35(2):93–112.
2. Simpson VM. Diagnosis and initial managment of subarachnoid hemorrhage. OA Emergency Medicine. 2013;1:1–11.
3. Fontanarosa PB. Recognition of subarachnoid hemorrhage. Ann Emerg Med. 1989;18(11):1199–205.
4. Marcolini E, Hine J. Approach to the diagnosis and Management of Subarachnoid Hemorrhage. West J Emerg Med. 2019;20(2):203–11.
5. Aisiku I, Edlow JA, Goldstein J, Thomas LE. An evidence-based approach to diagnosis and management of subarachnoid hemorrhage in the emergency department. Emerg Med Pract. 2014;16(10):1–29. quiz -30
6. Cohen-Gadol AA, Bohnstedt BN. Recognition and evaluation of nontraumatic subarachnoid hemorrhage and ruptured cerebral aneurysm. Am Fam Physician. 2013;88(7):451–6.
7. Perry JJ, Stiell IG, Sivilotti ML, Bullard MJ, Lee JS, Eisenhauer M, et al. High risk clinical characteristics for subarachnoid haemorrhage in patients with acute headache: prospective cohort study. BMJ. 2010;341:c5204.
8. Connolly ES Jr, Rabinstein AA, Carhuapoma JR, Derdeyn CP, Dion J, Higashida RT, et al. Guidelines for the management of aneurysmal subarachnoid hemorrhage: a guideline for healthcare professionals from the American Heart Association/american Stroke Association. Stroke. 2012;43(6):1711–37.
9. Bederson JB, Connolly ES Jr, Batjer HH, Dacey RG, Dion JE, Diringer MN, et al. Guidelines for the management of aneurysmal subarachnoid hemorrhage: a statement for healthcare professionals from a special writing group of the stroke council, American Heart Association. Stroke. 2009;40(3):994–1025.
10. Ahmed AE, Ganaw AMT, Mohamed AO, Khair B. Aneurysmal subarachnoid hemorrhage. ICU book, Intechopen; 2017. p. 73–99.
11. Edlow JA, Caplan LR. Avoiding pitfalls in the diagnosis of subarachnoid hemorrhage. N Engl J Med. 2000;342(1):29–36.
12. Edlow JA, Panagos PD, Godwin SA, Thomas TL, Decker WW. American College of Emergency P. clin-

ical policy: critical issues in the evaluation and management of adult patients presenting to the emergency department with acute headache. Ann Emerg Med. 2008;52(4):407–36.
13. Yu DW, Jung YJ, Choi BY, Chang CH. Subarachnoid hemorrhage with negative baseline digital subtraction angiography: is repeat digital subtraction angiography necessary? J Cerebrovasc Endovasc Neurosurg. 2012;14(3):210–5.
14. Kwon HM, Baek JW, Lee SP, Cho JI. A fatal adverse effect of barbiturate coma therapy: Dyskalemia. Korean J Neurotrauma. 2016;12(2):156–8.
15. O'Neill J, McLaggan S, Gibson R. Acute headache and subarachnoid haemorrhage: a retrospective review of CT and lumbar puncture findings. Scott Med J. 2005;50(4):151–3.
16. Sidman R, Connolly E, Lemke T. Subarachnoid hemorrhage diagnosis: lumbar puncture is still needed when the computed tomography scan is normal. Acad Emerg Med. 1996;3(9):827–31.
17. Perry JJ, Spacek A, Forbes M, Wells GA, Mortensen M, Symington C, et al. Is the combination of negative computed tomography result and negative lumbar puncture result sufficient to rule out subarachnoid hemorrhage? Ann Emerg Med. 2008;51(6):707–13.
18. van der Wee N, Rinkel GJ, Hasan D, van Gijn J. Detection of subarachnoid haemorrhage on early CT: is lumbar puncture still needed after a negative scan? J Neurol Neurosurg Psychiatry. 1995;58(3):357–9.
19. Buruma OJ, Janson HL, Den Bergh FA, Bots GT. Blood-stained cerebrospinal fluid: traumatic puncture or haemorrhage? J Neurol Neurosurg Psychiatry. 1981;44(2):144–7.
20. Quattrone A, Bono F, Oliveri RL, Gambardella A, Pirritano D, Labate A, et al. Cerebral venous thrombosis and isolated intracranial hypertension without papilledema in CDH. Neurology. 2001;57(1):31–6.
21. McKinney AM, Palmer CS, Truwit CL, Karagulle A, Teksam M. Detection of aneurysms by 64-section multidetector CT angiography in patients acutely suspected of having an intracranial aneurysm and comparison with digital subtraction and 3D rotational angiography. AJNR Am J Neuroradiol. 2008;29(3):594–602.
22. McCormack RF, Hutson A. Can computed tomography angiography of the brain replace lumbar puncture in the evaluation of acute-onset headache after a negative noncontrast cranial computed tomography scan? Acad Emerg Med. 2010;17(4):444–51.
23. Brisman JL, Song JK, Newell DW. Cerebral aneurysms. N Engl J Med. 2006;355(9):928–39.
24. Park SH, Lee CY. Supraclinoid internal carotid artery fenestration harboring an unruptured aneurysm and another remote ruptured aneurysm: case report and review of the literature. J Cerebrovasc Endovasc Neurosurg. 2012;14(4):295–9.
25. Yuan MK, Lai PH, Chen JY, Hsu SS, Liang HL, Yeh LR, et al. Detection of subarachnoid hemorrhage at acute and subacute/chronic stages: comparison of four magnetic resonance imaging pulse sequences and computed tomography. J Chin Med Assoc. 2005;68(3):131–7.
26. Brown SC, Brew S, Madigan J. Diagnosis of suspected subarachnoid hemorrhage in adults. Praxis (Bern 1994). 2011;100(24):1493–7.
27. Agid R, Lee SK, Willinsky RA, Farb RI. terBrugge KG. Acute subarachnoid hemorrhage: using 64-slice multidetector CT angiography to "triage" patients' treatment. Neuroradiology. 2006;48(11):787–94.
28. Kaufmann TJ, Huston J 3rd, Mandrekar JN, Schleck CD, Thielen KR, Kallmes DF. Complications of diagnostic cerebral angiography: evaluation of 19,826 consecutive patients. Radiology. 2007;243(3):812–9.
29. Wang H, Li W, He H, Luo L, Chen C, Guo Y. 320-detector row CT angiography for detection and evaluation of intracranial aneurysms: comparison with conventional digital subtraction angiography. Clin Radiol. 2013;68(1):e15–20.
30. Fu FW, Rao J, Zheng YY, Song L, Chen W, Zhou QH, et al. Perimesencephalic nonaneurysmal subarachnoid hemorrhage caused by transverse sinus thrombosis: a case report and review of literature. Medicine (Baltimore). 2017;96(33):e7374.
31. Zheng SF, Yao PS, Yu LH, Kang DZ. Keyhole approach combined with external ventricular drainage for ruptured, poor-grade, anterior circulation cerebral aneurysms. Medicine (Baltimore). 2015;94(51):e2307.

Grading of Aneurysmal Subarachnoid Hemorrhage

6

Adel E. Ahmed Ganaw, Moad Ehfeda, Nissar Shaikh, Ejaz Salam Khan, M. Faisal Malmstrom, Ali O. Mohamed Bel Khair, Ali Ayyad, and Sirajeddin Belkhair

6.1 Introduction

Aneurysmal subarachnoid hemorrhage (aSAH) is considered as one of the most devastating neurosurgical emergencies which affects 10 per 100,000 with mortality rate of almost 60%. It is a heterogeneous disorder with a varied range of original presentations and final outcomes. The outcome of aSAH patients is affected by many factors related to the patients, disease, and medical interventions and it is timing. It has been observed that clinical features at initial presentation of aSAH have weighty prognostic implications. An extensive work has been made to develop clinically grading scale of aSAH to measure the severity of initial neurological insult, in order to aid treating physicians in making management decisions, predict the outcome, and standardize patient's evaluation throughout medical as well as research centers.

Bramwell proposed the first grading scheme for SAH when classified patients with aSAH into either apoplectic or paralytic forms. Since then, at least 40 SAH grading scales have been proposed such as Botterell, Nishioka, and Cooperative Aneurysm Study systems [1].

Nowadays, the most popular SAH grading scales are the World Federation of Neurological Surgeons (WFNS) Scale, Hunt and Hess Scale or a slightly modified version, the Fisher Scale and the Glasgow Coma Score [1–3].

6.1.1 Definition of Grading Scale

Grading scale is a sophisticated scheme of data classification based on directional axis; therefore, it is a system for gauging its primary axis. The primary axis of the most common SAH grading scales is clinical severity. The purpose of grading scales is early prediction of prognosis or

A. E. A. Ganaw (✉) · M. Ehfeda · N. Shaikh
M. F. Malmstrom · A. O. M. Bel Khair
Anesthesia, perioperative medicine and critical care department, Hamad General Hospital, Hamad Medical Corporation, Doha, Qatar
e-mail: aganaw@hamad.qa; MEhfeda@hamad.qa; mmalmstrom@hamad.qa; Akhair2@hamad.qa

E. S. Khan
Anesthesia Department, NYC Health + Hospital, Metropolitan, New York, NY, USA
e-mail: ejaz_hzai@hamad.qa

A. Ayyad
Neurosurgery, Hamad General Hospital, Hamad Medical Corporation, Doha, Qatar
e-mail: aayyad@hamad.qa

S. Belkhair
Neurosurgery, Hamad General Hospital, Hamad Medical Corporation, Doha, Qatar

Neurosurgery Department, Weil Cornell Medical College, Ar-Rayyan, Qatar

Neurosurgery Department, Michigan State University, East Lansing, MI, USA
e-mail: SBelkhair@hamad.qa

A. E. A. Ganaw et al. (eds.), *Management of Subarachnoid Hemorrhage*,
https://doi.org/10.1007/978-3-030-81333-8_6

devastating complications by conversion qualitative impression of SAH severity into quantitative measurements. Consequently, it aids treating physicians to take appropriate decisions or interventions on the right time to prevent complications and improve the outcome.

In addition, grading scales standardize patient evaluation for communication between health care providers and scientific study purposes. The ideal grading scale must fulfill the following criteria:

1. Grading scale must be easy to apply during acute phase by health care provider and researchers.
2. Grading scale should be completely free from intra- and inter-observer variability.
3. It should have significant association with the outcome and or devastating complications.
4. The adjacent grades must have different outcomes. The intergrade differences in the outcome are extremely important to avoid misleading conclusion in clinical studies. The absence of intergrade differences may lead to two types of errors;
   (a) Coexisting error occurs when subgroups with clearly different outcomes are assigned the same grades. For instance, Grade IV of WFNS scale includes a broad spectrum of GCS grades [7–12]. If a clinical trial included only WFNS grade IV group of patients and patients with GCS of 7 were assigned to a control group while patients with GCS of 12 were assigned to the intervention group, the researcher would falsely conclude that the intervention dramatically improved the outcome [4].
   (b) Over-splitting error occurs when subgroups with almost the same outcome are assigned to different grades. For example, Grade I and II Hunt and Hess grading scales where both grades are assigned a GCS of 15 with no significant difference in the outcomes [4, 5].
5. Grading scale should be applicable retrospectively.
6. Grading scale should be very sensitive even in small population [1, 4]

6.1.2 The Hunt and Hess Grading Scale

Hunt and Hess Scale was projected in 1968 as reformation of the older grading scale initially described by Botterell and colleagues (Table 6.1) [6]. The scale was proposed to stratify the surgical risk and to determine the appropriate time of intervention. The scale proposal was based on the judgment of its authors, who thought the following were the most vital clinical signs in SAH:

1. The severity of meningeal inflammatory reaction.
2. The intensity of neurological impairment.
3. Arousing level of the patients.
4. Comorbidities.

Consequently, this grading scale was generating according to the degree of intensity of the first

Table 6.1 Hunt and Hess and Botterell et al. grading scales [1]

Grade	Hunt and Hess	Botterell et al
I	Asymptomatic or minimal headache and slight nuchal rigidity	Conscious with or without signs of blood in the subarachnoid space
II	Moderate to severe headache, nuchal rigidity, no neurological deficit other than cranial nerve palsy.	Drowsy without significant neurological deficit
III	Drowsiness, confusion or mild focal deficit.	Drowsy with neurological deficit and probably intracerebral clot
IV	Stupor, moderate to severe hemiparesis, and possibly decerebrate rigidity and vegetative disturbances.	Major neurological deficit, deteriorating because of large intracerebral clots or older patients with less severe neurological deficit but pre-existing cerebrovascular disease
V	Deep coma, decerebrate rigidity, moribund appearance	Moribund or near moribund with failing vital centers and extensor rigidity

Table 6.2 Modified Hunt and Hess scale [6]

Grade	Clinical description
0	Unruptured aneurysm
I	Asymptomatic or minimal headache and slight nuchal rigidity
Ia	No acute meningeal/brain reaction, but with fixed neuro-deficit
II	Moderate to severe headache, nuchal rigidity, no neurological deficit other than cranial nerve palsy
III	Drowsiness, confusion, or mild focal deficit
IV	Stupor, moderate to severe hemiparesis, possibly early decerebrate rigidity and vegetative disturbances
V	Deep coma, decerebrate rigidity, moribund appearance

3 clinical signs. The scale has five grades integrating all three axes, with distinction between grades made by illustrative terminology. Adjustment was added for serious comorbidities, which allocate the patients in the following highest severe grade. In 1974, the scale was modified by Hunt and Kosnik by adding two grades, 0 grade to describe patients with small unruptured cerebral aneurysms and 1a grade to describe patients with stable residual neurological impairment and do not have other signs of SAH (Table 6.2) [1, 7].

Despite its simplicity, popularity amongst the neuroscientific population and wide spread use in the literature, there are several limitations to the Hunt and Hess grading scale. Several terms used to define the grades (for instance stupor, drowsy, and deep coma) are ambiguous and subject to inconstant interpretation. Furthermore, consideration of three axes of clinical signs in one scale is confusing. If patient present at different points on the axes, treating physician must rely on his judgment to determine which axis is utmost important. For instance, a patient may present with thunderclap headache, fully conscious, and hemiplegic. On the arousal axis, the patient is fully conscious, no deficit and could be given grade 1. On the other hand, the patient is hemiplegic (severe neurological deficit), hence, could be given grade 4. In such a scenario, the treating physicians are forced to decide which axis should be considered to define the definitive grade. This uncertainty hazes the lines between adjoining grades and increases inter-rater reliability and weaken the prognostic strength of the grading scale.

In addition, the necessity to upgrade a patient's grade by one level in the presence of severe comorbidies or serious vasospasm on angigraphy reduces the inter-reliability of the scale. Because only some severe comorbidities are specified as well as the level of severity required for upgrading is vague. Moreover, some comorbidities such as diabetes has a lower impact on the course of SAH than others, such as hypertension [1].

Finally, there is over-splitting error in Hunt and Hess grading scale (no difference in outcome between grade I and II) which has negative impact on prognostic power of Hunt and Hess grade [8].

6.1.3 Fisher Scale

The Fisher Scale was projected by C.M Fisher (1980) to expect cerebral vasospasm in SAH patients (Fig. 6.1). The scale based on pattern of blood as well as the amount of blood seen on admission computed tomography (Table 6.3). It was validated prospectively in a limited number of cases (46 patients). Nevertheless, there are many limitations of the fisher scale. Fisher scale was created while quality of radiological image had almost one-tenth of the resolution recently existing. The measurements used in Fisher trial were real measurements on printed CT scan films which did not reflect the actual cloth thickness. Consequently, subarachnoid clot of <1 mm in real thickness is very rare as is the finding of no blood on initial CT scan, therefore grades1 and 2 were essentially be very rare. Moreover, in the original scale described by authors, grade IV included patients with diffuse thin SAH and intraventricular or intracerebral hemorrhage. There is uncertainty regarding grading patients

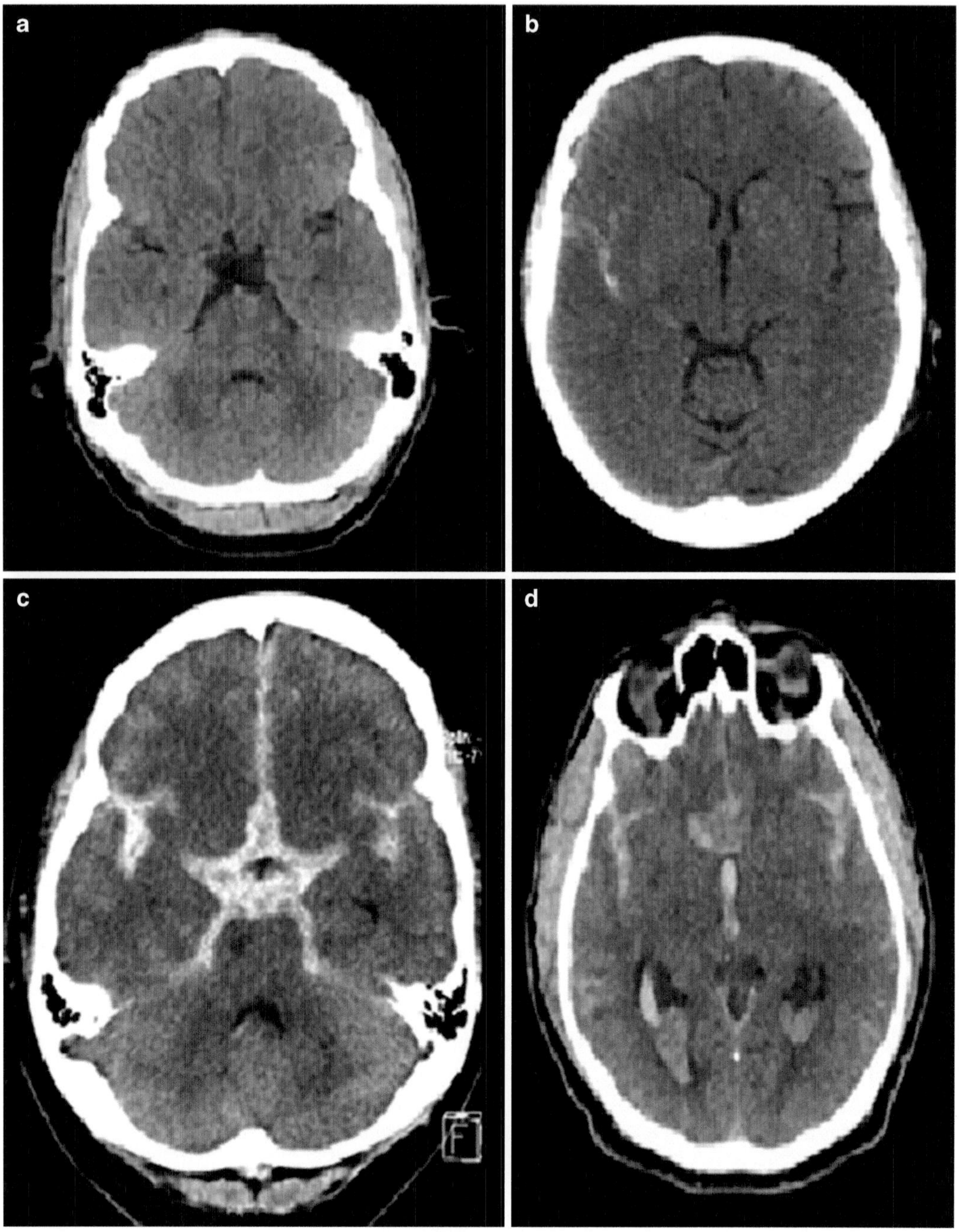

Fig. 6.1 show Different Fisher grading scales; (**a**) grade I fisher scale (no SAH or IVH detected, the incidence of vasospasm is 21%). (**b**) grade II Fisher scale (diffuse thin (<1 mm) SAH, no clots, the incidence of vasospasm is 25%). (**c**) grade III (localized clots and/or layers of blood >1 mm in thickness, no IVH, the incidence of symptomatic vasospasm is 37%). (**d**) grade IV Fisher scale (diffuse or no SAH, ICH, or IVH present, the incidence of symptomatic vasospasm is 31%). (Courtesy Dr. Adel E. Ahmed Ganaw)

Table 6.3 Fisher grade scale [6]

Group	Blood on CT scan
I	No subarachnoid detected
II	Diffuse or thin vertical layer <1 mm thick
III	Localized subarachnoid clot and /or vertical layer >1 mm thick
IV	Intra ventricular or intra-parenchymal clot with diffuse or no SAH

Table 6.4 Fisher revised scale [1]

Group	Blood on CT scan.
0	No SAH or IVH (intra ventricular hemorrhage).
I	Minimal /thin SAH, no IVH in either lateral ventricle.
II	Minimal /thin SAH, with IVH in both lateral ventricles.
III	Dense SAH (completely filling ≥1cistern or fissure, no IVH in either lateral ventricle.
IV	Dense SAH, with IVH in both lateral ventricles.

with thick SAH and intracerebral or intraventricular hemorrhage or just intraventricular hemorrhage. Furthermore, the grading scale is subjective. However, Ogilvy et al. reported high inter-rater reliability of high fisher grades (III, IV) [1, 9, 10].

In addition, important factors for instance clot density as well as percentage of daily cloth clearance, which are important predictors of cerebral vasospasm, are completely ignored in the grading scale [11].

Finally, Fisher Scale is not useful to operate as primary grading scheme for SAH, because it is not adequately comprehensive. It has been incorporated with other grading scales such as Hunt and Hess scale and added other factors like aneurysm size and location in Ogilvy grading scale [10].

Ogilvy grading scale gives one point for each of the following variables:

- Age greater than 50.
- Hunt and Hess grade 4–5 (in coma).
- Fisher grade score 3–4.
- Aneurysm size >10 mm.
- An additional point is added for a giant posterior circulation aneurysm (≥25 mm).

The total score ranges from 0–5, corresponding to grades 0–5 [10].

Ogilvy et al. proposed to predict the outcome for patients with aSAH who are surgically treated. It gave all factors equivalent weight. The most important limitations of Ogilvy scale are validated only in patients treated with surgical interventions and using the original Hunt and Hess grade, even if the patients grade changed before surgery [1].

6.1.4 Fisher Revised Scale

Revised Fisher scale was proposed to predict cerebral vasospasm and delayed neurological deficit post SAH (Table 6.4). Fisher revised scale is divided into five categories with stepwise increase in likelihood of developing cerebral ischemia with increasing the grade of revised Fisher scale.

Fisher Revised Scale has greater correlation with delayed neurological deficit and vasospasm than fisher scale. The main limitation is the subjective dichotomization of thin and thick SAH as no official description was provided or used during its derivation [12].

6.1.5 Hijdra Scale

The amount of subarachnoid blood on admission CT scan is associated with cerebral vasospasm, delayed cerebral ischemia, and poor outcome. To limit subjectivity in assessment amount of the subarachnoid blood, Hijdra et al. proposed a technique to grade amount of blood in subarachnoid

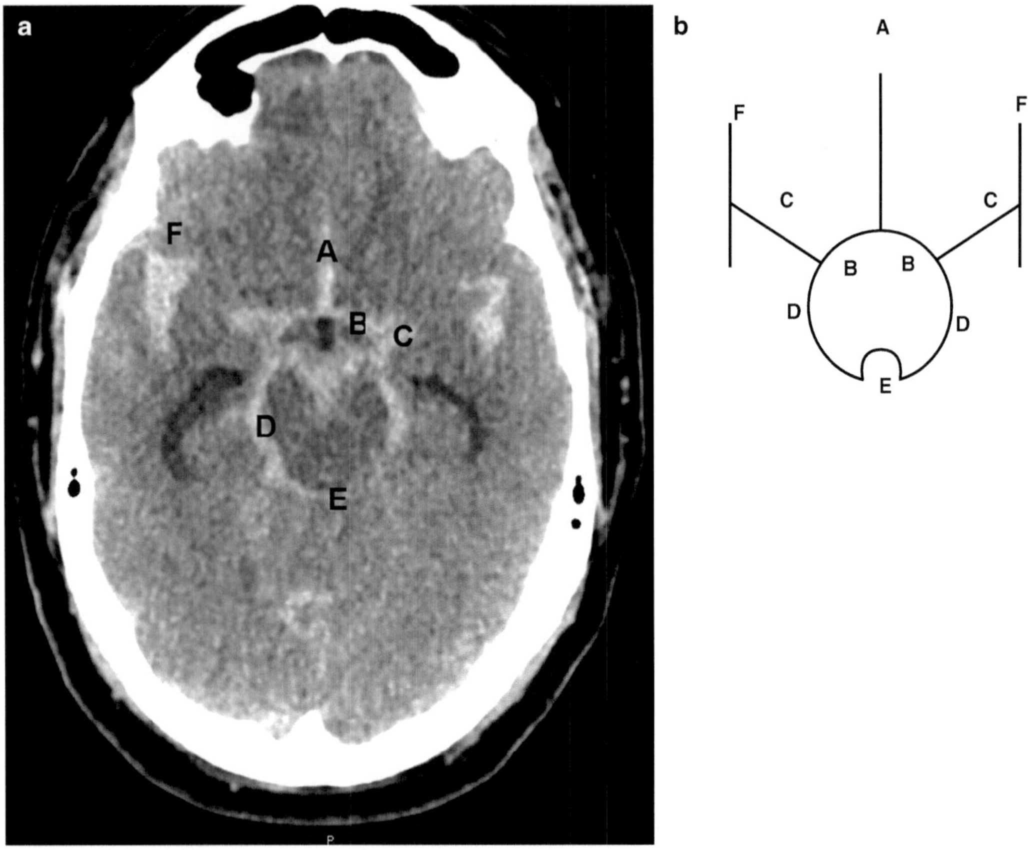

Fig. 6.2 (**a**) 10 Cisterns and Fishers in brain CT scan. (**b**) 10 Cisterns and Fishers in brain diagram (Courtesy Dr. Adel E. Ahmed Ganaw). A- Frontal hemispheric fissure; B- Suprasellar cisterns; C- Basal Sylvian fissures; D- Ambient cisterns; E- Quadrageminal cistern; F- Lateral Sylvian fissures

blood on admission CT scan, they graded amount of extravasated blood in each of ten cisterns and fissures (2 lateral Sylvian fissures, 2 basal Sylvian fissures, frontal hemispheric fissure, 2 Suprasellar cisterns, 2 Ambient cisterns and Quadrageminal cistern. Figure 6.2 independently on a semiquantitative scale as the following; [1, 13].

1. No blood =0
2. Small amount of blood = 1
3. Moderate filled with blood =2
4. Completely filled with blood = 3

They graded the clots that expanded the original size of fissure or cisterns and they did not consider clot density in their score. Calculated entire amount of subarachnoid blood (sum score) by adding the 10 scores and ranges 0–30. They used average score if cistern or fissure was inadequately visualized.

The followed same pattern to grade amount of blood in four ventricles;

1. No blood = 0
2. Sedimentation of blood in posterior part =1
3. Partially filled with blood = 2
4. Completely filled with blood =3

The total amount of ventricular blood (sum score) was the total amount of four scores and ranged from 0 to 12.

Hijdra et al. reported that their scale had high interobserver reliability with κ-values between 0.35 and 0.75 [1, 13].

J. S. Bretz et al. reported that the Hijdra scale was essentially useful prognostic instrument for

Table 6.5 Glasgow coma scale [1]

Motor	Verbal	Eye opening
6 Obeys verbal commands		
5 Localizes to noxious stimuli	5 Fully oriented	
4 Normal flexion to noxious stimuli	4 Disoriented	4 Open eyes spontaneously.
3 Abnormal flexion to noxious stimuli	3 Voice inappropriate wards	3 Open eyes to verbal commands.
2 Extension to noxious stimuli	2 Make incomprehensible sounds.	2 Open eyes to noxious stimuli.
1 No response to noxious stimuli	1 No vocalization	1 No eye opening

Table 6.6 Glasgow outcome scale [19]

Grade	Neurological status
5	Good recovery; resumption of normal life
4	Moderately disabled; independent lifestyle
3	Severely disabled patient; dependent on others to get through daily activities
2	Vegetative survival
1	Dead

prediction of functional outcome within Fisher grade III aSAH [14].

6.1.6 The Glasgow Coma Scale

The Glasgow Coma Scale (GCS) was proposed by neurosurgeon in Glasgow (1974). It is well known, easy to administer and calculate. It was initially created as bedside scheme for grading consciousness in head injury cases. The inter-rater reliability of the GCS in assessment of conscious level is greater than other schemes of consciousness assessment. Original GCS based on three axes: eye opening, verbal response, and motor response (Table 6.5). The GCS score is the sum of the numeric scores in these three axes, it converts a qualitative impression of disturbance of conscious level into a quantitative measurement. It ranges between 3 and 15 [1, 15, 16]. There are relative importance of each axis in GCS. For instance, patient with GCS 14 due to drop in conscious level has poorer outcome than it is for who has same GCS 14 due to reduced eye opening. One of the important limitations of GCS scale is that verbal axis represents major component of GCS scale, nevertheless, large proportion of SAH are early intubated during their clinical course. Some authors proposed grading scale for SAH that excluded verbal axis from GCS. Despite, prognostic strength, it has failed to gain popularity [17].

The psychometric features of the GCS have been stated to be inadequate due to possibility of overlapping of different scores, such as between 13 and 14, and 14 and 15, that may significantly affect outcome prediction. Therefore, some authors recommend a simplification of the GCS in SAH patient by compressing the 15-point scale to 5 points and called Glasgow outcome scale (Table 6.6). Simplified Glasgow outcome scale has statistically significant difference in outcome between the 5 grades [18, 19].

6.1.7 Prognosis on Admission of Aneurysmal Subarachnoid Hemorrhage (PAASH)

PAASH is five grading scoring scheme which based entirely on the preoperative GCS. The cut-off points between consecutive grades were carefully chosen by analyzing at which point two following grades matched to a statistically significant difference in outcome at 6 months.

Grade I (GCS -15), grade II (GCS 11–14), grade III (GCS -8-10), grade IV (GCS 4–7), and Grade V (GCS -3) [8].

PAASH grading scale was created to predict the outcome. It is simple, easy to remember, to apply as well as it is almost completely free from observer variability, because it was derived from well-known grading scheme (GCS). (Table 6.7) [20].

Table 6.7 Two SAH grading scales with criteria per grade and relation with outcome [20]

Grade	Criteria	Proportion of Patient with Poor outcome
I	GCS 15	14.8%
II	GCS 11–14	41.3%
III	GCS 8–10	74.4%
IV	GCS 4–7	84.7%
V	GCS 3	93.9%

Table 6.8 World federation of neurosurgeons SAH scale [6]

WFNS scale	GCS	Motor deficit, aphasia+/− hemiparesis or hemiplegia
I	15	Absent
II	14–13	Absent
III	14–13	Present
IV	12–7	Present/absent
V	6–3	Present/absent

6.1.8 World Federation of Neurosurgeons SAH Scale (WFNS)

The original World Federation of Neurosurgeons Scale (o-WFNS) of SAH was proposed in 1988 by expert opinion committee to predict the outcome of SAH. The committee members suggested that a SAH grading system (WFNS) should include five categories be based on Glasgow Coma scale (GCS) together with the presence of focal neurological deficit. In WFNS, GCS is compressed to 5 categories to improve intergrade differences in the outcome. WFNS has four axes, three GCS axes (eye opening, verbal response, and motor response) and the added fourth axis is neurological deficit to distinguish between grade II and III (GCS 13–14 patients without/with neurological deficits are classified into grade II and III, respectively, Table 6.8). Although the degree of extra prognostic power of adding focal neurological deficit is unknown [1, 6].

WFNS is superior to the Hunt and Hess Scale because it uses objective expressions and grades each of its axis separately. However, there are several limitations of o-WFNS grading scales. There are conflicting data about the reliability of o-WFNS in outcome prediction. Despite the stepwise increase in the possibility of poor outcome with increasing WFNS grade was reported by many studies, in many studies, o-WFNS failed to predict differences in outcome between adjacent grades especially between o-WFNS II and III or III and IV or IV and V [3, 18, 19].

Furthermore, large proportion of most severe SAH patients (grade V) have favorable outcome and improve dramatically after aggressive resuscitation. The o-WFNS based mainly on GCS which may drop significantly due to reversible causes such as seizures, anti-convulsant, and hydrocephalus. Therefore, r-WFNS was suggested, grading of SAH should be performed after resuscitation and correction of all reversible causes. In addition, neurological manifestations of brain stem herniation such as Oculomotor nerve (third nerve) palsy or loss of brain stem reflexes are not included in o-WFNS. Nakagawa et al. reported that prognosis of SAH patients with o-WFNS Grade V who did not have Oculomotor palsy was significantly better than those who had Oculomotor nerve palsy [21–23].

In o-WFNS, the authors did not describe the method for determining the GCS breakpoints. A wide range of GCS scores in some categories especially IV (GCS 7–12) may lead to coexisting error. Moreover, sometimes identification of neurological deficit is very difficult. Furthermore, there is inter-rater variability in application of the o-WFNS scale due to uncertainty in identifying the presence of neurologic deficits. Many attempts have been tried to modify the o-WFNS to improve its reliability in prediction of prognosis.

A modified o-WFNS was introduced by Fung et al. to improve prognostic power of grade V in o-WFNS. They proposed a herniation grading model (h-WFNS) by include clinical signs of brain stem dysfunction or herniation in o-WFNS scale. It is similar to o-WFNS but they assigned as grade IV all SAH who were formerly assigned as grade IV on the o-WFNS as well as patients with GCS 3–6 but do not show any positive sign of brain stem dysfunction or herniation such as posturing (decorticate and decerebrate posture), anisocoria, bilateral dilated pupils and no corneal reflexes. In grade V, they only assigned SAH with positive signs brain stem dysfunction or herniation. Therefore, the misleading effect of sedation and postictal status was eliminated, and prognostic power of grade V was significantly improved [21, 22].

Another modification of WFNS (m-WFNS) has been suggested by the WFNS Cerebrovascular Diseases and Treatment Committee (WFNS CVD and T committee) and Japan neurosurgical society to increase prognostication reliability of WFNS grade II and III. They assigned patients with GCS 14 to grade II and those with GCS 13 to grade III regardless of the presence of neurological deficit (Table 6.9). The superiority of m-WFNS to o-WFNS in outcome prediction was reported by multicenter prospective observational study recruited 1656 SAH patients [24].

6.1.9 VASOGRADE

The VASOGRADE was created to predict delayed cerebral ischemia (DCI). It is a practical grading scheme, semiquantitative, simple, easy to remember and to apply.

Table 6.9 original WFNS versus modified WFNS grading scale [24]

Grade	m-WFNS	o- WFNS
I	GCS 15	GCS 15
II	GCS 14	GCS 13–14 without focal neurological
III	GCS 13	GCS 13–14 with focal neurological
IV	GCS 7–12	GCS 7–12
V	GCS 3–6	GCS 3–6

VASOGRADE divides patients into three color coded categories according to the WFNS score after initial resuscitation and modified Fisher score at admission (Table 6.10). VASOGRADE-Green (modified Fisher scale 1 or 2 and WFNS 1 or 2), VASOGRADE-Yellow (modified Fisher 3 or 4 and WFNS 1–3), and VASOGRADE-Red (WFNS 4 or 5, irrespective of modified Fisher grade). Patients who classified as VASOGRADE- Green have lowest risk of DCI or Vasospasm, and those who classified as VASOGRADE – Red have highest risk of DCI and vasospasm. The prediction of DCI helps treating doctors to use the resources wisely and effectively [25].

VASOGRADE-Green (law risk group of DCI) patients may be monitored less aggressively than VASOGRADE-Yellow and VASOGRADE-Red patients. Frequent neurological examination may be enough as well as frequent expensive imaging can be avoided if not clinically indicated. Moreover, VASOGRADE-Green patients without medical complication of SAH may transferred to neurosurgery ward by the end of the first week to reduce to cost of staying in critical care [25].

While VASOGRADE-Red (high risk group of DCI) patients require close observation and frequent neurological evaluation by bedside nurses as well as neurological surveillance such as transcranial Doppler, CT perfusion, continuous electroencephalography. Both VASOGRADE – Red and VASOGRADE – Yellow patients should be admitted in high dependent or intensive care unit for at least 14 days. Furthermore, VASOGRADE-Red patients may benefit from invasive hemodynamic monitoring, aggressive strategies to avoid hypovolemia and hyponatremia.

Table 6.10 VASOGRADE scale [25]

VASOGRADE	Modified Fisher Scale	WFNS
Green	1-2	1-2
Yellow	3-4	1-3
Red	Any	4-5

VASOGRADE can be used for prognostication, risk stratification, communication between medical practitioners, standardization of management protocols, and enrollment criteria for academic activities [25].

6.2 Conclusion

Subarachnoid hemorrhage grading is critically important scheme to convert qualitative data of SAH severity into a numerical measurement with the intention of early prediction of prognosis and likelihood occurrence of serious complications such as vasospasm and delayed cerebral ischemia. Consequently, the treating physicians and family members can have proper anticipation for outcome. Grading scales also help clinicians in making appropriate management decisions in appropriate time, tracking patients status, follow up the patients response to the management and properly use of medical resources. Moreover, the grading scales facilitate the communications between the clinicians in different health care centers, as well as aid the academician to compare similar groups of patients in multicenter studies. The ideal grading scale should be simple, easy to remember, easy to apply and associated significantly with outcome or devastating complications. More than 40 grading scales have been proposed and modified to improve their reliability in predictions of devastating complications and outcome of SAH. But there are number of limitations in almost all scoring scales and all treating physicians should be aware of these limitations. Clinical grading scales should be performed after resuscitation and correction of all reversable causes. Although combination of grading scales may complicate the grading scale, it improves the prediction power of grading scale. Further studies are still required to establish powerful grading scale.

References

1. Rosen DS, Macdonald RL. Subarachnoid hemorrhage grading scales: a systematic review. Neurocrit Care. 2005;2(2):110–8.
2. Steiner T, Juvela S, Unterberg A, Jung C, Forsting M, Rinkel G, et al. European stroke organization guidelines for the management of intracranial aneurysms and subarachnoid haemorrhage. Cerebrovasc Dis. 2013;35(2):93–112.
3. Rosen DS, Macdonald RL. Grading of subarachnoid hemorrhage: modification of the World Federation of Neurosurgical Societies Scale on the basis of data for a large series of patients. Neurosurgery. 2004;54(3):566–76.
4. Takagi K, Tamura A, Nakagomi T, Nakayama H, Gotoh O, Kawai K, et al. How should a subarachnoid hemorrhage grading scale be determined? A combinatorial approach based solely on the Glasgow coma scale. J Neurosurg. 1999;90(4):680–7.
5. Hunt WE, Hess RM. Surgical risk as related to time of intervention in the repair of intracranial aneurysms. J Neurosurg. 1968;28(1):14–20.
6. Ahmed AE, Ganaw AMT, Bel Khair AOM. Aneurysmal Subarachnoid Hemorrhage. ICU book, Intechopen; 2017. p. 73–99.
7. Hunt WE, Kosnik EJ. Timing and perioperative care in intracranial aneurysm surgery. Clin Neurosurg. 1974;21:79–89.
8. Kiyoshi Takagi AT, Nakagomi T, Nakayama H, Gotoh O, Kawai K, Taneda M, Yasui N, Hadeishi H, Sano K. How should a subarachnoid hemorrhage grading scale be determined? A cominatorial approach based solely on the Glasgow Coma Scale. J Neurosurg. 1999;90(4):680–7.
9. Fisher CM, Kistler JP, Davis JM. Relation of cerebral vasospasm to subarachnoid hemorrhage visualized by computerized tomographic scanning. Neurosurgery. 1980;6(1):1–9.
10. Ogilvy CS, Carter BS. A proposed comprehensive grading system to predict outcome for surgical management of intracranial aneurysms. Neurosurgery. 1998;42(5):959–68. discussion 68-70
11. Reilly C, Amidei C, Tolentino J, Jahromi BS, Macdonald RL. Clot volume and clearance rate as independent predictors of vasospasm after aneurysmal subarachnoid hemorrhage. J Neurosurg. 2004;101(2):255–61.
12. Oliveira AM, Paiva WS, Figueiredo EG, Oliveira HA, Teixeira MJ. Fisher revised scale for assessment of prognosis in patients with subarachnoid hemorrhage. Arq Neuropsiquiatr. 2011;69(6):910–3.
13. Hijdra A, Brouwers PJ, Vermeulen M, van Gijn J. Grading the amount of blood on computed tomograms after subarachnoid hemorrhage. Stroke. 1990;21(8):1156–61.
14. Bretz JS, Von Dincklage F, Woitzik J, Winkler MKL, Major S, Dreier JP, et al. The Hijdra scale has significant prognostic value for the functional outcome of Fisher grade 3 patients with subarachnoid hemorrhage. Clin Neuroradiol. 2017;27(3):361–9.
15. Teasdale G, Jennett B. Assessment of coma and impaired consciousness. A practical scale. Lancet. 1974;2(7872):81–4.

16. Teasdale G, Knill-Jones R, van der Sande J. Observer variability in assessing impaired consciousness and coma. J Neurol Neurosurg Psychiatry. 1978;41(7):603–10.
17. Jagger J, Torner JC, Kassell NF. Neurologic assessment of subarachnoid hemorrhage in a large patient series. Surg Neurol. 1989;32(5):327–33.
18. Gotoh O, Tamura A, Yasui N, Suzuki A, Hadeishi H, Sano K. Glasgow Coma Scale in the prediction of outcome after early aneurysm surgery. Neurosurgery. 1996;39(1):19–24. discussion 5
19. Oshiro EM, Walter KA, Piantadosi S, Witham TF, Tamargo RJ. A new subarachnoid hemorrhage grading system based on the Glasgow coma scale: a comparison with the Hunt and Hess and world Federation of Neurological Surgeons Scales in a clinical series. Neurosurgery. 1997;41(1):140–7. discussion 7-8
20. van Heuven AW, Dorhout Mees SM, Algra A, Rinkel GJ. Validation of a prognostic subarachnoid hemorrhage grading scale derived directly from the Glasgow coma scale. Stroke. 2008;39(4):1347–8.
21. Wang AC, Heros RC. Editorial: subarachnoid hemorrhage grading scales. J Neurosurg. 2016;124(2):296–8. discussion 8
22. Fung C, Inglin F, Murek M, Balmer M, Abu-Isa J, Z'Graggen WJ, et al. Reconsidering the logic of world Federation of Neurosurgical Societies grading in patients with severe subarachnoid hemorrhage. J Neurosurg. 2016;124(2):299–304.
23. Nakagawa M, Sugiu K, Tokunaga K, Sakamoto C, Fujiwara K. The proposal of subgroups for grade V on world Federation of Neurologic Surgeons grading for subarachnoid hemorrhage. J Neurosurg Sci. 2013;57(4):303–6.
24. Sano H, Inamasu J, Kato Y, Satoh A, Murayama Y, Diseases WC, et al. Modified world federation of neurosurgical societies subarachnoid hemorrhage grading system. Surg Neurol Int. 2016;7(Suppl 18):S502–3.
25. de Oliveira Manoel AL, Jaja BN, Germans MR, Yan H, Qian W, Kouzmina E, et al. The VASOGRADE: a simple grading scale for prediction of delayed cerebral ischemia after subarachnoid hemorrhage. Stroke. 2015;46(7):1826–31.

Anesthetic Management of Aneurysmal Subarachnoid Hemorrhage (aSAH)

7

Adel E. Ahmed Ganaw, Ahamed Lafir Aliyar, Moad Ehfeda, and Nabil A. Shallik

7.1 Introduction

Aneurysmal subarachnoid hemorrhage (aSAH) due to a ruptured cerebral aneurysm is a devastating disease with significant multi-organ implications. Intracranial aneurysm rupture is the leading cause of non-traumatic subarachnoid hemorrhage. Worldwide, the prognosis is still very poor with a mortality as high as 35%. Among those survivors 33% need life-long care, another 33% suffer from impaired cognitive function which can affect their quality of life and functional status. Therefore, immediate diagnosis as well as early and appropriate management is paramount to improve outcome. Endovascular coiling or surgical clipping are the standard treatment options, anesthetic management of these patients is challenging due to their unstable physiology and associated severe neurological as well as medical complications such as re-bleeding, life-threatening obstructive hydrocephalus, hypertension, coma, myocardial dysfunction, hypotension, arrhythmia, pulmonary edema, cerebral edema, cerebral vasospasm, and electrolyte disturbances. Anesthesiologists must be aware of strategies to relax the brain while at the same time be able to preserve acceptable cerebral perfusion and oxygenation, accommodate requests for deliberate hyper−/hypotension as well as management of surgical emergencies like aneurysm rupture during any intervention [1–3].

A. E. A. Ganaw (✉) · A. L. Aliyar · M. Ehfeda
N. A. Shallik
Anesthesia, Perioperative Medicine and Critical Care Department, Hamad General Hospital, Hamad Medical Corporation, Doha, Qatar
e-mail: aganaw@hamad.qa; aaliyar1@hamad.qa; MEhfeda@hamad.qa; nshallik@hamad.qa

7.2 General Principles of Anesthesia

Anesthetic concerns for cerebral aneurysm clipping and coiling are comparable with noticeable differences being the venue, extent of blood loss, and the need for brain relaxation.

7.2.1 The Primary Goals of Anesthetic Management Are

- Maintain cerebral perfusion pressure (CPP) > 60 mmHg to prevent cerebral ischemia and maintain adequate collateral blood flow during the application of temporary clips.
- CPP = MAP—ICP or CVP whichever is greater
- The following factors that can cause a rise in ICP should be avoided or promptly treated:
  - Hypoventilation and hypercarbia—maintain $PaCO_2$ at low normal ~35mmhg.
  - hypoxia,
  - Seizures.

A. E. A. Ganaw et al. (eds.), *Management of Subarachnoid Hemorrhage*,
https://doi.org/10.1007/978-3-030-81333-8_7

   - Hyperthermia (ICP increases as cerebral compliance is reduced and compensation mechanisms are exhausted in SAH) [4].
   - pain,
- Hypotension must be avoided and if present must be treated with inotropes or vasopressors.
- Maintain normoglycemia and euvolemia. For more details, please refer to Chap. 3 (Central Nervous System Neurophysiology).
- Control of the transmural pressure gradient (TMPG) of the aneurysm to avoid sudden aneurysmal rupture which can be considered as central to the anesthetic management of intracranial aneurysms. The aneurysm's transmural pressure gradient (TMPG) is equal to the pressure within the aneurysm (mean arterial blood pressure MAP) minus the pressure outside/around the aneurysm (intracranial pressure ICP), i.e. TMPG = MAP-ICP. Noteworthy, both TMPG and CPP are affected by same variables (MAP and ICP). The main goal is to maintain the CPP as high as required to afford enough cerebral oxygenation, and TMPG as law as possible to decrease the jeopardy of aneurysm rupture. While changes in MAP and ICP lead to the same changes in TMPG and CPP, and as CPP and TMPG values are mathematically same, it always comes down to the choice between an ideal TMPG and the best CPP. The dilemma is balancing the jeopardy of inadequate cerebral perfusion against jeopardy of rupture of the cerebral aneurysm. Maintaining CPP and TMPG at preoperative baseline values through the surgery is the ideal solution. However, this target is hardly attainable.
- Adequate preparation to manage potential intraoperative complications [5].

This highlights the dilemma of balancing acceptable cerebral perfusion versus the risk of aneurysmal rupture. Therefore, until the aneurysm is secured, systolic blood pressure (SBP) should not be allowed to increase above 160 mmHg while the aim should be to maintain the preoperative baseline. At the same time hypotension (SBP < 110 mmhg) must be avoided to ensure adequate cerebral perfusion. Moreover, sudden reductions in ICP as can be seen with insertion of life saving external ventricular drain (EVD) insertions or aggressive osmotherapy should be avoided as this can increase the aneurysm's TMPG and cause rupture of the aneurysm [5].

- Anticipate and obtund painful stimuli, such as intubation and head pin placement.
- Provide a compliant brain to minimize retraction pressure.
- Rapid and smooth emergence, to allow early postoperative neurological assessment [5].

7.3 Preoperative Evaluation and Optimization

Patients with aSAH usually present with a "thunderclap" headache often described as the worst headache of their lives. This can be associated with nausea, vomiting, neck stiffness, neurological deficits, seizures, reduced consciousness, hemodynamic instability, and rarely cardiac arrest. The most important factor associated with a poor outcome is the preoperative level of consciousness [2].

If the patient is acutely ill at presentation, an ABC (Airway, Breathing, and Circulation) approach should be adopted to achieve cardiorespiratory stability ensuring cerebral perfusion and oxygenation while minimizing the risk of rebleeding. The airway should be secured, and cardiovascular support started as dictated by the clinical situation.

Once the patient has been stabilized, a thorough and systematic preoperative evaluation is paramount, as these patients can present with significant multi-organ dysfunction (Table 7.1) [6, 7] and comorbidities. However, delaying surgery/intervention to optimize the patient should be balanced against the urgency of surgery/intervention. Depending on the patient's neurological status, the history may have to be obtained from the family.

Preoperative assessment should include comorbidities (Hypertension, diabetes mellitus, ischemic heart disease, COPD, cerebral aneurysms can be associated with polycystic kidney disease and coarctation of aorta) [8] and associated medication history, allergies, previous anesthetics, smoking/alcohol

Table 7.1 Neurological and non-neurological complication [5, 10]

Neurological complications	Non- neurological complications
1. Hydrocephalus 2. Intracranial hypertension 3. Re-bleeding 4. Vasospasm and delayed cerebral ischemia(DCI) 5. Seizures	1. Pulmonary complications (pulmonary edema either cardiac or neurogenic, aspiration pneumonia) 2. Cardiac complications (QT – Prolongation, repolarization abnormalities, T wave changes, life-threatening arrhythmias, myocardial ischemia, elevated cardiac troponin, and neurogenic stunned myocardium) 3. Electrolyte disturbance (hyponatremia, hypomagnesemia, hypokalemia, hypocalcemia) 4. Hematological complications (Anemia, coagulopathy, leukocytosis) 5. Endocrine disturbance (hyperglycemia, hypothalamopituitary dysfunction) 6. Fever (infectious or central)

history, and fasting status. A thorough examination of the central nervous system, cardiovascular system, and respiratory system is essential as aSAH patients can have significant cardiac and respiratory dysfunction secondary to the catecholamine storm caused by the hemorrhage. The patient's baseline vitals and neurological status including size and reactivity of pupils, GCS, and deficits must be noted.

Preoperative investigations should be requested depending on the background history, the systemic examination, and expected complications (Table 7.2) [7, 9]. Patient's investigations and imaging must be reviewed.

The size, character, number, and location of the aneurysm, extent of subarachnoid hemorrhage, and the presence of features suggestive of raised ICP should be made note of. Biochemical disturbances if present should be corrected, especially in the presence of ECG changes and cardiac dysfunction. Maintaining euvolemia, normothermia, and normoglycemia is essential.

Patient or family should be informed of the possible anesthetic complications, rare but disastrous aneurysm rupture or re-bleeding, blood trans-fusions, and postoperative intubation.

Table 7.2 preoperative investigations for aSAH [5, 7]

Investigations	Comment
Full blood count	Exclude anemia
Coagulation screening	Exclude coagulopathy
Serum urea/ creatinine and electrolytes	Assess kidney function and exclude any electrolytes abnormalities
Serum glucose	Exclude hypoglycemia and hyperglycemia (associated with poor outcome)
Chest X ray	Exclude aspiration pneumonia, pulmonary edema (if clinically indicated)
12 leads ECG	Exclude arrhythmia and myocardial ischemia
Serum cardiac biomarker	Exclude myocardial injury (indicated if there is arrhythmia or pulmonary edema or hemodynamically unstable)
Transthoracic Echo	Exclude myocardial dysfunction (indicated only if patient. Hemodynamically unstable or if there is pulmonary edema).
Arterial blood gas	Assess oxygen delivery, $PaCO_2$, PaO_2, lactate level
CT brain	Assess intracerebral hemorrhage, hydrocephalus and high ICP
CT-angiography	- Identify site, size, and number of aneurysms

Various grading scales are available to assess and evaluate aSAH patients. These include the World Federation of Neurological Surgeons (WFNS) grades, modified Hunt and Hess clinical grades, and the Fisher Grades for CT findings. These grades allow assessment of surgical risk and prognosis, inter-physician communication about the patient's condition and conduct of scientific studies. For more details, please refer to Chap. 6 (Grading of aneurysmal subarachnoid hemorrhage).

7.4 Premedication

Premedication in patients with subarachnoid hemorrhage must be individualized. It is prudent to avoid preoperative sedative medications whenever possible to allow assessment of patient's neurological status and continued neuromonitoring. However, anxiety can increase the blood pressure and put the patient at increased risk of re-bleeding. This must be balanced against the use of sedatives that may lead to respiratory depression and an increase in $PaCO_2$ leading to a raised intracranial pressure (ICP). Consequently, the decision for premedication, type of premedication, and dosage of premedication is determined by clinical grade, respiratory rate, co-morbidity, chronic medication, and the level of ICP. Anxious patients with good Hunt and Hess grades (I and II) may receive smaller doses of oral benzodiazepines. Poor grade patients (III-V) may already be in ICU, intubated and sedated.

All vasoactive medications administered to maintain adequate cerebral perfusion should be continued. Moreover, patients should receive their regular doses of anticonvulsants and nimodipine. Anti-acid and anti-emetic should be considered as part of premedication and should be given before induction of anesthesia at the appropriate time [5].

7.5 Anesthesia for Surgical Clipping of Cerebral Aneurysm

Following a craniotomy and after careful surgical dissection, aneurysm obliteration is achieved by placing a clip at the junction of the aneurysm and the parent artery preventing blood flow into it. A relaxed brain is essential for optimal surgical exposure and to avoid excessive brain retraction, particularly in deep seated aneurysms. MRI compatible titanium clips are generally used.

7.5.1 Monitoring

7.5.1.1 Standard Monitoring

Standard monitoring includes pulse oximetry, noninvasive blood pressure (NIBP), 5 lead electrocardiogram (ECG), capnography, temperature, neuromuscular block, and urine output [11].

7.5.1.2 Hemodynamic Monitoring

Placement of arterial line under local anesthesia before induction of anesthesia is important to address any hemodynamic changes during induction and airway management. An arterial line is also essential to maintain hemodynamics intraoperatively and for frequent blood sampling. Central venous access is dependent on patient's general status, it is essential in poor grade patients or patients with significant cardiovascular dysfunction to titrate vasopressor or inotrope therapy. Central line should be inserted under guidance of ultrasound to reduce risk of puncture of carotid artery which needs manual compression which may impair cerebral blood flow. Currently, pulmonary artery catheter is rarely used to assess and monitor cardiac output, especially after introduction of reliable less invasive techniques to monitor and assess myocardial function and preload such as transpulmonary thermodilution techniques. In poor grade SAH patients, bedside transpulmonary thermodilution monitoring reduces the incidence of pulmonary edema, the consequences of DCI, and improves the clinical outcome [11–13].

7.5.1.3 Neuromonitoring

ICP Monitoring

ICP can be easily measured in patients with intraventricular drain. ICP monitoring may help anesthesiologists in the blood pressure management especially during induction and emergence from anesthesia. It should be considered in patients who have poor neurological status or patients with hydrocephalus as they often have intracranial hypertension [5]. For more details, please refer to Chap. 3 (Central Nervous System Neurophysiology).

Jugular Venous Bulb Monitoring

Indeed, monitoring brain oxygenation is extremely useful in anesthetic management of SAH. Cerebral venous oxygen saturation (SjvO2) can be measured by the retrograde insertion of a catheter in the jugular bulb. It reflects the balance between cerebral metabolic supply and demand in presence of stable cerebral metabolic rate. It resembles to mixed venous saturation in the assessment of the balance between systemic supply and demand. It may be helpful in the early detection of reduced cerebral perfusion due to hyperventilation or, in the perioperative blood pressure management, in determination adequacy of cerebral perfusion during temporary clipping, and in the recognition of hyperemia and luxury perfusion. Matta et el, reported that SjvO2 monitoring was helpful in more than 50% of their SAH patients. Sudden drop in SjvO2 may be an indication of aneurysmal rupture. However, recurrent SjvO2 fluctuations may occur without clear reasons. Furthermore, cannulation of internal jugular vein may decrease cerebral venous drainage and increase ICP [5, 6, 14].

Near-Infrared Spectroscopy

Near-infrared spectroscopy (NIRS) permits uninterrupted monitoring of brain regional oxygen saturation. Nevertheless, NIRS signal interference from extracranial source may affect accuracy of the readings, therefore, anesthesiologists cannot rely on NIRS to guide therapeutic intervention during surgical intervention [11, 15].

7.5.1.4 Neurophysiology Monitoring

Patient coughing, bucking, or moving during the procedure can lead to disastrous consequences like increase in ICP and aneurysm rupture. Consequently, adequate neuromuscular blockade should be ensured by continuously monitoring the depth of block using an appropriate neuromuscular transmission monitor(NMT).

Monitoring ICP through intraventricular catheters in patients with hydrocephalus or poor grade SAH can guide blood pressure management and aid in draining excess CSF perioperatively.

Bispectral Index (BIS) monitoring is essential in patients anesthetized using the total intravenous anesthesia(TIVA) technique. They can also guide propofol or thiopentone administration during periods when burst suppression is required. Although, the use of burst suppression has been questioned as the hemodynamic consequences of administering these drugs have a more deleterious effect than the neuroprotection provided by this technique with no overall outcome benefit [5, 16].

7.5.2 Induction

A smooth induction avoiding any sudden changes in blood pressure is paramount. An acute increase in blood pressure can increase the TMPG and cause aneurysm rupture. Whereas a precipitous drop in blood pressure can cause a dangerous reduction in cerebral perfusion, especially in patients with raised ICP and high grade aSAH. Although no single induction agent is superior to another, careful titration to achieve a smooth induction is essential.

Numerous agents have been used to blunt the intubation response, including high dose opioids like Fentanyl (5–10mcg/kg) or Sufentanil (0.5-1mcg/kg), Lidocaine (1.5–2 mg/kg), Esmolol (0.5 mg/kg), Labetalol 10–20 mg, and a second dose of Propofol (0.5-1 mg/kg) or Thiopental (1–2 mg/kg) [17].

Using a target-controlled infusion system, the concentration of Remifentanil to blunt the hemodynamic response to noxious stimuli is usually between 4 and 6 ng/ml. The concentration has to be decreased rapidly upon cessation of the painful stimulus to avoid hypotension. A continuous infusion of Remifentanil is particularly useful when a difficult airway is anticipated because it allows long-lasting suppression of laryngoscopy response with hemodynamic stability.

A non-depolarizing muscle relaxant (NDMR) is preferably used to facilitate endotracheal intubation and controlled mechanical ventilation as it has no effect on ICP or cerebral blood flow. The depolarizing muscle relaxant succinylcholine is associated with a transient rise in ICP, although this increase in ICP is not seen when the patients are under deep anesthesia, or when the succinylcholine is preceded by a small dose of non-depolarizing muscle relaxant. Moreover, Succinylcholine has been used effectively in many SAH patients without reported complications. It may be considered when difficult intubation is suspected or rapid sequence induction is indicated. Although Rocuronium (0.9–1.2 mg/kg) is a suitable alternative if the specific reversal agent Sugammadex is available [18, 19].

7.5.3 Maintenance

Common maintenance techniques include TIVA, inhalational with opioids or a combination of both. Although TIVA remains a popular choice due to its inherent effect on the cerebral blood flow, there is no evidence to suggest that one technique is superior to the other.

Propofol causes cerebral vasoconstriction and decreases cerebral metabolic rate leading to a decrease in ICP. Sevoflurane, isoflurane, and desflurane can also be used in concentrations less than 1 MAC (minimum alveolar concentration), concentrations greater than 1MAC can cause cerebral vasodilation and a consequent increase in ICP. Abrupt increase in desflurane concentration can increase ICP due to its effect on the sympatho-adrenal system.

Intraoperative analgesia can be provided either by intermittent boluses or continuous infusion of opioids. Intense stimulations such as pin insertion (Figs. 7.1 and 7.2), surgical incision or elevation of periosteum, and dural incision must be anticipated and treated by administering supplementary doses of opioids and deepening the planes of anesthesia to avoid hypertension and rupture of the aneurysm [1, 5].

Sevoflurane is a better choice than isoflurane because it is associated with faster recovery, especially after long-lasting procedures. Desflurane may be used but is a more potent cerebral vasodilator than sevoflurane [9, 20].

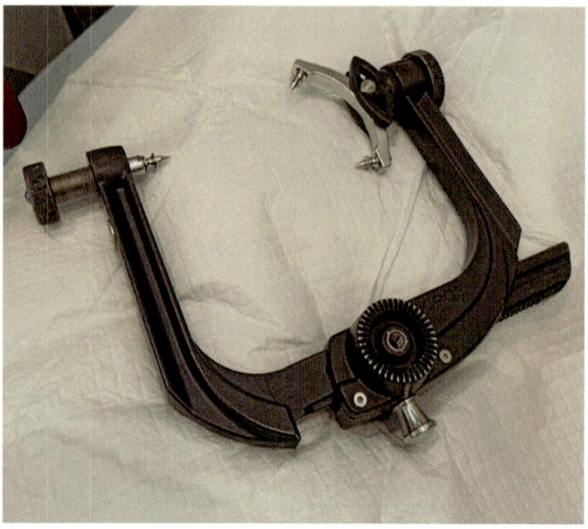

Fig. 7.1 Mayfield to fix the head with sharp pins of the patients. (Courtesy of Dr. Saleh Safi)

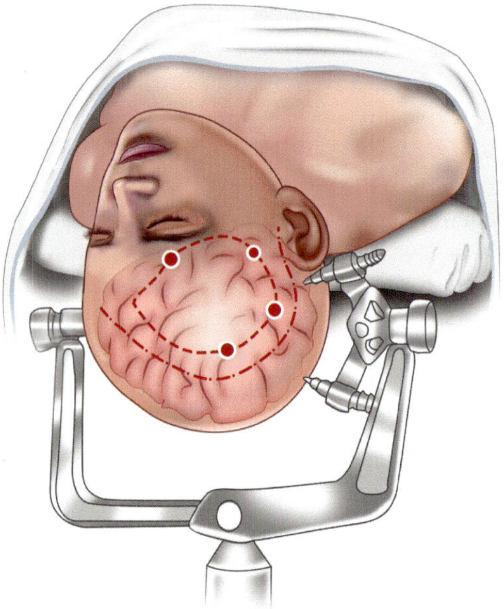

Fig. 7.2 Positioning of patient in 3-pin head clamp with incision marking with burr holes and extent of craniotomy in a standard pterional craniotomy

7.5.4 Brain Relaxation

Current guidelines recommend early surgery to secure the aneurysm as the risk of rebleed and its consequent complications is highest in the first 72 h. As a result, a greater proportion of patients presenting for surgery tend to have raised ICP and cerebral edema. Optimum brain relaxation techniques are essential to optimize surgical exposure, reduce brain retraction, and facilitate clipping of the aneurysm [1].

Sudden reduction in ICP raises the TMPG and increases the risk of aneurysm rupture. This reduction in ICP should be performed cautiously before Dural opening. Following agents/maneuvers can been used to facilitate brain relaxation:

7.5.4.1 Positioning

Head up position (15–30°) is the ideal position for SAH patients as it reduces venous bleeding in the surgical field. The neck must be in the neutral position, excessive flexion or rotation of the neck

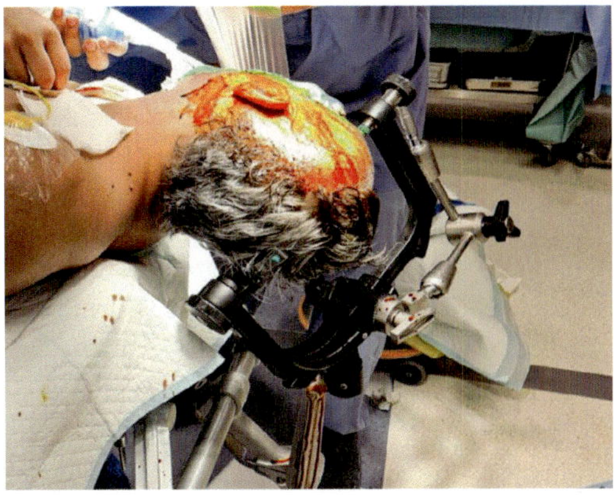

Fig. 7.3 Patient positioning for surgical clipping. (Courtesy of Dr. Saleh Safi)

impedes jugular venous drainage, increase intracranial blood volume, and ICP. During positioning, the tracheal tube must be well secured, and should be taped instead of tying it around the neck. If taping proves difficult due to factors like facial hair, moist skin, etc. a neck tie can be used while ensuring that it is not too tight impeding venous drainage (Fig. 7.3) [21, 22].

7.5.4.2 Mannitol

Mannitol (20%) is a hyperosmolar solution which increases the osmolality of the intravascular space. Fluid moves from the brain to the vascular space down the osmolar gradient leading to a reduction in ICP. The maximum effect of the mannitol on brain edema and ICP appears around 30–45 min after starting mannitol infusion and the clinical effect of mannitol is judged by drop of the ICP and/or brain edema rather than by urine output. The initial drop in ICP following mannitol administration may reflect compensatory cerebral vasoconstriction in the area of the brain with preserved autoregulation in order to maintain cerebral blood flow at physiological levels.

Rapid infusion of mannitol may initially cause hypotension followed by increase in blood volume, filling pressure and cardiac output at the end of the infusion, which may lead to transient increase in cerebral blood flow and ICP. However, this transient increase in ICP is less likely with slaw infusion of mannitol with a concentration of not more than 20% and in patients with preexisting high ICP. Mild hyperventilation may prevent the initial increase of ICP in high-risk patients. Thirty minutes after administration of mannitol, blood volume decreases to its baseline, but filling pressure and cardiac output may decrease below baseline levels. The transient increase in blood volume associated with mannitol can potentially precipitate pulmonary edema in patients with poor cardiac and renal function.

Mannitol increases serum osmolality, decreases hematocrit, and may cause metabolic derangements such as hyponatremia, hyperkalemia, and metabolic acidosis due to dilution of bicarbonate which is extremely important in presence of renal impairment.

The dose of mannitol ranges between 0.25 and 2 g/kg body weight. Treating physicians usually administer 0.5–1 g/kg over 20–30 min. Higher dose (>1 g/kg) and faster administration are associated with faster and larger reduction in ICP and brain edema. However, it is associated with significant risk of hypotension, electrolyte disturbance, increase intravascular, volume and cerebral blood volume. Therefore, the dose and speediness of administration should be based on clinical status. Administration of second dose is unlikely to reduce ICP if the serum osmolality more than 330 mOsm/L.

Theoretically, mannitol should be administered after dural incision, because sudden drop in ICP increases TMPG of the aneurysm and aneurysmal rupture. Furthermore, rapid administration of mannitol leads to brain shrinkage which may lead to traction and tearing of bridging veins. However, in clinical practice, neurosurgeons repeatedly request administration of mannitol after positioning of the patients. In such scenario, mannitol should be infused slowly at rate 100-200 ml/hr. and infusion rate increased after opening of the dura [5, 21].

7.5.4.3 Furosemide

Furosemide (0.25–1 mg/kg) decreases formation of CSF as well as water and ion movement across the blood–brain barrier. Furosemide has a synergistic effect with mannitol. The sustained diuretic effect of high dose of furosemide may lead to sustained high plasma osmolality which potentiate the effect of the mannitol. Therefore, it should be administered at smaller dose with mannitol (5–20 mg). Administration of furosemide prior to mannitol my blunt the initial increase of ICP induced by mannitol. Furosemide may be considered in patients with renal or cardiopulmonary impairment, the jeopardy of hypervolemia, and electrolyte derangement may be reduced when furosemide used instead of mannitol. The main disadvantages of furosemide are the general clinical impression that it is not reliable and effective as mannitol in reducing brain bulk and ICP.

In addition, combination therapy may lead to hypovolemia and electrolyte disturbances especially hypokalemia. Therefore, assessment of volume status and potassium level are very important [5, 21, 23].

7.5.4.4 Hypertonic Saline

Hypertonic saline 3% is as effective as mannitol in treatment of high ICP. The hypertonic saline causes hyperchloremic acidosis which may have detrimental effect on the kidney function [30]. 3% saline maintains hemodynamics hence can be used in unstable patients. It can be used at a dose of 3-5 ml/kg over 10–20 min [21].

7.5.4.5 CSF Drainage

CSF drainage by using either a subarachnoid lumbar or ventricular drain is an effective technique of decreasing ICP and to achieve brain relaxation. Extreme caution should, however, be exercised during insertion of the drain to minimize CSF loss and a prompt drop in ICP, so as to prevent a sudden increase in TMP and aneurysm rupture.

Lumbar drainage of CSF can cause brainstem herniation in patients with intracerebral hematoma; therefore, insertion of lumbar drainage should be avoided in those patients.

Theoretically, free drainage should be allowed only after dura incision to prevent re-bleeding; but in clinical practice 20–30 mL of CSF is frequently drained immediately before opening of the dura to facilitate dura incision. The drain is frequently left open throughout the surgery, till the aneurysm is clipped or until the dura closure [5, 21].

7.5.4.6 Hyperventilation

Hyperventilation is a quick and effective method of lowering ICP, however, overzealous hyperventilation may induce cerebral ischemia through intense cerebral vasoconstriction particularly in poor grade patients. Therefore, hyperventilation should only be used as a temporizing measure in patients with impending herniation. During the surgical procedure the target PaCO2 should be low normal (30–35mmhg) [21].

7.5.5 Fluids and Electrolytes

Maintenance of euvolemia and normal circulating blood volume is recommended to prevent DCI, therefore fluid administration should be guided by a combination of clinical assessment, invasive monitors such as CVP, PiCCO, and dynamic variables of fluid responsiveness like pulse pressure and stroke volume variation.

Fluid administration should be restricted to glucose free isotonic crystalloids (normal saline), plasmalyte or colloid solution. Hyperglycemia aggravates ischemic brain injury and must be avoided [21].

7.5.6 Temporary Clipping

Temporary clipping of feeder/parent vessels is commonly used to ensure good visualization of the surgical field and to avoid intraoperative rupture during surgical dissection of aneurysms. Temporary clipping substituted the use of global hypotension to reduce pressure gradient across the aneurysm wall and bleeding in the surgical field.

The main recommendations during temporary clipping are:

Blood pressure maintained at high normal levels to ensure adequate collateral circulation. Phenylephrine or noradrenaline can be used to induce hypertension.

Metabolic suppression by using Propofol or Barbiturates (thiopentone) to induce burst suppression and subsequently reduce energy consumption by brain cells allowing ischemia to be better tolerated during the application of temporary clips. The suppressing agents should be administered prior to clipping. However, the evidence behind this is lacking and there is a concern that the hemodynamic instability produced by high doses of thiopentone can be more detrimental than the benefits they offer. Therefore, adequate hemodynamic support to ensure collateral blood flow is essential.

FiO_2 increased to 100%.

Clamping time should not be longer than 20 min.

Induced hypothermia to decrease cerebral metabolic rate and energy consumption, however, induced hypothermia is associated with coagulopathy, arrhythmia, wound infection, shivering which leads to increase oxygen consumption and postoperative ventilation due to decrease in drug metabolism. A conservative recommendation would be mild hypothermia (34–35 °C) untill closing is started, followed by active rewarming. Although the evidence for this approach is limited [22, 24].

7.5.7 Intraoperative Aneurysmal Rupture

Intraoperative aneurysmal rupture is associated with high mortality and morbidity, the risk of intraoperative rupture is about 19%. It is associated with poor prognosis especially if the rupture occurs during induction. The intra-op rupture is usually due to sudden increase in the aneurysm's TMPG or due to surgical manipulation or dissection. Bleeding can be severe enough to cause hemorrhagic shock. The anesthetic management varies from center to center; however, the primary goal is to aid the surgeon in controlling the bleed.

Temporary occlusion of the feeder artery is the ideal technique to control the bleeding. When this is not possible, mean arterial pressure (MAP) should be briefly dropped to 40–50 mmHg to reduce arterial wall shear stress, reduce bleeding, facilitate surgical orientation, improve the surgical field, and simplify clipping of the ruptured aneurysm. However, a combination of hypovolemia and hypotension may induce cerebral ischemia.

One described technique is to induce cardiac arrest with adenosine, infused rapidly into a large vein, while the operative field is suctioned and temporary clips (so-called pilot clips) are placed. There is no consensus on the optimal dose or method of adenosine administration. We recommend that local guidelines are followed for this. One described regimen is the administration of 0.3–0.4 mg/kg of adenosine to achieve a temporary arrest of approximately 45 seconds, however, controlled studies are needed to validate this technique [5, 21, 25, 26].

Induced flow arrest with rapid ventricular pacing, using transcutaneous pacing pads provide similar benefits seen with adenosine arrest. Sometimes manual compression of the ipsilateral carotid artery is helpful especially if there is large and uncontrolled premature rupture. Some clinicians administer a bolus dose or continuous infusion of thiopental because of its cerebro-vasoconstrictive and neuro protective properties. However, thiopental administration may affect hemodynamic stability and delay recovery [21].

7.5.8 Emergence

At the end of the operation, the anesthesiologist should maintain a normal blood pressure and $PaCO_2$, which will help the surgeon identify any bleeding or brain edema before closing the dura. Massive brain edema following the surgery may require the bone flap to be left out, insertion of ICP monitor, and postoperative sedation and ventilation. Early extubation facilitating early postoperative neurological evaluation is preferred after uncomplicated surgery in patients who presented with a low WFNS grade(I,II). Mild hypertension (10–20% above the baseline) may augment cerebral perfusion particularly in patients with vasospasm. Blood pressure > 20% of baseline can be treated with Labetalol, Esmolol, or Hydralazine as extreme increases in blood pressure may lead to postoperative hemorrhage. If the patient fails to recover to the expected GCS in postoperative period, urgent (non-contrast) brain CT scan is required to exclude intraoperative bleeding.

Poor grade patients (Hunt and Hess grades III–V) or who have had intraoperative complications should be admitted in the intensive care unit for postoperative ventilation, continuous ICP monitoring, and frequent neurological assessment. Intravenous Paracetamol and Codeine are most commonly used for analgesia, long-acting opioid such as Morphine should be used carefully to avoid respiratory depression, CO_2 retention and postoperative nausea and vomiting. In addition, Morphine may affect postoperative neurological assessment. Non-steroid anti-inflammatory drugs (NSAID) may increase risk of bleeding and should be avoided. Prophylactic anti-emetics such as Ondansetron should be administered. Antiepileptic prophylaxis should be considered for cases with temporal or frontal hematoma. All patients are at risk of venous thromboembolism; therefore, stockings should be applied with intermittent calf compression devices throughout the perioperative period. Pharmacological prophylaxis with low-molecular-weight heparin should be started on the second postoperative day if there are no contraindications [5, 11, 25, 27].

7.6 Anesthesia for Interventional Neuroradiology (INR)

Endovascular treatment of cerebral aneurysm can be achieved by depositing electrically detachable platinum coils within the aneurysmal sac reducing blood flow into the aneurysmal sac and ultimately causing secondary thrombosis. When the aneurysm is wide necked, balloon assisted, or stent assisted coiling is performed to prevent the coils from herniating out into the parent vessel. One other method is to insert flow diverter stents to direct blood flow away from the aneurysm resulting in progressive thrombosis of the aneurysm. The interventional radiologist generally selects a trans-femoral arterial approach, placing a large 6 French femoral sheath followed by a catheter. This is then directed into the Carotid (for anterior circulation) or Vertebral artery (for posterior circulation). A micro-catheter is introduced through this into the cerebral circulation. Then detachable platinum coils are advanced into position and the coils deployed into the aneurysmal sac until an optimal seal is achieved [5]. For more details please refer to Chap. 8 (Subarachnoid hemorrhage coiling and intervention).

7.6.1 Anesthetic Concerns Include

- Remote site anesthesia.
- Radiation safety.
- Managing anticoagulation.
- Inadequate lighting (Fig. 7.4).
- Maintaining patient immobility.
- Maintain physiological stability.
- Manipulating systemic and regional blood flow.
- Handling unanticipated complications during the intervention like hemorrhage or vascular occlusion [5].
- Contrast related complications.
- Hypothermia management.
- Transport of critically ill patients to and from radiology suites.
- Smooth as well as rapid recovery for neurological evaluation [28, 29].

7.6.1.1 Remote Site Anesthesia

Anesthesia for INR is normally performed in the neuroradiology suite outside the operating theater complex. Non-operating room anesthesia (NORA) procedures, compared to procedures performed in the operating room, have a higher frequency of severe injury and death [4–6]. This can be attributed to limited workspace, inadequate lighting, unfamiliar equipment, lack of skilled anesthesia support staff, limited patient access during the procedure, and unavailability of immediate senior help when necessary.

The INR suite is an inconvenient place for the anesthetist as it is an environment established for the needs of the radiologist, equipped with multiple bulky equipment. This is made worse by the movement of the C-arm around the patient. Consequently, access to the patient is very

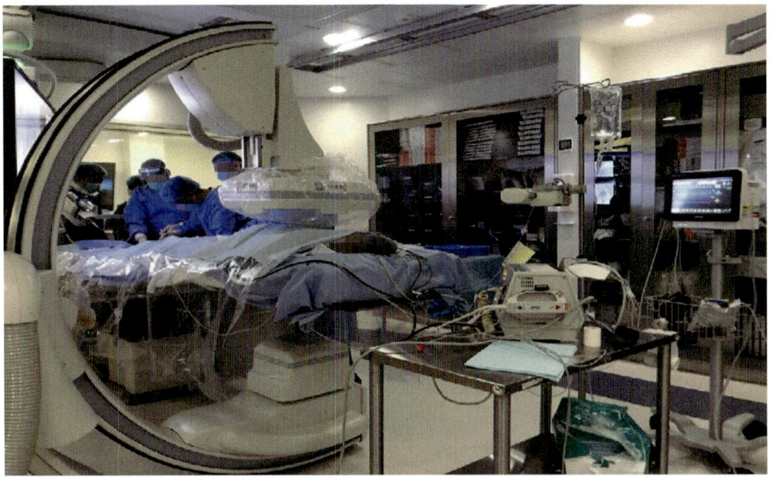

Fig. 7.4 Crowded interventional radiology room with limited work space, limited patient access, inadequate lightning, C-arm around patient's head. (Courtesy of Dr. Shakeel)

restricted during the procedure. Therefore, it is very important to make sure the airway and intravenous (I.V) and arterial lines are carefully secured, and long anesthesia circuits and lines are utilized. Moreover, temperature monitoring and patient warming is very important as the need for low INR suite temperatures to ensure proper functioning of the radiological equipment exposes the patient to hypothermia (Fig. 7.2).

The anesthetist should make himself familiar with the environment and equipment and should ensure that appropriate drugs and support are available before starting a case at the neuroradiology suite [30].

7.6.1.2 Radiation Safety

Patients and staff are exposed to high doses of ionizing radiation at the INR suite. Digital subtraction angiography delivers considerably higher radiation than fluoroscopy. Since radiation exposure poses a significant health risk, conscious measures must be taken to minimize exposure risk. Therefore, during the whole procedure, all staff in the radiology suit should minimize their exposure by wearing protective lead aprons of at least 0.5 mm thickness, thyroid shields, eye protection, radiation exposure badges and stay as far away from the radiation source as possible. Recent evidence suggests that anesthetists may be exposed to a significant amount of scattered radiation, which increases the risk of cataract formation [21, 31, 32].

7.6.1.3 Anticoagulation

The persistent decrease in morbidity and mortality by dual antiplatelet agent therapy in coronary artery thrombosis patients experiencing percutaneous coronary intervention (PCI) has drawn interest for their use in endovascular interventions of the central nervous system (CNS). Careful management of anticoagulation is paramount to prevent thromboembolic complications during and after the procedure. The procedure itself is inherently thrombogenic due to the insertion of various catheters, thrombogenic nature of material instilled and the subsequent endothelial trauma. Therefore, all INR patients should be anticoagulated with I.V unfractionated Heparin (70 IU/kg) to obtain a 2–3 fold increase in Activated Clotting Time (ACT 250 s) [21].

Antiplatelet agents are being increasingly utilized for anticoagulation in INR procedures. The glycoprotein IIb/IIIa inhibitors like Abciximab are used for management of acute thromboembolic complications during the procedure. Rescue therapy with GpIIb/IIIa inhibitors is associated with significant less morbidity and mortality when compared to thrombolytic agents.

I.V. Aspirin is also used in combination with Heparin and Abciximab to avoid vascular occlusion secondary to thromboembolism, it is used pre-, intra-, and post-procedure at the request of the radiologist [33].

The Thienopyridine derivative, Clopidogrel is added to Aspirin as part of a dual antiplatelet regimen if it is planned to place a device like stent or flow divertor, primarily in patients with unruptured aneurysms. Aspirin 75 mg daily is usually continued for life and Clopidogrel 75 mg daily for 3 months to reduce the incidence of thromboembolic complications. For more details please refer to Chap. 8 (Subarachnoid hemorrhage coiling and intervention).

7.6.2 Pre-Intervention Assessment

Detailed pre-anesthesia assessment as well as understanding underlying neurological pathology are extremely important. Pre-anesthesia assessment should include baseline vital signs (blood pressure, heart rate respiratory rate, temperature, and oxygen saturation at room air) as well as full neurological examination to identify baseline Glasgow Coma Scale (GCS) and to recognize any neurological deficit. All neurological images should be reviewed. Possibility of a difficult airway should be actively sought as additional airway equipment and help may not be immediately available in the intervention suite. If risk of a difficult airway is present, the necessary arrangements must be made.

Careful cardiovascular and respiratory evaluation is mandatory for all SAH patients. Anesthesiologists should assess functional capacity and cardiovascular reserve of these patients. Special consideration should be given to baseline renal parameters to assess the risk of possible contrast induced Nephropathy (CIN). Preoperative anticoagulation therapy must be noted. Allergy history especially to shellfish, iodine, and protamine is important and should be documented and anticipated prior to the intervention [5, 21, 28].

7.6.3 Monitoring

In addition to standard monitoring, invasive arterial line is required for accurate blood pressure monitoring and frequent blood sampling for ACT, electrolytes, and blood gas analysis.

Accurate invasive blood pressure monitoring is essential as significant hemodynamic changes can be encountered during the procedure. Moreover, specific blood pressure targets can be requested by the radiologist depending the clinical situation. It is preferable to place the SPO_2 probe on the toe of the leg which has the femoral artery catheter inserted by the radiologist. This may allow detection of femoral artery obstruction or thromboembolism. At least 2 large bore IV cannulas are required for rapid administration of fluid and medications.

A central venous line is not routinely inserted but can become necessary in acutely ill patients requiring inotropes or vasopressors. Serious complications can arise from extravasations of contrast from central lines, as a result peripheral IV lines are preferred for contrast injection unless the central line is confirmed to be power injectable.

Insertion of un urinary catheter is mandatory due to the significant volume of heparinized flush solution and radiographic contrast that can be used along with the possible administration of Mannitol and Furosemide as discussed before, Temperature monitoring is vital to avoid hypothermia which can occur in the neuroradiology suite due to the cold environment and potentially long procedures [5, 21].

7.6.4 Anesthetic Technique

Although there is limited evidence to support the superiority of any one anesthetic technique over the other for INR cases, practice should follow local hospital guidelines. In general, diagnostic procedures are done under monitored anesthesia care or sedation if the clinical state of the patient permits, while therapeutic procedures like aneurysm coiling and stent/flow divertor insertion are done under general anesthesia [28].

7.6.4.1 Sedation for Only Diagnostic Procedure

For a diagnostic procedure to be successful under sedation, selecting the right patient is paramount. This requires a well informed and cooperative patient. Consequently, patients presenting with confusion, low GCS or high WFNS grades are not candidates for sedation. Propofol infusion or midazolam with intermittent boluses of opioids are the most commonly employed techniques. While dexmedetomidine can be considered as an alternative, it should be avoided or used with caution in hemodynamically unstable patients. The usual complications of sedation like aspiration, hypoventilation, hypoxia, and hypercapnia can have disastrous consequences in aSAH patients. Airway equipment and emergency drugs must be checked and kept ready for all cases. The patient must be helped to obtain a final comfortable position, as this can help the patient tolerate long periods of lying motionless and reduce anesthetic requirements [21, 34].

7.6.4.2 General Anesthesia

General anesthesia with endotracheal intubation is the most commonly employed technique for therapeutic procedures. It provides an immobile patient necessary to obtain the best image, reduce motion artifacts and minimize catheter related complications. Anesthetic management should follow the same principles employed in the care of a patient with intracranial aneurysms. The main disadvantages of general anesthesia are the inability to examine the patient's neurological status during the procedure, hemodynamic changes associated with induction of anesthesia and consequence of endotracheal intubation and extubation like hypertension, coughing, and straining which can lead to raised ICP and re-bleeding. The laryngeal mask airway (LMA) can be considered for airway management as it permits airway control with less hemodynamic stress as well as smooth recovery from anesthesia although airway protection can be a concern in full stomach patients and in patients who develop intraprocedural complications necessitating more invasive procedures or prolonged mechanical ventilation [28].

Propofol, desflurane, and sevoflurane are the most common anesthetic agents used in general anesthesia, which can provide rapid control in depth of anesthesia, and a smooth and rapid emergence.

Nitrous oxide should be avoided, as it may lead to expansion of micro-air emboli which may accidently introduced during injection of contrast and irrigation fluid [28].

Deliberate hypertension can be requested by the neuroradiologist in an attempt to improve collateral circulation during acute arterial occlusion or vasospasm. In a sleep patient where the effect of deliberate hypertension cannot be assessed with an improvement in the patient's neurological status, the blood pressure is usually increased by 20–30% above baseline. The first line agent used for inducing hypertension is phenylephrine. Nor-epinephrine may be considered when phenylephrine is ineffective. ECG changes like ST and T wave changes should be monitored for possible cardiac ischemia. The benefit of deliberate hypertension to improve blood flow should be weighed against the potential risk of intracranial hemorrhage. This requires excellent communication with the interventional radiologist.

7.6.5 Complications of INR Procedures

The complications of INR procedures can be acute and catastrophic, good communication between the neuroradiologist, anesthetist, and the radiographer will facilitate systematic and rapid management of such disasters. The primary role of the anesthesia team is to protect the airway, maintain adequate ventilation, and manipulate hemodynamics according to the clinical situation and institute ICP reducing measures as appropriate. The complications can be divided into CNS- and non-CNS complications. CNS complication can be either hemorrhagic or occlusive, while non-CNS complications include contrast medium reaction, contrast induced nephropathy, hematomas at puncture site [21].

7.6.5.1 Hemorrhagic Complications

Hemorrhagic complications are considered one of the most catastrophic complications that require immediate intervention as well as good communications between anesthesiologist and the interventional radiologist. Primary roles of anesthesiologist are securing airway and maintain adequate cerebral perfusion. Patients may tolerate minor leaks. Nevertheless, in significant bleeding, anesthesiologist should secure the airway, PaCO2 should be maintained between 30 and 35 mmHg. Furthermore, brain edema should be treated with either mannitol or hypertonic saline.

Immediate reversing of heparin with protamine should be considered (1 mg Protamine /100 IU Heparin given in the last 2 h). Antihypertension medications should be reserved for patients with clinical evidence of worsening end-organ deterioration and extremely high blood pressure in order to maintain adequate cerebral perfusion in areas with a loss of autoregulation. It is sensible to retain the blood pressure at the same level before the re-bleeding. Aneurysm perforation can be treated via packing the defect with coils. If the coiling fails, emergency craniotomy should be considered. New SAH may complicated with acute hydrocephalus which requires emergency EVD [21, 32].

7.6.5.2 Occlusive Complications

Vascular occlusion may cause cerebral infarction if not promptly treated. It may be caused by thrombosis, vasospasm, or mal position of equipment like coils, stents, or microcatheters.

Anesthesiologists should raise arterial blood pressure (160–180 mmHg in secured aneurysm, 140–160 in unsecured aneurysm) to increase collateral blood flow. Furthermore, avoiding hyperventilation is extremely important to avoid cerebral vasoconstriction. Angiographically noticeable thrombus is cured via mechanical lysis by the radiologist using a guide wire or local saline infusion [21].

Thrombolytic agents such as tissue plasminogen activators (tPA) may be considered to cure intraoperative thrombosis, however, there is no strong evidence to support routine use of tPA. The recanalization success rate of local intra-arterial tPA was 44% [21, 35]. Intravenous or intra-arterial antiplatelet has shown promising results with less morbidity and mortality than thrombolytic therapy [36]. Intervention radiologist may play a major role in clearing the parent artery by removing Mal-positioned coils. If endovascular trial fails, craniotomy should be considered [5, 21]. Vasospasm treated with maintain high perfusion pressure, good hydration, nimodipine, and balloon angioplasty. For more details, please refer to Chap. 10 (complications and critical care management).

7.6.5.3 Contrast Reactions

Contrast reactions are usually caused by hypertonicity, direct cardiac depression, idiosyncratic anaphylactoid reaction. Prophylactic steroids and antihistamine should be considered for patients who had previous reaction to contrast [5, 37]. The incidence of anaphylactoid reaction is law with nonionic contrast. However, the incidence of lethal reactions was comparable with ionic contrast (1:10.000) [21, 38].

7.6.5.4 Contrast Induced Nephropathy (CIN)

It is defined as an increase of Serum Creatinine by 25% above the baseline by 48 h or an absolute increase of >0.5 mg/dl [39, 40].

This is one of the most common causes of renal failure. The risk factors include diabetes mellitus, high dose of contrast, volume depletion, co-administration of nephrotoxic medications, and preexisting renal disease Table 7.3.

Table 7.3 risk factors of CIN [39]

Modifiable risk factors	Non-modifiable risk factors
Volume of infused contrast.	Diabetes mellitus.
Concomitant administration of nephrotoxic agents.	Chronic kidney disease (CKD).
Recent exposure to contrast.	Shock /refractory hypotension.
	Elderly (>75 years)
	Advanced congestive heart failure.

Pre-Procedural Management for High-Risk Patients

Volume Repletion

a. Adequate hydration with isotonic saline (normal saline) is strongly recommended. Infusion of normal saline (1 L) should be started 3 h before the intervention at rate 100–150 ml/hr. and continued 6–8 h after the procedure [39].

b. Infusion of isotonic Sodium bicarbonate (154 mEq/l) at rate 3 ml/kg/h for 1 h before contrast infusion, then reduced to 1 ml/kg/h for 6 h post the intervention. However, only one study supported using sodium bicarbonate over normal saline and further studies required to support use sodium bicarbonate [41].

Patient Medication

Avoiding potentially nephrotoxic drugs such as non-steroidal anti-inflammatory drugs (NSAID), Aminoglycoside antibiotics.

Intraoperative Management for High-Risk Patients

- Minimize contrast volume, literatures [42]
- Low- or iso-osmolar contrast agents.
- Maintain euvolemia.
- Maintain perfusion pressure [39].

Postoperative Management

- Follow-up for 48 h post intervention.
- Hold nephrotoxic medications till renal function returns to normal.
- Maintain euvolemia [39]

7.6.6 Postoperative Care

All patients should be admitted to a high dependency unit after the procedure, unless there is indication for intensive care admission. Continuous neurological assessment is mandatory to identify any new neurological deficit which can herald the onset of an intracranial complication like vasospasm, cerebral edema, or hydrocephalus.

In order to avoid femoral hematoma, Hip flexion on the side of the femoral catheter should be avoided and patient should be kept at reverse Trendelenburg position for at least 3 h post-catheter removal and direct pressure should be applied on femoral artery for at least 20 min after catheter removal.

In patients with occlusive conditions or vasospasm, high mean arterial pressures are required to maintain cerebral perfusion pressure as well as continued treatment with nimodipine for 3 weeks.

Reevaluation for aneurysm re-growth and development of a new aneurysm are strongly recommended at 6 months post-intervention, then another reassessment at 18 months from initial intervention is suggested [5, 28, 43].

7.7 Conclusion

A neuro-anesthesiologists may play a major role in improvement of the outcome of subarachnoid hemorrhage patients by maintaining overall hemostasis and adequate cerebral perfusion pressure, preventing or limiting the fluctuations in transmural pressure gradient, brain edema, cerebral vasospasm during all phases of anesthesia. Anesthesiologists should be familiar with pathophysiology, management of subarachnoid hemorrhage and its neurological as well as non-neurological complications. Prediction, early recognition, and immediate proper management of the complications are vital to improve the outcome of subarachnoid patients. Endovascular management is a rapidly expanding field, anesthesiologists should be aware of all the challenges of non-operating room anesthesia.

References

1. Kundra S, Mahendru V, Gupta V, Choudhary AK. Principles of neuroanesthesia in aneurysmal subarachnoid hemorrhage. J Anaesthesiol Clin Pharmacol. 2014;30(3):328–37.
2. Passier PE, Visser-Meily JM, van Zandvoort MJ, Post MW, Rinkel GJ, van Heugten C. Prevalence and determinants of cognitive complaints after aneu-

rysmal subarachnoid hemorrhage. Cerebrovasc Dis. 2010;29(6):557–63.
3. de Gans K, Nieuwkamp DJ, Rinkel GJ, Algra A. Timing of aneurysm surgery in subarachnoid hemorrhage: a systematic review of the literature. Neurosurgery. 2002;50(2):336–40. discussion 40-2
4. Stretti F, Gotti M, Pifferi S, Brandi G, Annoni F, Stocchetti N. Body temperature affects cerebral hemodynamics in acutely brain injured patients: an observational transcranial color-coded duplex sonography study. Crit Care. 2014;18(5):552.
5. Priebe HJ. Aneurysmal subarachnoid haemorrhage and the anaesthetist. Br J Anaesth. 2007;99(1):102–18.
6. Matta BF, Lam AM, Mayberg TS, Shapira Y, Winn HR. A critique of the intraoperative use of jugular venous bulb catheters during neurosurgical procedures. Anesth Analg. 1994;79(4):745–50.
7. Al-Shahi R, White PM, Davenport RJ, Lindsay KW. Subarachnoid haemorrhage. BMJ. 2006;333(7561):235–40.
8. Connolly ES Jr, Rabinstein AA, Carhuapoma JR, Derdeyn CP, Dion J, Higashida RT, et al. Guidelines for the management of aneurysmal subarachnoid hemorrhage: a guideline for healthcare professionals from the American Heart Association/american Stroke Association. Stroke. 2012;43(6):1711–37.
9. Matta BF, Mayberg TS, Lam AM. Direct cerebrovasodilatory effects of halothane, isoflurane, and desflurane during propofol-induced isoelectric electroencephalogram in humans. Anesthesiology. 1995;83(5):980–5. discussion 27A
10. Lecours MG. Anesthesia for the surgical treatment of cerebralaneurysms. Anestesiaparael Tratamien to Quirúrgicode Aneurismas Cerebrales. Rev Colomb Anestesiol. 2015;43:45–51.
11. Nicolas Bruder SB, Velly L. In: Ali HPZ, editor. Textbook of Neuroanesthesia and Neurocritical Care. Singapore: Springer; 2019. 15 p.
12. Mutoh T, Kazumata K, Ishikawa T, Terasaka S. Performance of bedside transpulmonary thermodilution monitoring for goal-directed hemodynamic management after subarachnoid hemorrhage. Stroke. 2009;40(7):2368–74.
13. Mutoh T, Kazumata K, Terasaka S, Taki Y, Suzuki A, Ishikawa T. Early intensive versus minimally invasive approach to postoperative hemodynamic management after subarachnoid hemorrhage. Stroke. 2014;45(5):1280–4.
14. Clavier N, Schurando P, Raggueneau JL, Payen DM. Continuous jugular bulb venous oxygen saturation validation and variations during intracranial aneurysm surgery. J Crit Care. 1997;12(3):112–9.
15. Ter Minassian A, Poirier N, Pierrot M, Menei P, Granry JC, Ursino M, et al. Correlation between cerebral oxygen saturation measured by near-infrared spectroscopy and jugular oxygen saturation in patients with severe closed head injury. Anesthesiology. 1999;91(4):985–90.
16. Kamath S, Gadhinglajkar SV. Can changes in BIS provide clue to lower limit of cerebral autoregulation? J Neurosurg Anesthesiol. 2008;20(2):152.
17. Woods AW, Allam S. Tracheal intubation without the use of neuromuscular blocking agents. Br J Anaesth. 2005;94(2):150–8.
18. Petersen KD, Landsfeldt U, Cold GE, Petersen CB, Mau S, Hauerberg J, et al. Intracranial pressure and cerebral hemodynamic in patients with cerebral tumors: a randomized prospective study of patients subjected to craniotomy in propofol-fentanyl, isoflurane-fentanyl, or sevoflurane-fentanyl anesthesia. Anesthesiology. 2003;98(2):329–36.
19. Kovarik WD, Mayberg TS, Lam AM, Mathisen TL, Winn HR. Succinylcholine does not change intracranial pressure, cerebral blood flow velocity, or the electroencephalogram in patients with neurologic injury. Anesth Analg. 1994;78(3):469–73.
20. Matta BF, Heath KJ, Tipping K, Summors AC. Direct cerebral vasodilatory effects of sevoflurane and isoflurane. Anesthesiology. 1999;91(3):677–80.
21. Lin BF, Kuo CY, Wu ZF. Review of aneurysmal subarachnoid hemorrhage--focus on treatment, anesthesia, cerebral vasospasm prophylaxis, and therapy. Acta Anaesthesiol Taiwanica. 2014;52(2):77–84.
22. Randell T, Niemela M, Kytta J, Tanskanen P, Maattanen M, Karatas A, et al. Principles of neuroanesthesia in aneurysmal subarachnoid hemorrhage: the Helsinki experience. Surg Neurol. 2006;66(4):382–8. discussion 8
23. Schettini A, Stahurski B, Young HF. Osmotic and osmotic-loop diuresis in brain surgery. Effects on plasma and CSF electrolytes and ion excretion. J Neurosurg. 1982;56(5):679–84.
24. Nguyen HP, Zaroff JG, Bayman EO, Gelb AW, Todd MM, Hindman BJ, et al. Perioperative hypothermia (33 degrees C) does not increase the occurrence of cardiovascular events in patients undergoing cerebral aneurysm surgery: findings from the intraoperative hypothermia for aneurysm surgery trial. Anesthesiology. 2010;113(2):327–42.
25. Daniel C. Subarachnoid Haemorrage Disease and the Anaesthetist. S Afr J Anaesthesiol Analg. 2010;16(1):60–8.
26. Al-Mousa A, Bose G, Hunt K, Toma AK. Adenosine-assisted neurovascular surgery: initial case series and review of literature. Neurosurg Rev. 2019;42(1):15–22.
27. Collen JF, Jackson JL, Shorr AF, Moores LK. Prevention of venous thromboembolism in neurosurgery: a metaanalysis. Chest. 2008;134(2):237–49.
28. Varma MK, Price K, Jayakrishnan V, Manickam B, Kessell G. Anaesthetic considerations for interventional neuroradiology. Br J Anaesth. 2007;99(1):75–85.
29. Young WL, Pile-Spellman J. Anesthetic considerations for interventional neuroradiology. Anesthesiology. 1994;80(2):427–56.
30. Campbell K, Torres L, Stayer S. Anesthesia and sedation outside the operating room. Anesthesiol Clin. 2014;32(1):25–43.
31. Anastasian ZH, Strozyk D, Meyers PM, Wang S, Berman MF. Radiation exposure of the anesthesiolo-

gist in the neurointerventional suite. Anesthesiology. 2011;114(3):512–20.
32. Lakhani S, Guha A, Nahser HC. Anaesthesia for endovascular management of cerebral aneurysms. Eur J Anaesthesiol. 2006;23(11):902–13.
33. Brinjikji W, McDonald JS, Kallmes DF, Cloft HJ. Rescue treatment of thromboembolic complications during endovascular treatment of cerebral aneurysms. Stroke. 2013;44(5):1343–7.
34. Arain SR, Ebert TJ. The efficacy, side effects, and recovery characteristics of dexmedetomidine versus propofol when used for intraoperative sedation. Anesth Analg. 2002;95(2):461–6. table of contents
35. Hahnel S, Schellinger PD, Gutschalk A, Geletneky K, Hartmann M, Knauth M, et al. Local intra-arterial fibrinolysis of thromboemboli occurring during neuroendovascular procedures with recombinant tissue plasminogen activator. Stroke. 2003;34(7):1723–8.
36. Schulenburg E, Matta B. Anaesthesia for interventional neuroradiology. Curr Opin Anaesthesiol. 2011;24(4):426–32.
37. Goldberg M. Systemic reactions to intravascular contrast media. A guide for the anesthesiologist. Anesthesiology. 1984;60(1):46–56.
38. Steinberg EP, Moore RD, Powe NR, Gopalan R, Davidoff AJ, Litt M, et al. Safety and cost effectiveness of high-osmolality as compared with low-osmolality contrast material in patients undergoing cardiac angiography. N Engl J Med. 1992;326(7):425–30.
39. Schweiger MJ, Chambers CE, Davidson CJ, Blankenship J, Bhalla NP, Block PC, et al. Prevention of contrast induced nephropathy: recommendations for the high risk patient undergoing cardiovascular procedures. Catheter Cardiovasc Interv. 2007;69(1):135–40.
40. Thomsen HS, Morcos SK. Contrast media and the kidney: European Society of Urogenital Radiology (ESUR) guidelines. Br J Radiol. 2003;76(908):513–8.
41. Merten GJ, Burgess WP, Rittase RA, Kennedy TP. Prevention of contrast-induced nephropathy with sodium bicarbonate: an evidence-based protocol. Crit Pathw Cardiol. 2004;3(3):138–43.
42. Mehran R, Aymong ED, Nikolsky E, Lasic Z, Iakovou I, Fahy M, et al. A simple risk score for prediction of contrast-induced nephropathy after percutaneous coronary intervention: development and initial validation. J Am Coll Cardiol. 2004;44(7):1393–9.
43. Meyers PM, Schumacher HC, Higashida RT, Derdeyn CP, Nesbit GM, Sacks D, et al. Reporting standards for endovascular repair of saccular intracranial cerebral aneurysms. AJNR Am J Neuroradiol. 2010;31(1):E12–24.

Subarachnoid Hemorrhage Coiling and Intervention

8

Ahamed Lafir Aliyar
and Ayman Zakaria Ahmed Mohamed

8.1 Introduction

Interventional neuroradiology is an integral part of any neuroscience service and helps in the progresses of understanding vascular diseases in the central nervous system (CNS) [1]. Aneurysmal subarachnoid hemorrhage (SAH) remains a devastating and often fatal condition. In patients who survive the initial ictus, the aneurysm is targeted for obliteration to prevent re-bleeding and its consequent complications. Endovascular treatment by coiling has emerged as a less invasive alternative to conventional surgical clipping of the aneurysm [2]. The first endovascular attempt to treat a cerebral aneurysm was attempted by Luessenhop and Velasquez in 1964 where a silicon balloon was used to occlude the aneurysm [3]. Endovascular coiling, as we know now was pioneered by Guglielmi et al. 1991, using what was called the Guglielmi detachable coils (GDC coils) [4]. Now, this has been replaced with newer and more advanced coils from different manufacturers.

The initial results of the International Subarachnoid Aneurysm Trial (ISAT) of neurosurgical clipping versus simple endovascular coiling in 2143 patients with ruptured intracranial aneurysms were originally published in 2002 and was conducted to establish comparative outcomes in a prospective randomized fashion in patients equally suitable for either endovascular coiling or surgical treatment [5]. For such patients, the absolute reduction in death and morbidity was 6.9% and the relative risk reduction was 23% [6]. A complete analysis at 1 year revealed that the absolute and relative risk reductions had increased to 7.4 and 24%, respectively [5]. This trial had a dramatic impact on the management of aneurysmal SAH, resulting in an increase in the proportion of patients treated by endovascular coiling [7].

Interventional Neuroradiology (INR) is a subspecialty of neurology, neurosurgery, and radiology where minimally invasive imaging based techniques are utilized for the treatment of diseases of the central nervous system. Conditions in the past that would have required major surgical intervention can now be treated using a minimally invasive endovascular approach.

Endovascular surgical neuroradiology, neurointerventional surgery, interventional neuroradi-

A. L. Aliyar (✉)
Department of Anesthesiology, ICU and Perioperative Medicine, Hamad Medical Corporation, Doha, Qatar
e-mail: aaliyar1@hamad.qa

A. Z. A. Mohamed
Radiology, Cairo University Hospitals, Interventional Neuro-Radiology (INR), Neuro-Radiology Department, Doha, Qatar

A. E. A. Ganaw et al. (eds.), *Management of Subarachnoid Hemorrhage*,
https://doi.org/10.1007/978-3-030-81333-8_8

ology and endovascular neurosurgery are different names given to the same service practiced by physicians having different medical backgrounds. In Europe it is mostly performed by interventional neuro-radiologists, in North and South America it is shared mainly by neurosurgeons and neuro-radiologists, while in Japan most procedures are performed by neurosurgeons. This multidisciplinary aspect of the filed has resulted in tremendous vitality and richness in terms of evidence and techniques.

Currently endovascular treatment is recommended for the following:

1. All aneurysms associated with subarachnoid hemorrhage (especially the posterior circulation and cavernous carotid aneurysms) as it is less invasive and associated with a shorter stay in ICU/hospital and quicker patient recovery.
2. Non-ruptured aneurysms associated with increased bleeding risks (e.g. large irregular size, comorbidities) justifying their treatment.
3. High risk patients with multiple co-morbidities. (old age, bad neurological status) [8].

The main disadvantage of aneurysm coiling is that it has a high rate of recurrence reaching 6% in large aneurysms (10 mm up to 25 mm in size) and 30% in giant aneurysms (more than 25 mm in size). A majority of these recurrences needs a complementary treatment [9]. Moreover, the cost of endovascular treatment is higher, when compared to surgical clipping.

This chapter aims to provide the reader with a basic overview of the concepts of endovascular treatment, procedures, possible complications, and outcome in the endovascular management of ruptured cerebral aneurysms.

8.2 Concept of Treatment

A cerebral aneurysms requires two factors to develop; first a defective vessel wall whether congenital (collagen diseases), degenerative (atherosclerotic), infective (mycotic) or traumatic (dissection). This weak wall when exposed to the second factor of continuous sheer stress of blood flow starts to yield and dilate secondary to the vortices and eddy currents developing inside until it ruptures resulting in subarachnoid hemorrhage (Fig. 8.1).

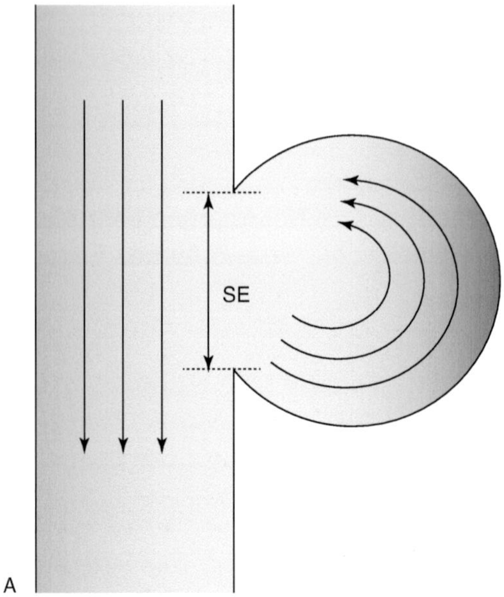

Fig. 8.1 A drawing showing the two etiological factors developing cerebral aneurysms; Point of wall weakness and the sheer stress on walls by the blodd flow. SE: sac entrance. Yongxue Zhang et al. Total Endevascular Repair of Thoracoabdominal Aortic Aneurysms With Non-Customized Stent Grafts. Ann Thorac Surg; 2014; 98:1606–12

The shape of the aneurysm is determined by the surrounding subarachnoid septations and spaces, we can always define a fundus, sac, and neck for every aneurysm. The largest diameter (dome) defines the size of the aneurysm (Small <10 mm, large 10–25 mm and Giant >25 mm) while the neck is considered small if <4 mm and wide if >4 mm or greater than 50% of the dome [10] (Fig. 8.2).

There are two approaches to the endovascular treatment of cerebral aneuryrsms—either to exclude the aneurysm from the circulation by filling the fundus, sac, and neck with thrombogenic material (e.g. coils or liquid embolic material) while preserving the patency of the parent artery or by diverting the blood flow away from the aneurysm by placing a flow diverter in the parent artery (endo-luminal diversion) or disrupting the flow inside the aneurysmal sac by placing a small device inside (Intra-saccular diversion). In both types of diversion, gradual and spontaneous thrombosis of the aneurysm occurs.

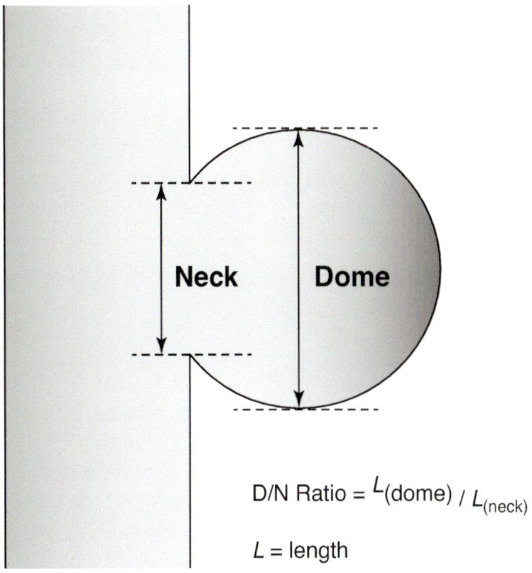

Fig. 8.2 The dome (maximum dimension)/neck relation in any aneursym weather smaller or larger than two should determine the strategy of endo-vascular treatment. Yongxue Zhang et al. Total Endovascular Repari of Thoracoabdominal Aortic Aneurysms With Non-Customized Stent Grafts. Ann Thorac Surg; 2014; 98:1606–12

8.3 Equipment and Materials

8.3.1 The Angio Suite

Angiography is the process of visualizing a blood vessel's lumen and blood flow characteristics using digital subtraction technique after injecting a contrast dye. Most modern angiography suites have a biplane machine, which utilizes two X-Ray tubes capable of simultaneously acquiring two image planes. The arms of the biplane have the ability to move over a wide area, warranting careful patient positioning and organization of patient monitors, lines, wires, tubing, etc. to avoid any injury, disconnection or mishap. The new generation of angio suites are equipped with softwares that make detection and visualization of vascular anomalies much easier, thereby assisting the physician in obtaining the best views and to develop the best strategy to manage the lesion (Fig. 8.3).

Fig. 8.3 Modern angio suite with a biplane machine and a complete setup for general anestheisa

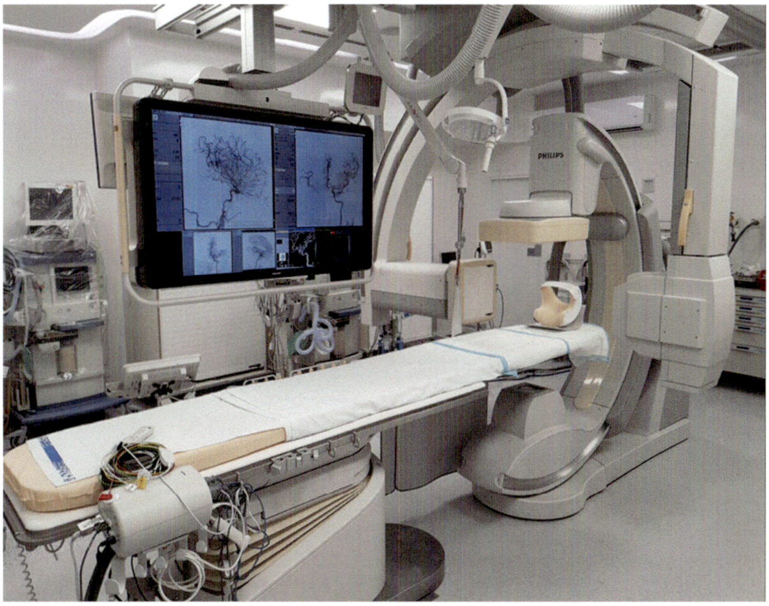

8.3.2 Introducers (Sheaths)

A sheath is a small tube that is inserted through the skin and subcutaneous tissue to acquire vascular access. Commonly used sizes are 4Fr up to 9Fr that can vary in length from 3 cm to 90 cm. The arterial access can be from the femoral artery, radial artery or less commonly the carotid artery in the neck.

8.3.3 Catheters

Vascular catheters are categorized as either diagnostic or guiding catheters. Both diagnostic and guide catheters have different head shapes to choose from. Diagnostic catheters commonly used range from 4Fr to 6Fr in adults and are used for diagnostic angiogram. Guiding catheters range from 6Fr to 8Fr in adults with a stainless steel braided core that gives the extra stiffness necessary for passing other equipment like micro catheters and guide wires inside. Guiding catheters can only be passed as high up as cervical carotids but they are too stiff to be safely placed intracranially. All diagnostic and guiding catheters are advanced inside the vessels over guide wires. The most commonly used guide wire is the 0.035 inch hydrophilic wires (Fig. 8.4).

8.3.4 Microcatheters

Microcatheters are small catheters usually less than 3Fr that can be navigated into intracranial vessels. They require the use of micro wires inside them to steer and guide their way into the cerebral vessels.

8.3.5 Micro-Guide Wires

Micro-guide wires are used to guide microcatheters, stents, and balloons to target intracranial vessels. It is smaller than regular guide wires with a diameter of 0.014 inch having pre-shaped or shapeable distal ends.

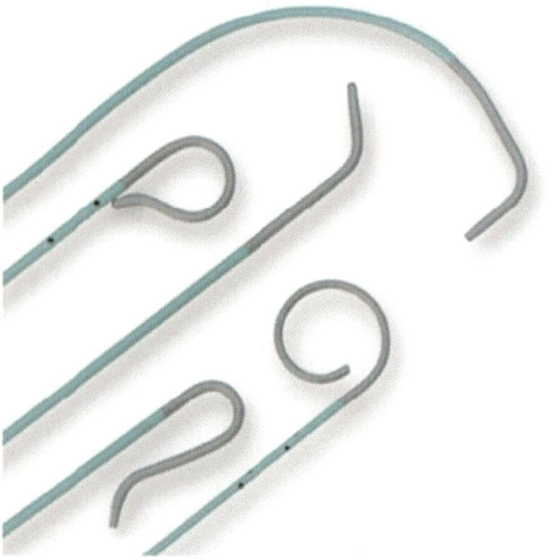

Fig. 8.4 Different types of diagnostic catheters for cerebral angiogram. Boston Scientific. "Imager™ II." *Imager™ II Angiographic Catherer—Baston Scientific*, www.bostonscientific.com/en-US/products/catheters%2D%2Ddiagnostic/imager-ii-angiographic-catheter.html

8.3.6 Torque Device

Torque devices are used at the operator end to effectively translate torque from the user end to the tip of the wire in the patient.

8.3.7 Balloons

Endovascular balloons are of two types–compliant and non-compliant. Compliant balloons are low pressure balloons that when inflated take the shape of the vessel in which they are inflated making them useful for temporary vessel occlusion or balloon assisted aneurysm coiling. On the other hand, non-compliant balloons are stiff and expand to a particular shape and size at a given pressure, making them best suited for angioplasty.

8.3.8 Stents

Stents are intravascular structures that can either have an open cell, closed cell or braided construction. The cells of a closed cell stent are

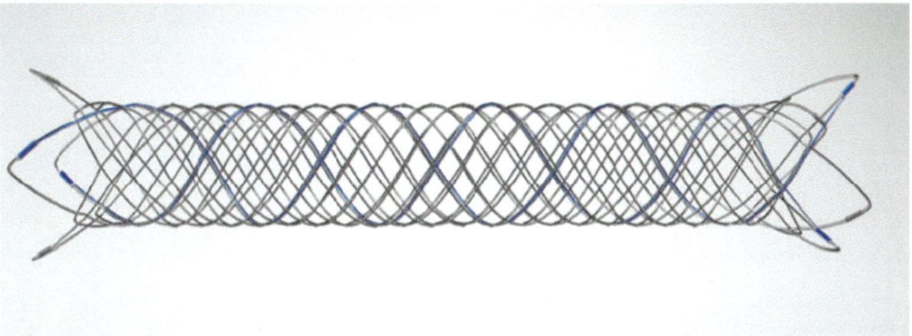

Fig. 8.5 ELVIS stent (Microvention) having have a woven or interlaced metal fiber microarchitecture. Microventin. "MicroVention." *Microvention*. www.mircoventin.com/emea/product/lvis-family

completely surrounded by struts, whereas the cells of an open cell stent are only partially surrounded by struts. Consequently, closed cell stents are stiffer and have a lower incidence of embolic complication. However, the open cell stents are better suited for stent assisted aneurysm coiling. Flexibility and scaffolding are key characteristics derived from stent designs Braided stents on the other hand have a woven or interlaced metal fiber microarchitecture, which usually forms the basis of flow diverter stents. The stents can be broadly classified as balloon mounted or self-expanding stents. Balloon mounted stents are loaded on to a non-compliant balloon which when inflated, simultaneously expands, and deploys the stent. The self-expanding stents are made from a metal alloy (Nitinol) with a shape memory. They are preloaded on a delivery catheter and are deployed by pulling back the delivery catheter and holding the stent in place with a pusher device (Fig. 8.5).

8.3.9 Flow Diverting Stents

Flow diverters are special types of stents which are woven tightly, having sub- millimeter spaces between its metal elements (struts) and acts more like a tube than a regular stent passing 90% of the inlet flow through the outlet opening with only 10% escaping through the side walls. Flow diverters are placed across the neck of the aneurysm in the parent vessel with the aim of diverting blood flow away from the aneurysmal sac and greatly reducing chances of aneurysm rupture and allowing the aneurysm to undergo spontaneous thrombosis. All types of stents require the patient to be pre-medicated with an antiplatelet regimen that continues up to 1 year after stent placement. This regimen will be further discussed later (Fig. 8.6).

8.3.10 Coils

Cerebral aneurysm coils are generally thin platinum wires which come in various sizes and shapes and sometimes with certain bioactive materials incorporated into them to enhance thrombosis. These coils are wound in a tight helix called the primary wind. These can then be coiled into another helix or predetermined 3D structure. Although a detailed review of the different types of coils is beyond the scope of this book, the following are a few types of coils.

8.3.10.1 Helical Coils

GDC was the first helical coil that was FDA approved for treating intracranial aneurysms. The coil is made of platinum attached to a stainless steel pusher. Once the coils are placed in position, they can be detached from the stainless steel pusher electrolytically. They are no longer used and replaced by other brands from different companies.

8.3.10.2 3D Coils/360 Coils

Framing coils or primary coils–these coils attain complex 3D structures once deployed, which can be then used as a frame to insert other coils within it to enhance aneurysm packing (Fig. 8.7).

8.3.10.3 Hydrogel Coils

These coils are incorporated with hydrogel which is a highly absorbent polymer which expands

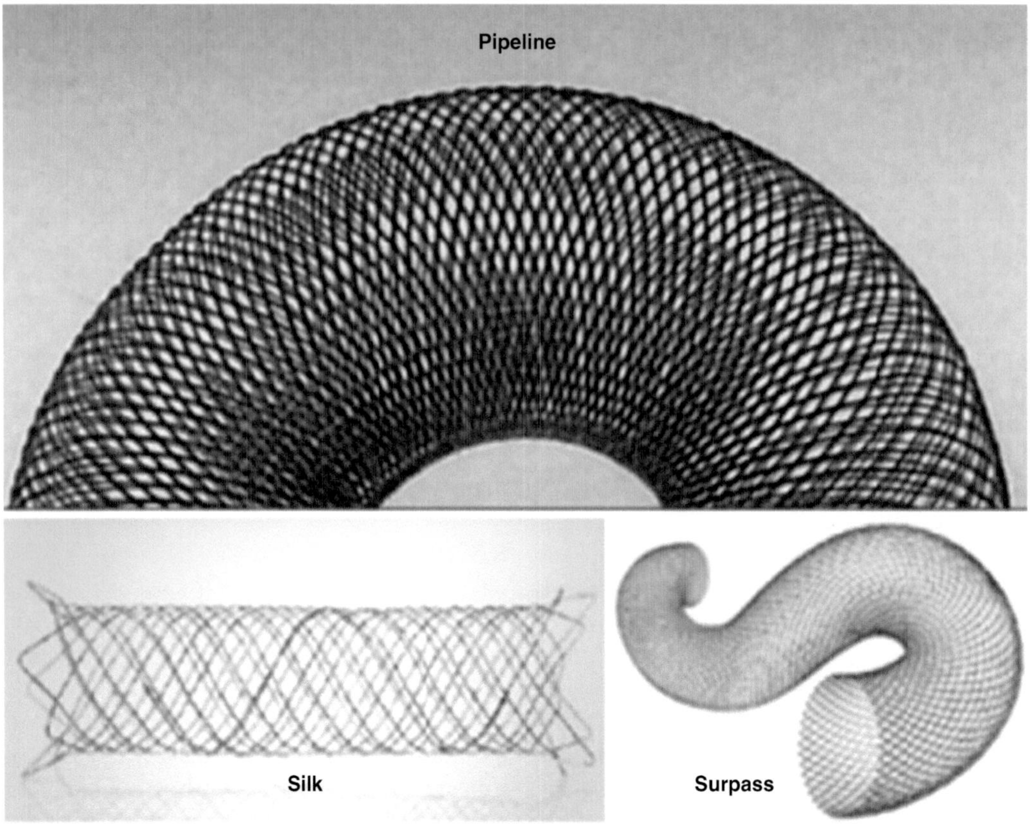

Fig. 8.6 Different brands of endo-luminal flow diverters for the treatment of wide neck aneurysms. Ghobani. Mohammad, et al. "Flow diverter Embolization Device for Endovascular Treatment of Rupured Blister and Wide Necked Very Small Aneurysms." *Heliyon*, vol. 5, no. 9, 2019, https://doi.org/10.1016/j.heliyon.2019.e02241

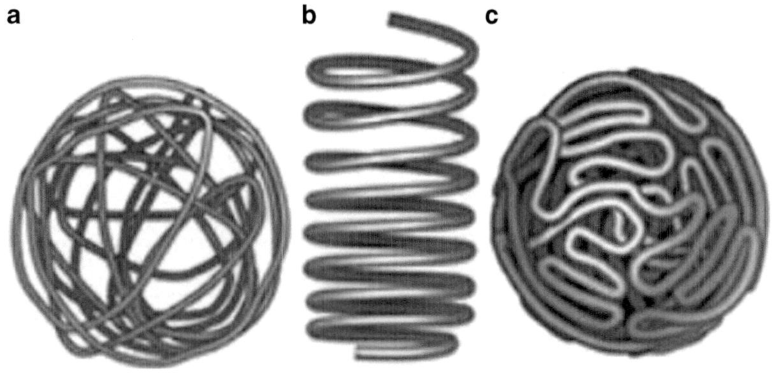

Fig. 8.7 Demonstrating the difference between (**a**) complex 3-D coils, (**b**) Helicals coils and (**c**) large volume coils. *Themes, UFO. "Intracranial Aneurysms." Radiology Key, 3 Dec. 2016, radiologykey.com/intracranial-aneurysms/*

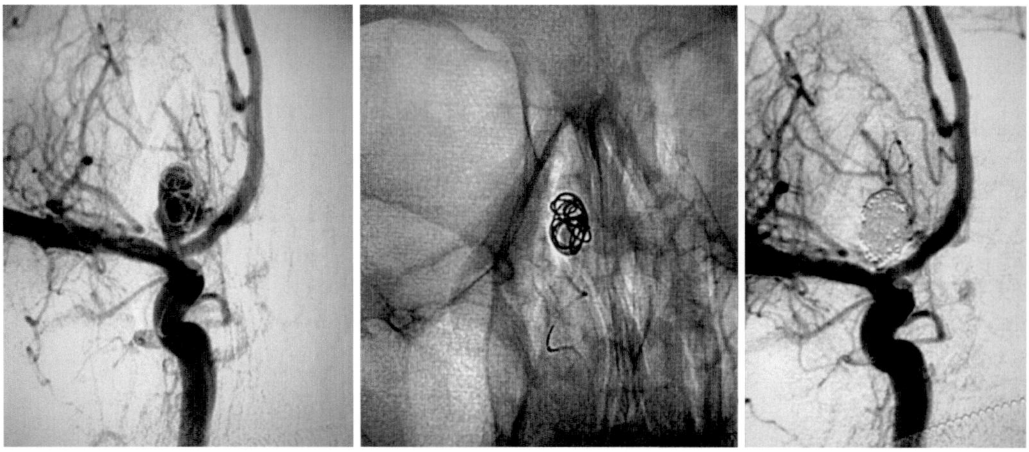

Fig. 8.8 Simple coiling of ruptured right internal carotid tip aneurysm. *Courtesy by Dr. Ayman Z. Ahmed*

when it come into contact with fluids like blood. This improves aneurysm packing and also supports thrombosis (Fig. 8.8).

8.3.11 Intra-Saccular Diversion Devices

The intra-saccular aneurysm embolization system is a permanent Nitinol (nickel titanium) self-expanding mesh ball implant. The implant is placed into the sac of the intracranial aneurysm and designed to disrupt blood flow entering the aneurysm and help promote thrombosis. It is provided in several sizes and models to cater to the size of different aneurysms and unlike regular flow diverters or stent do not require antiplatelet premedication, which favors them in the acute treatment of ruptured cerebral aneurysms.

8.4 Procedures and Techniques

8.4.1 Anesthesia

General anesthesia (GA) is usually preferred to achieve complete immobilization of the patient to avoid intracerebral trauma that can occur if the patient moves while instrumentation is being attempted. Moreover, a vascular road-mapping technique is used to guide coil delivery during the procedure, this becomes inaccurate due to motion artifacts if the patient moves after a road-map has been created. GA would also allow better hemodynamic and ventilatory control of patients during the procedure. This becomes more important in patients with a ruptured aneurysm and subarachnoid hemorrhage. While GA is the preferred anesthetic technique, care should be taken to avoid the hemodynamic disturbances that commonly occur during induction and intubation.

8.4.2 Access

Classically these procedures have been performed through the femoral arterial approach due to their large caliber, rich lower limb collaterals, easy access, and distance from the angio machine. The femoral artery is the distal extension of the external iliac artery as it travels deep to the inguinal ligament. It is bound by the femoral vein medially and the femoral nerve laterally. Distally, it bifurcates into the superficial and deep femoral arteries.

The radial arterial or direct carotid approach can be used in patients who have atherosclerotic femoral arteries, local infection or lesions of the iliac artery or aorta.

8.4.3 Simple Coiling

Simple coiling is suitable for all intracranial aneurysms with sac-to-neck ratios >2.0 [11]. The greater this ratio, the easier it becomes for coil deposition and coil stability within the lesion. Simple coiling refers to trans-arterial advancement of a micro catheter into the aneurysmal sac with the help of micro-guide wire followed by the delivery of detachable coils to achieve dense packing and induce blood clot formation within the aneurysmal sac, hence isolating it from active circulation [12]. Tight coil packing with density of at least 20–25% is known to be important for preventing recanalization after embolization of cerebral aneurysms. However, the most important risk factor for recanalization is residual volume and not packing density. The larger the aneurysm volume, the greater the packing density has to be to minimize the residual volume and risk of recanalization [13].

Large series confirmed the feasibility of aneurysm coiling (96.9% in ruptured aneurysms and 94.0% in non-ruptured aneurysms), with acceptable procedural mortality (1.4% in ruptured aneurysms and 1.7% in non-ruptured aneurysms), and morbidity rates (8.6% in ruptured aneurysms and 7.7% in non-ruptured aneurysms) [14, 15] (Fig. 8.12).

8.4.4 Treatment of Wide Neck Aneurysms

An aneurysm is considered to have a wide neck if the diameter of the neck is greater than 4 mm or a fundus: neck diameter ratio of two or less. The smaller the ratio the greater the chances of a coil herniating back into the parent vessel lumen. Despite the advances in coils and techniques, endovascular coiling of wide necked aneurysms remains a challenge due to reasons like coil herniation, coil compaction, low volumetric filling, and recanalization. The following are techniques used to overcome this problem (Fig. 8.2).

8.4.4.1 Balloon Assisted Coiling (BAC)

In this technique both a microcatheter and a silicon balloon are simultaneously used either through a single large guide catheter or two guide catheters. This silicon balloon is advanced up to the level of the aneurysm neck followed by introduction of the microcatheter into the aneurysm. This is followed by slowly deploying the coil into the aneurysm. If the coil has a tendency to herniate out, the balloon is gently inflated to hold the coil within the aneurysm. After the coil is completely introduced in the aneurysm, the balloon is deflated and the coil observed to ensure that it is stable before detachment. This process can be repeated with multiple coils until adequate filling of the aneurysm is achieved. Although the balloon modeling technique has allowed us to coil wide neck aneurysms, it does not come without complications. Balloon inflation against an unsecured aneurysm can cause neck deformation or aneurysm rupture. At the same time inflation in smaller vessels can cause vessel rupture or thrombosis. In non-ruptured aneurysms, the rate of thromboembolic events was not higher in the BAC group as compared with coiling alone (5.4% versus 6.2%) with a similar clinical outcome in both groups. In ruptured aneurysms, the rate of thromboembolic events was also similar in both groups (12.7% in the coiling group and 11.3% in the BAC group). The treatment morbidity was 3.9% in the coiling group and 2.5% in the BAC group, and treatment mortality 1.2% in the coiling group and 1.3% in the BAC group [16, 17] (Fig. 8.9).

8.4.4.2 Stent Assisted Coiling (SAC)

This technique is similar to that of BAC except here a stent with an open cell construction is first placed to cover the aneurysm neck followed by introduction of a microcatheter into the aneurysm through one of the stent cells. The coil is then deployed into the aneurysm while the stent acts as a scaffold holding the coils within the aneurysm. In patients with un ruptured aneurysms, the stent can be left in place along with the coils, provides the patients are premedicated with

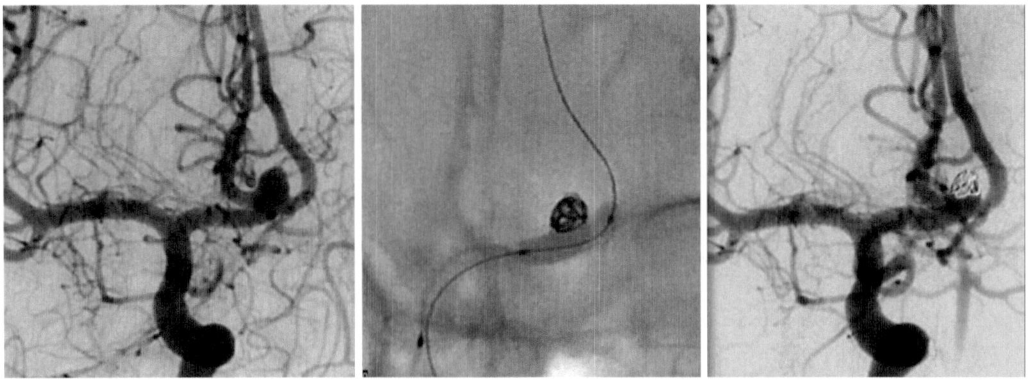

Fig. 8.9 Balloon assisted coiling (BAC) of ruptured anterior communicating artery aneurysm. *Courtersy by Dr. Ayman Z. Ahmed*

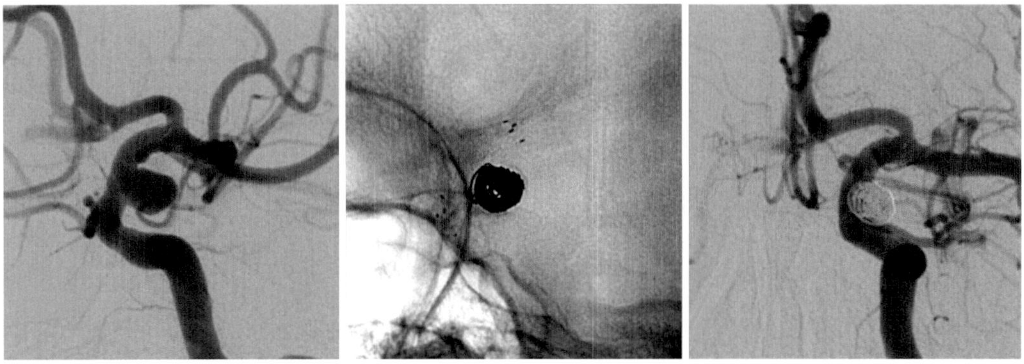

Fig. 8.10 Stent assisted coiling (SAC) of wide neck non-ruptured Left cavernous aneurysm. *Courtesy by Dr. Ayman Z. Ahmed*

antiplatelet agents. In ruptured aneurysms, where antiplatelet agents cannot be used as a primary option, the stent can be retrieved again through the deployment microcatheter and removed after successful coil placement. In a multicenter registry, a total of 107 patients with 107 aneurysms were enrolled that were treated with SAC. The complete occlusion rate after the procedure was 66.4%. An additional 14% of the treated aneurysms showed a progressive occlusion at 12–18 months follow-up; aneurysm recurrence rate was 9.7%. Subsequently, 4% of the aneurysms were retreated. The peri-procedural thromboembolic rate was 3.7%; delayed thromboembolic events were observed in 3%. The overall mortality rate at 12–18 months was 1%, and the permanent morbidity rate was 1% [18] (Fig. 8.10).

8.4.4.3 Three-Dimensional Coils (3D Coils)

These 3D coils assume a complex shape once they exit the microcatheter and enter the aneurysm. The idea is that these 3D coils cover the aneurysm neck and prevent subsequently deployed coils (3D or regular) from herniating out of the aneurysm (Fig. 8.11).

8.4.4.4 Simultaneous Coil Deposition

In this technique two coils are deployed into the aneurysm simultaneously (by two micro-catheters) with the goal of achieving a complex shape that covers the aneurysm neck and at the same time the intermingling of the two coils prevent each other from herniating out.

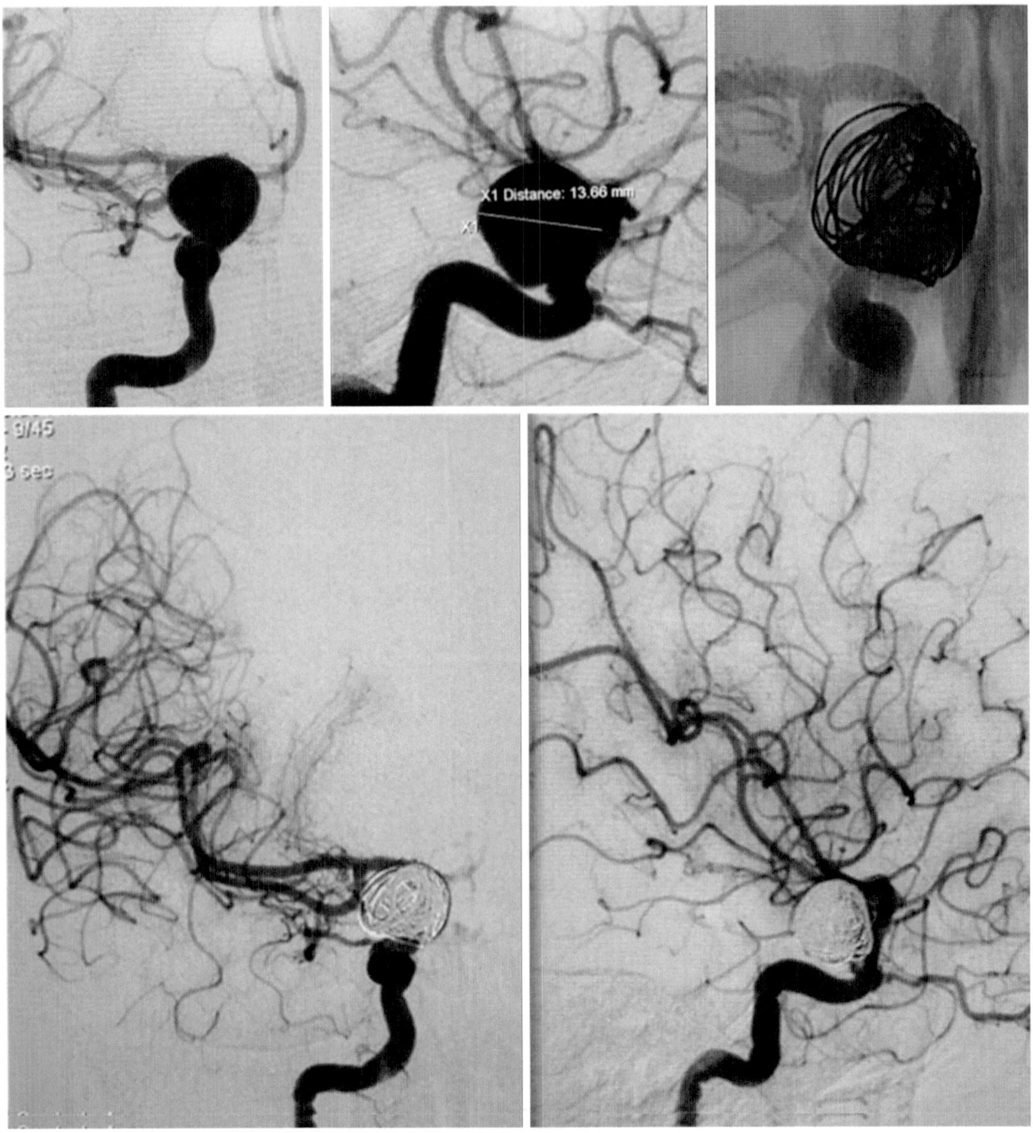

Fig. 8.11 Large 3D coils for endovascular treatment of wide neck aneurysms. *Courtesy by Dr. Ayman Z. Ahmed*

8.4.4.5 Liquid Embolic Agents

Liquid embolic agents (e.g. Onyx Medtronic-USA) could be directly injected into the aneurysm through a microcatheter while having a balloon deployed against the aneurysm neck to prevent its leakage into the parent vessel. These liquid embolic agents solidify immediately on contact with blood. Theoretically these agents can completely fill the aneurysm thus reducing the incidence of aneurysm recurrence.

8.4.4.6 Partial Embolization

Although a controversial topic, incomplete aneurysm embolization could be the only feasible option in certain situations like ruptured large aneurysms with a large neck or ruptured aneurysms at the bifurcation of the middle cerebral artery owing to the complex relationship of the fundus or neck of the aneurysm to afferent or efferent vessels. The idea is that partial embolization will provide some security against a second bleed and allows

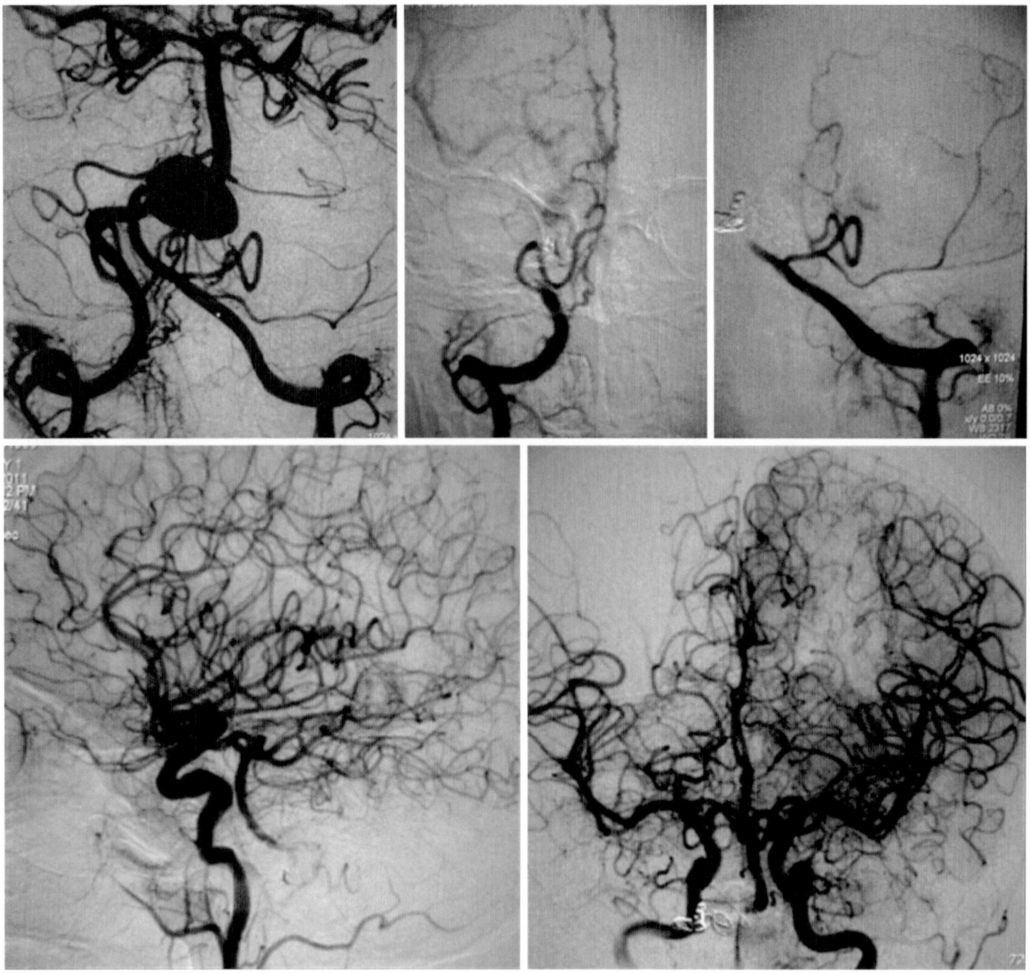

Fig. 8.12 Parent artery occlusion (PAO) of both distal vertebral arteries to treat non-ruptured large vertebra-aneurysm. Patent circle of Wills filling the basilar artery in a retrograde pattern

the patient to recover out of the ictus phase thus providing further options to deliver a definitive treatment (e.g. using stents or flow diverters with antiplatelet coverage).

8.4.4.7 Deconstructive Treatment

If a particular aneurysm is dissecting in nature or has a wide neck involving the parent artery not amenable to any of the above techniques and the patient has good collateral circulation (around the circle of Willis or between anterior and posterior circulation of the brain), the option of parent artery occlusion together with the aneurysm can be considered to provide a definitive treatment and prevent recurrence (Fig. 8.12).

8.4.5 Flow Diverters

Flow diverters are a new generation of stents and devices for aneurysm treatment. These stents require premedication with antiplatelet agents. The flow diverter is placed in the parent artery (intraluminal flow diversion) at the level of the aneurysm neck diverting blood flow away from the aneurysm leading to gradual aneurysm thrombosis. In intra-saccular flow disruption, mesh of the flow disruptor is placed inside the aneurysmal sac to create blood flow stasis with subsequent thrombosis. Intra-saccular devices do not require antiplatelet premedication [19].

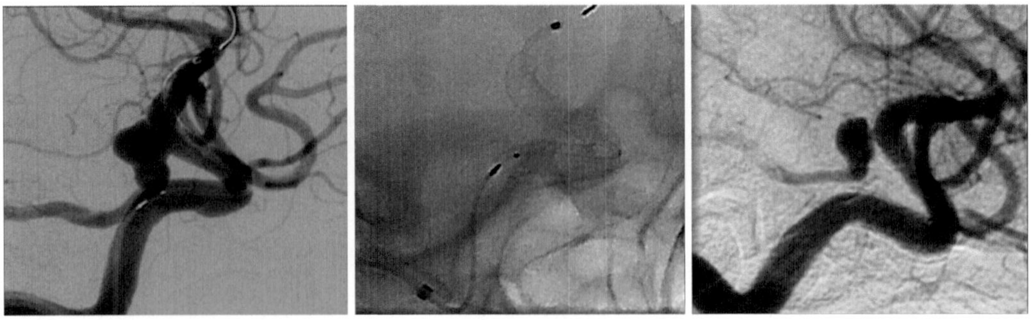

Fig. 8.13 Flow diverter treatment of non-ruptured right posterior communicating artery aneurysm. *Courtesy by Dr. Ayman Z. Ahmed*

Treatment with flow diverters is a feasible and effective technique for ruptured and non-ruptured aneurysms with complex anatomy (Giant, fusiform, dissecting, large neck, bifurcation with side branches) where coiling and clipping are difficult or impossible [20]. A satisfactory occlusion was achieved in almost 80% of cases after flow diverter treatment with a permanent-related serious event and mortality rates of 5.9% and 1.2% at 12 months, respectively [21] (Fig. 8.13).

8.4.6 Antiplatelets

If intracranial stenting or flow diversion is considered for the treatment of non-ruptured aneurysms, premedication with antiplatelets is mandatory. Aspirin, at a low-dose of 100 mg or high-dose of 300 mg daily in combination with Clopidogrel, at a dose of 75 mg daily is prescribed for 5 days before endovascular treatment [22]. In the case of high-risk aneurysms (large irregularly sized aneurysms or blister aneurysms) that need to be treated immediately, this combination can also be given as a single loading dose of 300 mg Aspirin with 300 mg Clopidogrel just before the procedure [23]. However, it must be noted that the bleeding risk is higher with the single loading dose regimen. Antiplatelets therapy (Aspirin 100 mg with Clopidogrel 75 mg) should be continued for 90 days after endovascular treatment.

About 4–50% of patients on clopidogrel are considered to be non-responders leading to thromboembolic events. Ticagrelor is another antiplatelet agent with low resistance rates that can be used as a single agent or in combination with aspirin. When administered alone, a loading dose of 180 mg followed by a maintenance of 90 mg BID for 90 days proved safe and effective in patients undergoing stent or flow diverter placement [24, 25].

8.5 Complications

The rate of complications with endovascular treatment of aneurysm can vary between 8.4% and 18.9%. Endovascular treatment of ruptured cerebral aneurysms in patients with subarachnoid hemorrhage is associated with a higher incidence of complications as opposed to unruptured aneurysms. More advanced techniques utilizing multiple endovascular devices like balloon or stent assisted coiling have also been reported to have a higher complication rate [8].

8.5.1 Thromboembolism

Thromboembolic complications in patients undergoing endovascular treatment of cerebral aneurysms have been reported to be as high as 5–10% [26–28]. A thrombus in the parent vessel or in a catheter leading to downstream embolization and stroke remains a significant problem. The presence of foreign material in the vasculature like catheters, guidewires, balloons or stents naturally predispose these procedures to thromboembolic complications. Large diameter aneurysms and coil protrusion are independent risk factors for post-procedural thrombosis.

Continuous flushing of catheters can help prevent clots and subsequent clot embolization. Heparin is the most commonly used agent to prevent thromboembolic complications. Heparin is administered at a dose of 70–100 IU/kg after arterial puncture. This is followed by top up doses to maintain an activated clotting time (ACT) of 200–250 (1.5–2 times baseline). Where point of care ACT is not available, heparin 1000 IU can be administered empirically every hour to maintain anticoagulation.

Aneurysm coil protrusion into the parent artery leaves a surface for potential thrombus formation. This can be managed by inflating a balloon in the parent artery to push the protruded coil back into the aneurysm with or without subsequent stent placement to prevent re-herniation. Partial coil protrusion or herniation not causing significant parent artery occlusion can be conservatively managed with antiplatelet medications.

Thromboembolic complications during endovascular management of cerebral aneurysms are cause for major morbidity. The main sources of embolism are presence of friable plaques, clots within the aneurysm or catheters, air bubbles, coils vascular stasis, and iatrogenic dissection of vessels.

Patients with a ruptured aneurysm are in a hypercoagulable state predisposing them to a higher risk of thromboembolic complications [29].

8.5.2 Aneurysm Rupture

Aneurysm rupture during coil deposition has been reported in up to 4–5% of cases [30–32]. This can occur at the aneurysmal sac or neck usually while depositing the first coil. The main risk factors are hypertension, small aneurysms, and middle cerebral artery aneurysms. If a rupture is suspected, attempts should not be made to withdraw the perforating coil as this helps to plug the hole and prevent further bleeding. Communication between the interventionist and the anesthetist is paramount during this period. Heparin should be reversed with protamine at a dose of 1 mg for every 100 IU of heparin administered. Protamine has to be infused through a peripheral line over 10–15 mins. Patients should be closely monitored for possible allergic reactions, hypotension, bronchospasm, and pulmonary hypertension. Rapid coiling of the aneurysm is essential to minimize further bleed. Once satisfactory coiling has been achieved a post-procedure CT head is required to assess the extent of bleed. An external ventricular drain may have to be inserted emergently in patients with significant bleed.

8.5.3 Vascular Injury

The utilization of endovascular devices like catheters, guidewires, stents, balloons, and coils and their intravascular manipulation can predispose the patient to significant vascular injuries like vessel dissection, vessel rupture, formation of Pseudoaneurysm, and retroperitoneal hematoma.

8.5.3.1 Pseudoaneurysm

A Pseudoaneurysm occurs when vessel injury leads to collection of blood within the outer two layers of the vessel wall (Tunica Media and Tunica Adventitia). They usually occur at the primary access site which is usually the femoral artery at the groin. They present as a pulsatile, erythematous, and tender mass. The most common cause being improper closure techniques like inadequate compression or poor post-closure care. Hip flexion should be avoided for at least 6 h post-procedure. If a patient presents with signs suggestive of an enlarging pseudoaneurysm post-angiography, an ultrasound must be requested immediately and referred to the primary interventionist or a vascular surgeon. Small pseudo aneurysms can be managed conservatively with manual compression. Whereas, larger lesions may need further evaluation by vascular surgeons and subsequent open or endovascular treatment.

8.5.3.2 Retroperitoneal Hematoma

A retroperitoneal hematoma or hemorrhage is a potentially life threatening complication of endovascular aneurysm coiling. It is usually the result of a puncture to the posterior wall of the femoral artery during cannulation. Multiple attempts, high insertion point above the inguinal ligament and anticoagulation therapy are potential risk factors to develop retroperitoneal bleeding. Patients can present with very non-specific symptoms like abdominal, back, hip or lower limb pain, and abdominal distension. The retroperitoneum is a potentially large space that can harbor a significant bleed until the patient presents with hemodynamic compromise. Hypotension not responding to fluids and a fall in hematocrit should prompt investigation with a CT abdomen. When diagnosed they need urgent treatment along with close patient monitoring and resuscitation.

8.5.3.3 Dissection or Rupture

Improper handling of endovascular devices can lead to vessel injury causing dissection or rupture which can become quickly life threatening if not immediately diagnosed and promptly treated. Retrograde dissections usually need no further intervention. However, anterograde dissections require emergency stenting and antiplatelet loading.

In the rare event, should a vessel rupture occur, heparin should be reversed immediately. A trial of intermittent balloon inflation at 3 min intervals may be attempted to arrest bleeding. If this fails, urgent vascular surgery referral must be sort and complete arterial occlusion may become necessary.

8.5.4 Vasospasm

Vasospasm is a common reversible complication that may occur 5–10 days after SAH. By-products of blood breakdown cause the walls of an artery to contract and spasm. Vasospasm narrows the inside diameter (lumen) of the artery and thereby reduces blood flow to that region of the brain, causing a secondary stroke. It is an indicator of poor outcome and a leading cause of morbidity and mortality in subarachnoid hemorrhage patients. Vasospasm most commonly occurs in the proximal vessels of the anterior and middle cerebral vessels, while less likely in the posterior circulation. Consequently, subarachnoid hemorrhage is best cared for in tertiary care centers with access to cerebral angiography. A high degree of suspicion for vasospasm is essential during ICU care, and any signs or symptoms suggestive of such must be investigated and treated immediately to avoid permanent stroke and neurologic deficit [33]. The primary aim is to restore adequate blood flow and prevent cerebral ischemia.

8.5.4.1 Diagnosis of Vasospasm

The gold standard radiographic test for diagnosis is cerebral angiography. However, this is an invasive test and it is not practical for daily surveillance in all cases. Up to 70% of patients with aneurysmal SAH show constriction of the cerebral arteries on angiography starting from day 3, but only about 50% of these patients have a neurologic deficit attributable to this and 20% of them will go on to develop infarction [34]. Trans-cranial Doppler (TCD) has been shown to be reliable in the MCA with sensitivity of 67%. The American Academy of Neurology conducted a systematic review of the literature and concluded that TCDs can be used reliably to screen for the presence of vasospasm in the MCA, but not other vessels [35, 36]. CT angiography has also been used in some centers for the detection of cerebral vasospasm. Several studies showed good correlation between CT angiogram (CTA) and digital subtraction angiography (DSA) in predicting vasospasm and that many unnecessary angiograms could be avoided by using CTA as a screening test [37] A meta-analysis found a sensitivity and specificity for CTA of 80 and 93%, respectively [38]. The only medical strategies for prevention of vasospasm with enough evidence to be included in the guidelines for SAH patients were maintenance of normal circulating blood volume, and Nimodipine. Hopefully this will change in the future as further randomized trials are conducted using newer preventive therapies [33].

8.5.4.2 Endovascular Management of Vasospasm

In the larger cerebral vessels (ICA, M1, and basilar), balloon angioplasty has been shown to

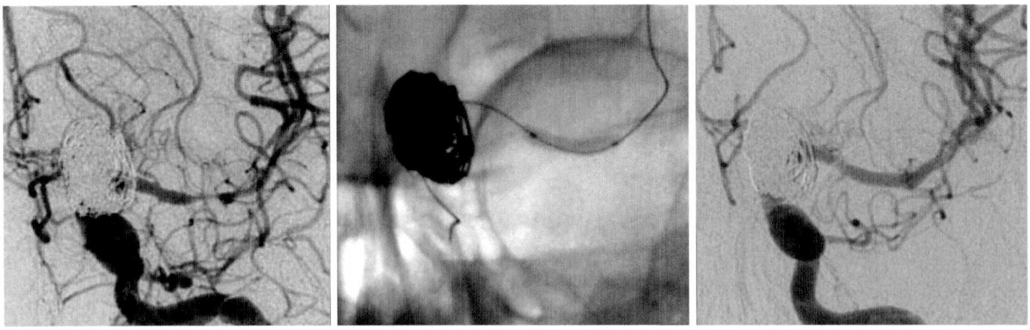

Fig. 8.14 Balloon angioplasty of vasospasm in the left middle cerebral artery 1 week after coiling of large cavernous aneurysm. *Courtesy by Dr. Ayman Z. Ahmed*

be very effective and may be more durable. Angioplasty is not generally considered to be safe beyond the carotid or M1 segments [39]. This may change with the introduction of newer balloon catheters that are safer in more distal segments. We use angioplasty with great caution in the A1 segment. Verapamil and Nimodipine are calcium channel blockers, either one can be used at a dose of 10 mg by slow intra-arterial injections into the spastic vessel, if there is no systemic hypotension, it is reasonable to increase to 20 or 30 mg in divided doses if the spasm is severe. The effect of these drugs on the patient's hemodynamics, intracranial pressure, and subsequently the cerebral perfusion pressure should be monitored while administering these drugs. Effective communication between the anesthesiologist and the interventionist is essential. One study compared the effectiveness of balloon angioplasty to intra-arterial nimodipine and found both therapies to be effective in radiographic resolution of vasospasm [33] (Fig. 8.14).

8.6 Conclusion

The endovascular management of cerebral aneurysms is a rapidly growing field. The continuous development of new techniques, sophisticated devices and more skilled interventionists has paved the way for more patients being managed endovascularly. Since surgical techniques have not seen major advancements for a long time, it is difficult to compare both methods or to conduct a randomized control trial for long-term results. Simply because by the time you can get a result comparing one technique of endovascular treatment with standard clipping, several other endovascular techniques would be available which may have better outcomes.

Since early reports for simple coiling showed some recanalization with large and giant aneurysms, regular follow-up at 6 months to 1-year intervals from the date of treatment for up to 3–4 years by angiography or other imaging modalities (e.g. MRA, CTA) is essential. This is particularly important for the early detection of recanalization and subsequent management.

The current guidelines for management of aneurysmal subarachnoid hemorrhage recommend that in patients with ruptured aneurysms technically amenable for both endovascular coiling and clipping, endovascular coiling should be considered first. Endovascular treatment should be approached with meticulous planning and preparation to minimize the risk associated with the procedure and maximize the success rates. The current trends suggest that the management of cerebral aneurysms with endovascular techniques will become the mainstay of treatment in the future.

References

1. Rodesch G, Picard L, Berenstein A, et al. Interventional Neuroradiology: a Neuroscience sub-specialty. Interv Neuroradiol. 2013 Sep;19(3):263–70.

2. Ahmed AZ, Zohdi AM, Zaghloul MS, ElSammanb AK. Endovascular coiling versus surgical clipping in the treatment of ruptured anterior communicating artery aneurysm in Cairo University Hospitals. EJRNM. September 2013;44: 3:523–30.
3. Luessenhop AJ, Velasquez AC. Observations on the tolerance of intracranial arteries to catheteri- zation. J Neurosurg. 1964;21:85–91.
4. Guglielmi G, Vinuela F, Dion J, Duckwiler G. Electrothrombosis of saccular aneurysms via endovascular approach. 2. Preliminary clinical experience. J Neurosurg. 1991;75:8–14.
5. Molyneux A, Kerr R, Stratton I, Sandercock P, Clarke M, Shrimpton J, et al. International Subarachnoid Aneurysm Trial (ISAT) of neurosurgical clipping versus endovascular coiling in 2143 patients with ruptured intracranial aneurysms: a randomized trial. Lancet. 2002;360:1267–74.
6. Raymond J, Guilbert F, Weill A, Georganos SA, Juravsky L, Lambert A, et al. Long-term angiographic recurrences after selective endovascular treatment of aneurysms with detachable coils. Stroke. 2003;34:1398–403.
7. Raper DMS, Allan R. International subarachnoid trial in the long run: critical evaluation of the long-term follow-up data from the ISAT trial of clipping versus coiling for ruptured intracranial aneurysms. Neurosurgery. June 2010;66(6):1166–9.
8. Harrigan MR, Deveikis JP. Intracranial aneurysm treatment. In: Handbook of cerebrovascular disease and neurointerventional technique. Cham: Springer. p. 189–238.
9. Ries T, et al. Long-term follow-up of cerebral aneurysms after endovascular therapy–prediction and outcome of retreatment. AJNR. 2007;28(9):1755–61.
10. Gonzalez N, Sedrak M, Martin N, Vinuela F. Impact of anatomic features in the endovascular embolization of 181 anterior communicating artery aneurysms. Stroke. 2008;39:2776–82.
11. Zhao J, Lin H, Summers R, et al. Current treatment strategies for intracranial aneurysms. March 2017. Angiology. 2018 Jan;69(1):17–30.
12. Lazareska M, Aliji V, Stojovska-Jovanovska E, et al. Endovascular treatment of wide neck aneurysms. J Med Sci. 2018 Dec 20;6(12):2316–22.
13. Sadato A, Hayakawa M, Adachi K, et al. Large residual volume, not low packing density, is the most influential risk factor for recanalization after coil embolization of cerebral aneurysms. PLoS One. 2016;11(5):e0155062.
14. Gallas S, Pasco A, Cottier JP, Gabrillargues J, Drouineau J, Cognard C, et al. A multicenter study of 705 ruptured intracranial aneurysms treated with Guglielmi detachable coils. AJNR Am J Neuroradiol. 2005;26:1723–31.
15. Gallas S, Drouineau J, Gabrillargues J, Pasco A, Cognard C, Pierot L, et al. Feasibility, procedural morbidity and mortality, and long-term follow-up of endovascular treatment of 321 unruptured aneurysms. AJNR Am J Neuroradiol. 2008;29:63–8.
16. Pierot L, Spelle L, Leclerc X, Cognard C, Bonafé A, Moret J. Endovascular treatment of unruptured intracranial aneurysms: comparison of safety of remodeling technique and standard treatment with coils. Radiology. 2009;251:846–55.
17. Pierot L, Cognard C, Anxionnat R, Ricolfi F, for the CLARITY group. The remodelling technique for endovascular treatment of ruptured intracranial aneurysms is more efficacious than standard coiling with a similar safety. Radiology. 2011;258:546–53.
18. Gentric JC, Biondi A, Piotin M, et al. Safety and efficacy of Neuroform for treatment of intracranial aneurysms: a prospective, consecutive, French Multicentric Study. AJNR Am J Neuroradiol. 2013 Jun-Jul;34(6):1203–8.
19. Pierot L, Wakhloo AK. Endovascular treatment of intracranial aneurysms. Stroke. 2013;44:2046–54.
20. Briganti F, Leone G, Marseglia M, et al. Endovascular treatment of cerebral aneurysms using flow-diverter devices: a systematic review. Neuroradiol J. 2015 Aug;28(4):365–75.
21. Gory B, Berge J, Bonafé A, et al. Flow diverters for intracranial aneurysms the diversion national prospective cohort study. Stroke. 2019;50:3471–80.
22. Ma N, Xu Z, Mo D, et al. Safety of low-dose aspirin in endovascular treatment for intracranial atherosclerotic stenosis. PLoS One. 2014;9(8):e105252.
23. Han YF, Dai QL, Chen XL, Xiong YY, et al. Emergent loading dose of antiplatelets for stenting after IV rt-PA in acute ischemic stroke: a feasibility study. Int J Neurosci. 2018;128(4):311–7.
24. Shariff U, Hassan A, Qureshi A. Safety and effectiveness of ticagrelor in patients with clopidogrel resistance undergoing angioplasty, stent or flow diverter placement. Neurology. 2018;90.
25. Narata AP, Amelot A, Bibi R, et al. Dual antiplatelet therapy combining aspirin and ticagrelor for intracranial stenting procedures: a retrospective single center study of 154 consecutive patients with unruptured aneurysms. Neurosurgery. 2019 Jan 1;84(1):77–83.
26. Horowitz M, Samson D, Purdy P. Does electrothrombosis occur immediately after embolization of an aneurysm with Guglielmi detachable coils? AJNR Am J Neuroradiol. 1997;18:510–3.
27. McDougall CG, Halbach VV, Dowd CF, Higashida RT, Larsen DW, Hieshima GB. Endovascular treatment of basilar tip aneurysms using electrolytically detachable coils. J Neurosurg. 1996;84:393–9.
28. Pruvo JP, Leclerc X, Ares GS, Lejeune JP, Leys D. Endovascular treatment of ruptured intracranial aneurysms. J Neurol. 1999;246:244–9.
29. Qureshi AI, Mohammad Y, Yahia AM, et al. Ischemic events associated with unruptured intracranial aneurysms: multicenter clinical study and review of the literature. Neuro- Surg. 2000;46(2):282–9. discussion 289–290
30. Pierot L, Cognard C, Anxionnat R, et al. Ruptured intracranial aneurysms: factors affecting the rate and outcome of endovascular treatment complications in a

series of 782 patients (CLARITY study). Radiology. 2010;256:916.
31. Sturiale CL, Brinjikji W, Murad MH, Lanzino G. Endovascular treatment of intracranial aneurysms in elderly patients: a systematic review and meta-analysis. Stroke. 2013;44:1897.
32. Renowden SA, Benes V, Bradley M, Molyneux AJ. Detachable coil embolisation of ruptured intracranial aneurysms: a single center study, a decade experience. Clin Neurol Neurosurg. 2009;111:179.
33. Bauer AM, Rasmussen PA. Treatment of intracranial vasospasm following subarachnoid hemorrhage. Front Neurol. 2014;5:72.
34. Bederson JB, Connolly ES, Batjer HH, Dacey RG, Dion JE, Diringer MN, et al. Guidelines for the management of aneurysmal subarachnoid hemorrhage: a statement for healthcare professionals from a special writing group of the stroke council, American heart association. Stroke. 2009;40(3):994–1025.
35. Washington CW, Zipfel GJ. Participants in the international multi-disciplinary consensus conference on the critical care management of subarachnoid hemorrhage. Detection and monitoring of vasospasm and delayed cerebral ischemia: a review and assessment of the literature. Neurocrit Care. 2011;15(2):312–710.
36. Sloan MA, Alexandrov AV, Tegeler CH, Spencer MP, Caplan LR, Feldmann E, et al. Assessment: transcranial Doppler ultrasonography: report of the therapeutics and technology assessment subcommittee of the American academy of neurology. Neurology. 2004;62(9):1468–8110.
37. Anderson GB, Ashforth R, Steinke DE, Findlay JM. CT angiography for the detection of cerebral vasospasm in patients with acute subarachnoid hemorrhage. AJNR Am J Neuroradiol. 2000;21(6):1011–5.
38. Greenberg ED, Gold R, Reichman M, John M, Ivanidze J, Edwards AM, et al. Diagnostic accuracy of CT angiography and CT perfusion for cerebral vasospasm: a meta-analysis. AJNR Am J Neuroradiol. 2010;31(10):1853–6010.
39. Zwienenberg-Lee M, Hartman J, Rudisill N, Madden LK. Effect of prophylactic transluminal balloon angioplasty on cerebral vasospasm and outcome in patients with Fisher grade III subarachnoid hemorrhage: results of a phase II multicenter, randomized, clinical trial. Stroke. 2008;39(6):1759–6510.

Surgical Management of Aneurysmal Subarachnoid Hemorrhage

9

Arshad Ali and Muhammad Mohsin Khan

9.1 Historical Background

The dawn of surgical treatment for cerebral aneurysm is based on proximal ligature of feeding vessel to induce thrombosis, first conceptualized by a Scottish surgeon, John Hunter in 1748 [1]. This transformative concept called Hunterian ligation was initially used in peripheral aneurysm and the first carotid ligation was done by Astley Paston Cooper to treat a cervical segment aneurysm in 1805 [2]. Victor Horsley performed the first surgery to expose a giant Internal Carotid artery (ICA) aneurysm and treated it by bilateral cervical carotid occlusion [3]. The Hunterian ligation was subsequently refined as "fractional ligation" that continued to be used but with modification of "gradual occlusion" to avoid complications of ischemic strokes and giving time for development of collateral cerebral circulation [4]. With this refinement, surgeons were able to place different types of vascular clamps (for example, Selverstone clamp) in the neck to occlude the artery gradually and progressively over period of days [5]. The Hunterian ligation subsequently extended to "trapping" of aneurysm by occluding the feeding artery proximal and distal to aneurysm [6]. In 1935, Walter E Dandy took the credit by successfully trapping a cavernous sinus aneurysm by ligating ICA proximally in the neck and distally intracranially [7].

The birth of direct aneurysm exposure and clipping was first performed on February 6, 1937 by Walter E Dandy by using the sliver clips at the John Hopkins Hospital. In 1944, he published the first monograph "Intracranial arterial aneurysm" in which he described his experience of 36 operations with 25% morality with "cure" rate of 55% [8]. Meanwhile, a Portuguese neurologist Egas Moniz [9] developed the ability to visualize cerebral aneurysm by angiography that facilitated a planned treatment. The results of direct surgical intervention remained a controversy among neurosurgeons due to the high morbidity and mortality associated with direct clipping until the next leap occurred with the introduction of microsurgical techniques and the use of operating microscope [10]. The greatest impact of the microscope was to effectively illuminate the surgical corridors, vivid visualization of aneurysm, better understanding of microsurgical anatomy, and refinements in operative techniques. Now over 200 years of history of technological advancements with improved details of microsurgical anatomy and remarkable micro-

A. Ali (✉)
Department of Neurosurgery, Hamad Medical Corporation, Doha, Qatar

Department of Academic Medicine, College of Medicine, Qatar University, Doha, Qatar

Department of Neurological Surgery, Weill Cornell Medicine-Qatar, Doha, Qatar
e-mail: AAli84@hamad.qa

M. M. Khan
Department of Neurosurgery, Hamad Medical Corporation, Doha, Qatar
e-mail: mkhan51@hamad.qa

A. E. A. Ganaw et al. (eds.), *Management of Subarachnoid Hemorrhage*,
https://doi.org/10.1007/978-3-030-81333-8_9

surgical experiences, a growing generation of dedicated cerebrovascular neurosurgeons have been produced that includes but not limited to, Drake, Sundt, Spetzler, Dolenc, and Yasargil [11–18].

9.2 Perianeurysmal Environment and Subarachnoid Spaces

The natural history of cerebral aneurysms can be divided into 3 stages: (1) aneurysm formation or initiation, (2) growth or enlargement, and (3) rupture [19, 20]. Different underlying mechanisms that controls evolution from one stage to next are multifactorial and these include hemodynamic loads, wall biomechanics, mechanobiology, and contacts with the perianeurysmal environment. The impetus to form aneurysm is based on the general concept of hemodynamic stress that induces focal damage in the endothelium and this weakening subsequently grows and enlarges, in due to course, ultimately manifesting as a rupture of vessel wall into subarachnoid spaces [21].

Aneurysms are located in the subarachnoid spaces and this space is compartmentalized into a variety of different fissures and cisterns that have been named according to their locations and proximity to important anatomical landmarks to describe the relationship of the cerebral vessels to the arachnoid spaces and to the numerous trabeculae or bands which suspend these vessels from the walls of the cisterns (Fig. 9.1). Some of the important subarachnoid spaces for aneurysmal anatomical locations are Sylvian fissure, interpeduncular cisterns, carotid cisterns, pontine cisterns, peri-mesencephalic cisterns, and foramen magnum cistern. The traditional definition of the subarachnoid space as consisting of a freely communicating channel for the flow of CSF is an inadequate explanation that does not fully explain the pathophysiology of aneurysmal development and does not correlate with operative findings. These subarachnoid spaces are lined by arachnoid bands that contribute in the development of a perianeurysmal environment [22].

Perianeurysmal environment is the term coined to explain the effects of all the structures and contents of subarachnoid spaces that are surrounding the individual aneurysm in a particular anatomical location. Although, increase in size of aneurysm is thought to occur from focal vessel wall weakening that yields to hemodynamic pressure but rupture occurs when "internal" wall stresses exceed strength [21, 23]. However, there is a growing body of evidence that "internal" mechanobiological stresses are not sufficient to explain the dynamic morphological changes noted in the course of aneurysm formation, growth and ultimately rupture but there are considerable constraint effects of possible interaction between aneurysm and surrounding anatomical architecture of arachnoid band webs with cisternal spaces that form the peculiar perianeurysmal environment [24], From microsurgical anatomical viewpoint, understanding of subarachnoid spaces with perianeurysmal arachnoid bands is crucial while doing exposure of the ruptured aneurysms. Knowledge of the cisternal anatomy allows precise exploration along the "cisternal pathways" [22].

9.3 Preoperative Assessment and Preparation

The aim of aneurysm treatment is to secure aneurysm to prevent rebleeding or enlargement while simultaneously minimizing injury to brain tissue and cranial nerves and preserving the normal vasculature.

9.3.1 Timing of Surgery

In the past there had been controversy whether the surgery for ruptured aneurysm should be performed early (<48–96 h) or delayed (>10–14 days) [25].

Following are arguments in favor of early surgery:

- Once aneurysm is clipped, rebleeding does not occur which is the leading cause of significant morbidity and mortality in SAH patients.
- Surgical clipping allows subsequent complications to be managed like vasospasm, seizures, and unstable blood pressure that can be

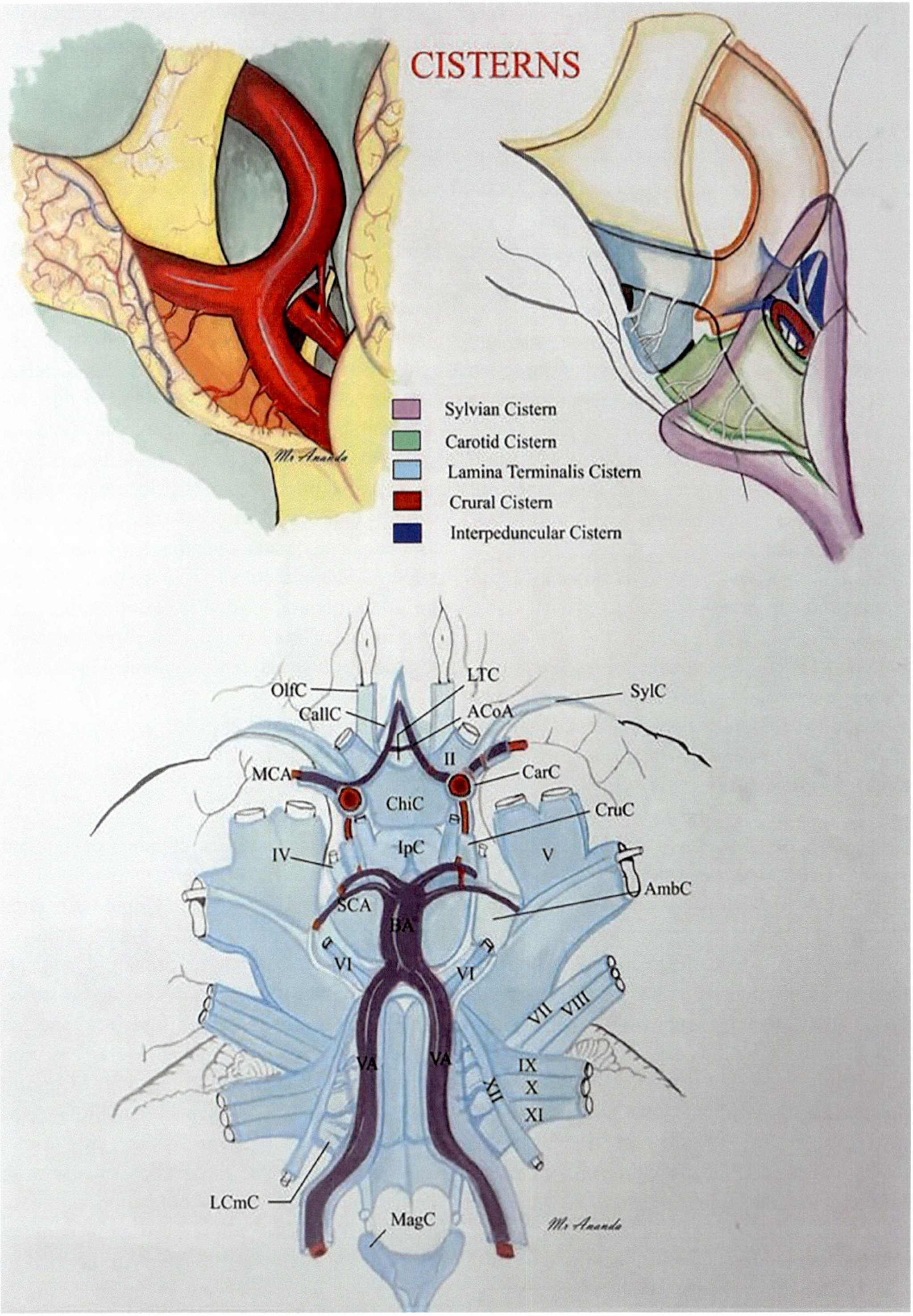

Fig. 9.1 Different nomenclatures of basal cisterns. SylC (Sylvian cistern), OlfC (Olfactory cistern), CallC (callosal vessels cistern), LTC (Lamina terminalis cistern), CarC (Carotid cistern), ChiC (Chiasmal cistern), IpC (Interpeduncular cistern), CruC (Crural cistern), Cr3C (third Cranial (Occulomotor) nerve cistern), (AmbC (Ambient cistern), MagC (Magnum cistern), LCmC (Lateral Cerebellomedullary cistern)

lethal in setting of an already devastating emergency.

- Surgery may also help prevent vasospasm by allowing for lavage of vasospasmogenic agents in blood from subarachnoid space.
- Overall mortality is reduced with early surgery.

Proponents of delayed surgery advocate so for the following reasons:

- Early after SAH, brain is edematous and inflamed which necessitates greater retraction of soft friable inflamed brain tissue prone to laceration.
- Incomplete lysis of the clot in subarachnoid space hampers surgery and may result in greater mechanical trauma to the blood vessels, hence promoting vasospasm.
- There is also greater risk of intraoperative rupture with early surgery.

In conclusion predominant evidence from literature favors that surgery or coiling should be performed as soon as possible to alleviate the risk of rebleeding in most patients with aneurysmal subarachnoid hemorrhage [26–28].

9.3.2 Preoperative Imaging

At the time admission, patients with ruptured cerebral aneurysm undergo computed tomographic (CT) scan along with CT angiography. In most of the cases CT angiography is sensitive enough to diagnose the cause of acute subarachnoid hemorrhage due to underlying aneurysm. However, a formal digital subtraction angiography (DSA) is carried out to further delineate the details of cerebral angioarchitecture including morpho-diagnosis of aneurysm. DSA study is studied in detail by neurosurgeons with highly valuable input provided by a neuroradiologist/neurointerventionist hence enabling the operating surgeon to formulate an imaginative strategy prior to actual proceedings of clipping. In addition to taking into consideration anatomical configuration and morphology, neck and dome/neck ratio, there is a need to understand the parent vessels, perforators as well as any vessels arising from the aneurysm and the whole vascular construct of collateral circulation surrounding the aneurysm [29].

9.3.3 Operating Microscope

Since 1960s, micro-neurosurgery has been revolutionized with the use of operating microscope [10]. It has become an essential armamentarium for aneurysmal surgery in particular as it provides advantage of properly illuminated surgical corridor, anatomical details under high magnification, and ease of approaching the surgical field from different angles for optimal access and exposure [30]. Operating microscopes must be assessed and prepared prior to each case that includes balancing, focus/orientation of the camera, and checking of automated functions before the sterile draping. The placement of microscope in the operating room is decided in relation to surgical positioning of patient, neurosurgeon's handedness, scrub nurse and other equipment location.

9.3.4 Aneurysm Clips

Historically, Walter Dandy was the first person who accomplished direct clipping of internal carotid artery aneurysm with malleable silver clip in 1937 [31]. Afterwards, aneurysm clips have been progressively undergoing improvement and refinement in terms of their biocompatibility, metallurgic properties, and designing as per need of cerebrovascular surgeons. There a variety of different aneurysm clips that has been designed and branded by manufactures according the need of the contemporary cerebrovascular surgeons including Yasargil, Drake, Sugita and Spetzler [32–34]. All these clips satisfactorily accomplish the aneurysm obliteration with ease in intraoperative use with respective clip applicator and have paramagnetic compatibility due to titanium metal for postoperative magnetic imaging [35]. The choice of size, shape, and angle depends upon done orientation, neck size, and visual angle of surgical corridor (Fig. 9.2). In terms of difference, temporary clips have less closing force at their blades as compared to per-

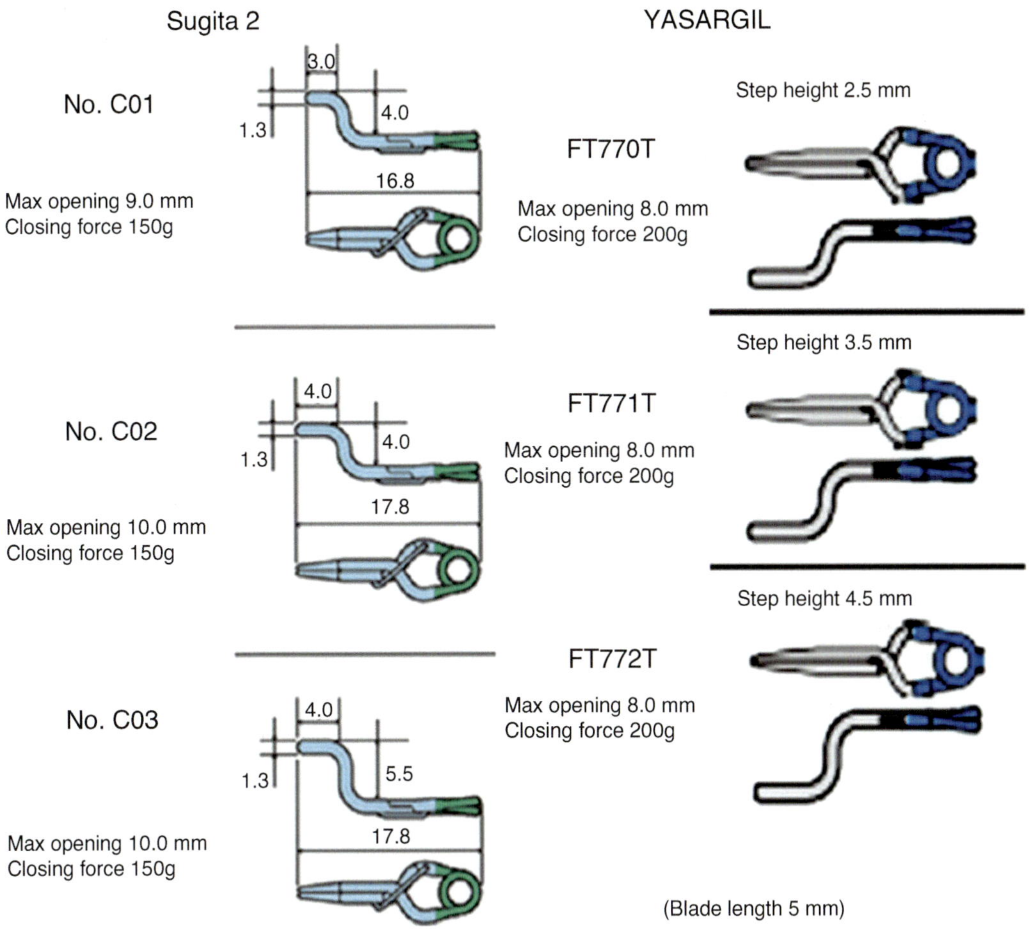

Fig. 9.2 Commercially available aneurysm clips. Sugita 2 clip (left). YASARGIL clip (right). The figure is modified from their catalogs. All the numbers are in millimeter (mm)

manent clip. Futuristic aneurysm (smart) clips are being aimed to design with nanotechnology with highly robust biocompatible materials equipped with "electronic sensing" technology at their tips to create a perioperative multidimensional angioarchitectural modeling combined with robotic application [34].

9.4 Surgical Positioning and Approaches

9.4.1 Surgical Positions

The surgical position is key to gain optimal access to a proper surgical corridor. After general anesthesia, the patient's head is fixed in a 3-point fixation head clamp (Mayfield ®device) and then positioned accordingly, depending on the location of the aneurysm. In addition to optimal access to specified surgical corridor, the principles for positioning involves the utilization of gravity in pulling lobes, or the brain, away from the skull base, therefore minimizing manual brain retraction during surgery. The head is elevated above the heart to achieve adequate venous drainage. The neck is then extended to achieve the gravitational displacement of brain away from the skull base. After that, the patient's head is rotated away from the side of the aneurysm (Fig. 9.3). For example, for most anterior circulation aneurysms, the head is rotated 15–30° away from midline to the contralateral side of aneurysm. Head rotation flexibil-

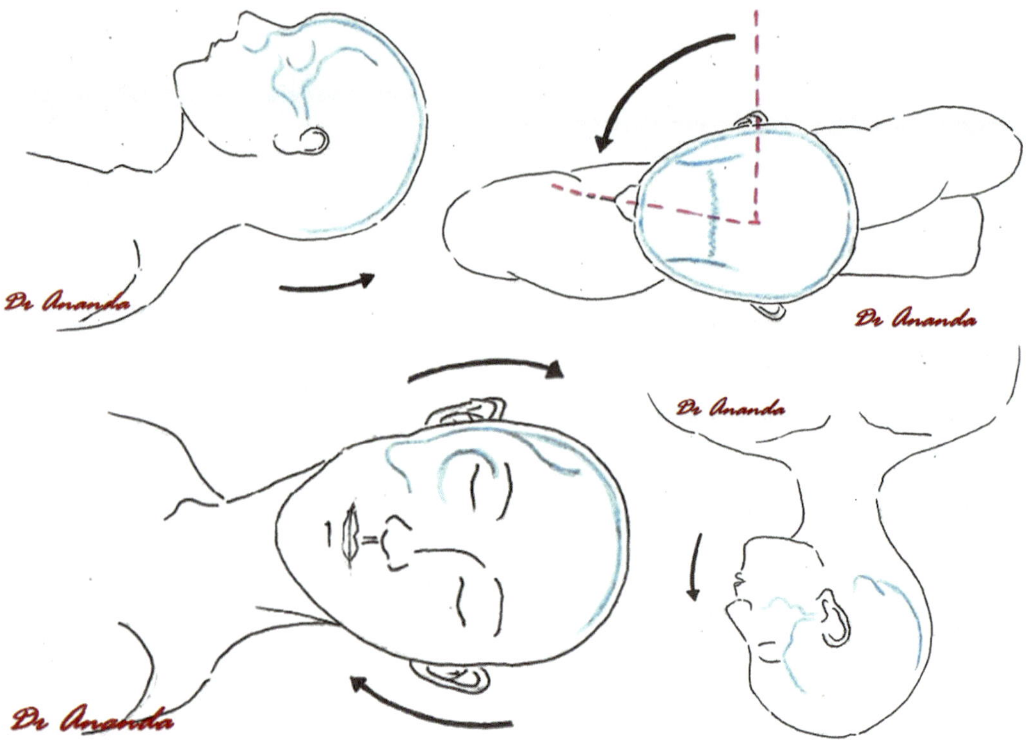

Fig. 9.3 The four important steps of patient positioning. (1) Elevation of head. (2) Rotation of 80–100° to the contralateral side until the zygomatic arch is in a horizontal position. (3) Head is lateroflexed to the contralateral side to support the gravity-related self-retraction of the temporal lobe. (4) The last step is to retroflex the head 15–20°

ity is assessed preoperatively, and an ipsilateral shoulder roll can help reduce cervical spine restricted mobility [36].

9.4.2 Surgical Approaches

9.4.2.1 Perianal Approach

The pterional craniotomy is the key approach for most of the aneurysms in the anterior circulation, as well as allowing an operative window for basilar tip aneurysms [37]. After fixing and positioning the head as described above in surgical positioning section, skin incision is marked with indelible marker (Fig. 9.4). Superficial temporal artery and at least one of the branches preferably preserved for their potential harvesting in the future vascular bypass. The temporalis muscle can be divided along its fibers from the base of zygomatic arch and dissected upwards to the superficial temporal line followed by its detachment from its insertion. Raising a single layer myofascial flap and interfacial dissection helps minimize cosmetic complications and prevent injury to the frontalis branch of the facial nerve [38].

Burr holes are placed in the squamous segment of the temporal bone, just beneath the superior temporal line and in the anatomical key burr site at the anterior end of zygomatic arch. The bone flap is raised by connecting these burr holes by using high-speed craniotome (Fig. 9.4). To achieve adequate access and exposure to the skull base, the lateral aspect of the sphenoid ridge is resected or drilled up to the level meningo-orbital band. After achieving optimal extradural hemostasis, dura mater is opened preferably in a curvilineal fashion with base reflected on lateral sphenoid wing and it is tacked back flushed with the inner table [36, 39].

At this stage, the neurosurgeon evaluates the brain relaxation by slightly lifting the frontal lobe

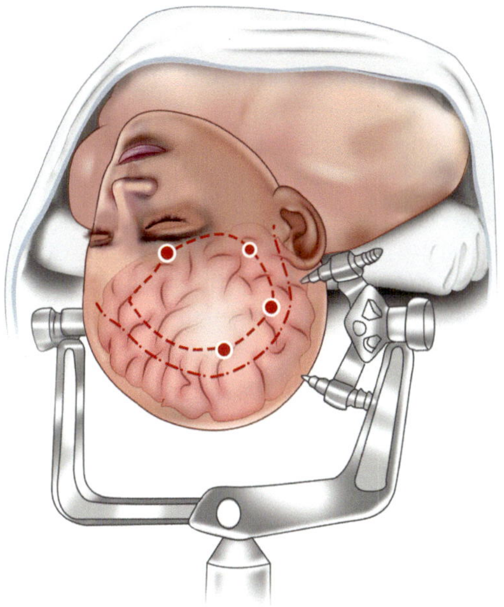

Fig. 9.4 Positioning of patient in 3-pin head clamp with incision marking with burr holes and extent of craniotomy in a standard pterional craniotomy, the most common approach for aneurysms of anterior circulation

and basal cistern is opened to allow egress of CSF to achieve further brain relaxation. In some situations, even after opening the cisterns, and application of adjunctive anesthetic measures, it may not be possible to achieve adequate brain relaxation. At this point, some neurosurgeons place a ventriculostomy catheter to drain CSF out directly accessing the ventricle in controlled manner. Once the adequate brain relaxation is attained, the operating microscope is brought in to start microsurgical dissection to proceed for aneurysmal exposure [36, 40].

9.4.2.2 Sub-Temporal Approach

The sub-temporal approach is frequently used to gain access to the interpeduncular fossa or lateral brainstem. This approach provides a surgical corridor to reach at or below the level of the posterior clinoid and can help surgeons for the Hunterian ligation of the basilar artery including clipping aneurysms of superior cerebellar, posterior cerebellar artery, and low-lying basilar bifurcation aneurysms. The key benefit of this approach is better visual recognition of the thalamoperforators, when approaching aneurysms of the basilar quadrification. For aneurysms originating from the P2 segment of the PCA, there is an advantage to have both proximal and distal control [29, 41].

To avoid surgical retraction injury to temporal lobe, right side is generally preferred. In preoperative planning, the location of vein of Labbe with its junction to transverse sinus is identified to avoid venous insults. This information also helps to know the limit of safe temporal lobe retraction. The patient should be in the decubitus position with head stabilized in the Mayfield head clamp. Standard temporal craniotomy is fashioned with "horseshoe" shaped incision. The nuanced point here is to gain access to skull base along the posterior temporal fossa floor by drilling down and flattening the squamous temporal bone. The mastoid air cells should be obliterated and then dura is opened, followed by gentle retraction of the temporal lobe to get visualization of medical edge of tentorium. Gradual and progressive elevation of uncus leads to the interpeduncular cistern covered by the membrane of Lilliquist. The identification of the third cranial nerve acts an important anatomical lead. Generally, the superior cerebellar artery might be tracked beneath the oculomotor nerve and dissection continued to the basilar trunk. The principles for achieving adequate functional brain relaxation are similar to those outlined in the pterional approach.

9.4.2.3 Far Lateral Retrosigmoid Approach

Far lateral retrosigmoid approach is adopted while accessing surgical exposure to posterior circulation aneurysm including the aneurysms of posterior inferior cerebellar artery, vertebrobasilar junction, anterior inferior cerebellar artery [39, 42]. The head is fixed in three-pin head clamp and patient is placed in lateral decubitus with neck flexed and head inclined to ease access to retrosigmoid territory. It is pertinent that ipsilateral shoulder may limit maneuverability of surgeon depending upon his/her handedness. This is usually compensated with tilt of operating table while accessing depth of surgical corridor and application of aneurysm clips.

A hockey-stick incision is placed starting at the level of the mastoid, goes upward toward the superior nuchal line, curving gently toward the inion in the midline and carried inferiorly to the finish at the level second cervical spinous process. The muscle tissue that happen to be there is detached in the midline raphae that is an avascular plane from the spinous process to the occipital and the mastoid area. Dissection is carried out till the identification of the posterior arch of the atlas. At this point, occipital triangle is identified that is bounded by rectus capitis posterior major, superior oblique muscle, and the inferior oblique muscles. Occipital triangle contains vertebral artery, a chief vascular structure is in this approach. The suboccipital triangular is opened up by simply removing the attachment of rectus capitis medially and on the superior oblique laterally. The vertebral artery is encircled with a venous plexus that may lead to bleeding during the procedure. The condylar emissary vein lead to identification of occipital condyle, another important key landmark in this approach. The suboccipital craniotomy is performed including the posterior rim of foramen magnum and laterally reaching up to the sigmoid sinus. After performing the C-1 hemilaminectomy, the last step in bone removal is drilling of the postero-medial third part of the occipital condyle. Identification and protection of vertebral artery is crucial during all this bony work to avoid any catastrophe. Rarely skeletonization to mobilize of vertebral artery from its contact with C1-lamina is required depending on its anatomical variation [42].

9.5 Proximal Vascular Control and Temporary Clipping

Proximal vascular control is considered the standard technique for microsurgical clipping of cerebral aneurysm [43, 44]. The key understanding is to get exposure of predominant parent or feeding artery that is providing the major hemodynamic flow to the aneurysm in advance. This all-time intermittent and temporary vascular control helps meticulous dissection in very close proximity of aneurysm and prompt control of the catastrophic bleeding in case of inadvertent premature rupture of aneurysm. This becomes particularly relevant tenet in case of giant or large aneurysm clipping. Temporary proximal occlusion softens the dome of aneurysmal sack in advance and aids preparation for permanent clipping [45]. The duration of temporary clipping is variable depending on size of the vessel involved. For smaller caliber vessels (like M1), it is recommended for as small duration as 2.5 min and larger vessels like ICA can be occluded as long as 20 min. The usual practice is to use intermittent occlusion ranging from 2.5 to 5 min depending upon pertinent surgical situation [46, 47].

To have adequate choice of proximal control, preoperative analysis of cerebral angiography is necessary to understand the predominance of vascular feeder to aneurysm and its hemodynamic relationship. Sometimes, the preference to the side of surgical approach may also depend on vascular dominance of feeder to the aneurysm. For example, assessing the vascular predominance of A-1 is important in case of anterior communicating artery aneurysm because in case of accidental aneurysmal rupture or at the time of dissecting the neck or dome of aneurysm, application of temporary clips at predominantly feeding A-1 can immediately help control the major vascular bleeding and can provide the necessary time for surgeon to take necessary steps efficiently. In certain aneurysm location (like ophthalmic segment), it is not possible to expose ICA proximal to aneurysm origin. In such situations, Internal carotid artery is exposed (before craniotomy) in the neck and vascular band is left in situ in case of emergent need to occlude ICA as mandated during the operative procedure. Proximal control strategies will further be discussed and elaborated in intraoperative aneurysmal rupture section below.

Cerebral protection strategies are frequently used during temporary clipping period. A bolus of thiopentone is usually given by the neuroanesthetist in consultation with operating neurosurgeon to decrease the cerebral metabolism. Cerebral protection helps the brain tissue survive in decreased perfusion states by allowing reduced metabolic rate. It is also sometimes combined with concurrent monitoring with EEG if a long temporary clipping is required, especially in a complex aneurysm surgery. Other neuroprotection techniques that help achieve lower rate of cerebral metabolism during the period of temporary clipping are hypothermia and now less favorable option of induced hypotension that may result in cerebral ischemia [47, 48].

9.6 Retractorless Technique

Self-retaining retractors have been routinely used in contemporary neurosurgical practice whenever neurosurgeons confront a deep intracranial lesion under the microscope especially in the approaches for skull base and cerebrovascular pathologies. Their use allows surgeons to gain access deep into the surgical bed, unhindered by tissues hanging over in the visual line of long and deep surgical corridor. This also avoided the need for holding over-hanging tissue away from surgical field with handheld retractors with an invariably sustained pressure by surgical assistants. The effective use of retractors has also played a significant role in microsurgical training as well [29, 43, 49]. Although, self-retaining retractors have been in use for many years, their use has been documented in association with complications including retractor-induced ischemic injury, brain swelling and inadvertent brain injury during manipulation and adjustment [49]. More fixed retractor systems require time and repeated readjustments as required during the course of surgical exposure and to align with angle of operating microscope field of vision [29, 50].

There are extensive studies that have shown the potential harmful effects based on cellular and molecular mechanisms associated with the use of sustained pressure on brain tissues by retractors both from animal and human studies [50, 51]. This is demonstrated by techniques such as autoradiography, mechanical transduction, somatosensory evoked potentials mapping, laser Doppler cerebral flow, tissue microdialysis, and intraoperative functional mapping that have used to trace the processes of metabolism, oxidation, and electrical events that preempt the reversible and irreversible injury to the underlying brain tissue induced by retraction. These experimental conditions have also been evaluated during the situations of induced hypotension to further understand the pathogenesis that are encountered during natural operating conditions [50, 52]. This data has forced surgeons to adopt techniques of intermittent retractor release on brain tissue in a cycle of 5–7 min and biomedical industry got indulge in inventing retractor systems such as sponge-based retractor systems, microballoon paddies, and rolled expanded polytetrafluoroethylene sheets with no significant adoption in contemporary neurosurgical practice [32, 53].

With established practice of endovascular treatment with reduced complications, there is a progressive refinement in microsurgical techniques complemented with experience and skill of cerebrovascular surgeons. Robert F Spetzler [54], a renowned retired skull base and cerebrovascular neurosurgeon at Barrow Neurological Institute, Phoenix-Arizona coined the term of "retractorless surgery" in a landmark publication. Although a gentle traction on cerebral tissue can be safe and effective but he proposed intermittent brain retraction instead of sustained fixed retraction. He introduced the use of this technique in all his cases undergoing for skull base or cerebrovascular lesions and demonstrated meticulous dissection of arachnoidal planes, careful placement of the handheld suction device and the operating instruments, patient positioning that enhances gravity-based retraction, and appropriate selection of the operative corridor all served to obviate the need for fixed retraction [54, 55]. Later studies published to clearly demonstrate the usefulness of retractorless surgical techniques exclusively used in aneurysm surgery and it has reduced the morbidity and mortality associated with microsurgical clipping [54–56].

9.7 Microsurgical Dissection and Clip Application

Microsurgical dissection of the aneurysm necessitates meticulous surgical skill and incorporates not only the aneurysm but also the exposure and identification of all surrounding vessels. The key tenet is sharp microsurgical dissection of the tissue around the aneurysm neck during which the aneurysm is freed from surrounding tissues or structures and is prepared for application of clipping. Microsurgical scissor is used with skillful maneuvers as its blades can be used for blunt tissues to make these free and at the same time cutting sharply using manual dexterity. In addition, arachnoid knife in different shapes along with sharp hooks are used as adjunct for sharp dissection throughout the surgical exposure in subarachnoid spatial exposure. Suction tip is also used to hold arachnoid or tissue bands clearly off the vital structures while cutting with sharp objects. Pial planes and normal anatomy is preserved by careful dissection under high magnification. Microsurgical, circumferential dissection of the aneurysm should be the goal of subarachnoid dissection [32]. This must be preceded by obtaining proximal arterial control. Here comes the utilization of proximal temporary control as it facilitates the precision of sharp dissection of adherent arachnoid and fibrous tissues. Any kind of blunt dissection or pulling or having traction can inadvertently lead bleeding in surgical field or may in certain case result in premature aneurysm rupture [32, 43]. Another specialized maneuver that can be of help especially when operating giant aneurysm is so called "Dallas technique" or a suction decompression. In this technique, cervical segment of ICA is exposed in advance in anticipation before starting the intracranial dissection. It is also possible to use endovascular alternative of this maneuver if surgery is being performed in the hybrid operating room with facility of intraoperative cerebral angiography. Applying suction decompression can facilitate the tissue dissection as well reconstruction of the vessel wall for wide neck aneurysm with successive placement of aneurysm clips [57, 58].

The principle of applying an aneurysm clip involve forming a natural vascular construct that the blades of clips should be abutting along the axis of wall of parent artery without causing any stenosis or entrapping any adjoining branching or feeders arising in close proximity to the aneurysm neck. While choosing the approach size clip, a general principle is that the length of aneurysm blades should be 1.5 times the size of the neck of aneurysm. Surgeon's intuition and experience is key at this stage in selecting the appropriate angle and number of clips. While applying the aneurysm clip, surgeon remain vigilant and visualize meticulously the tip of the blades of aneurysm clips all along on both sides, making sure that blades completely encompasses the entire length of aneurysm neck and at the same time no perforating vessels or any branch is entrapped or kinked due to clips in place (Fig. 9.5). The clip application is considered the most anxious moment of aneurysm surgery and it is possible that a rapid and uncontrolled closure may lead to inaccurate application [22, 32, 43].

Post-clip application, the dome of the aneurysm is carefully examined if there is still any pulsation visible. If aneurysm is still filling despite application of clip, a second tandem clip is placed parallel to first clip. Persistent filling following initial clip application can be the result of residual distal neck, increased aneurysm thickness, intrasaccular thrombus or atheroma/calcification of the proximal neck. In such situations, surgeon uses different techniques including temporary proximal occlusion, suction decompression or induced transient cardiac arrest using adenosine (discussed later) to achieve an optimal placement of clips for complete obliteration. In rare situations, if the neck of aneurysm is still challenging the optimal closure of blades of clip, then surgeon may shape the neck of aneurysm with bipolar diathermy use at a low power to cause some shrinking of aneurysm wall. The maneuver involves surgeon experience and level of confidence and his/her surgical manual dexterity.

These techniques are applicable to all aneurysms irrespective of their locations. However, aneurysm location, dimensions, and configuration, anatomical arrangements of aneurysm-parent artery complex, angle of surgical exposure, condition of brain tissue and experience of surgeon all dictate further nuances of operating techniques and steps. Simulations are being used now by surgeons and trainees to virtually rehearse the technique and surgical approach before actu-

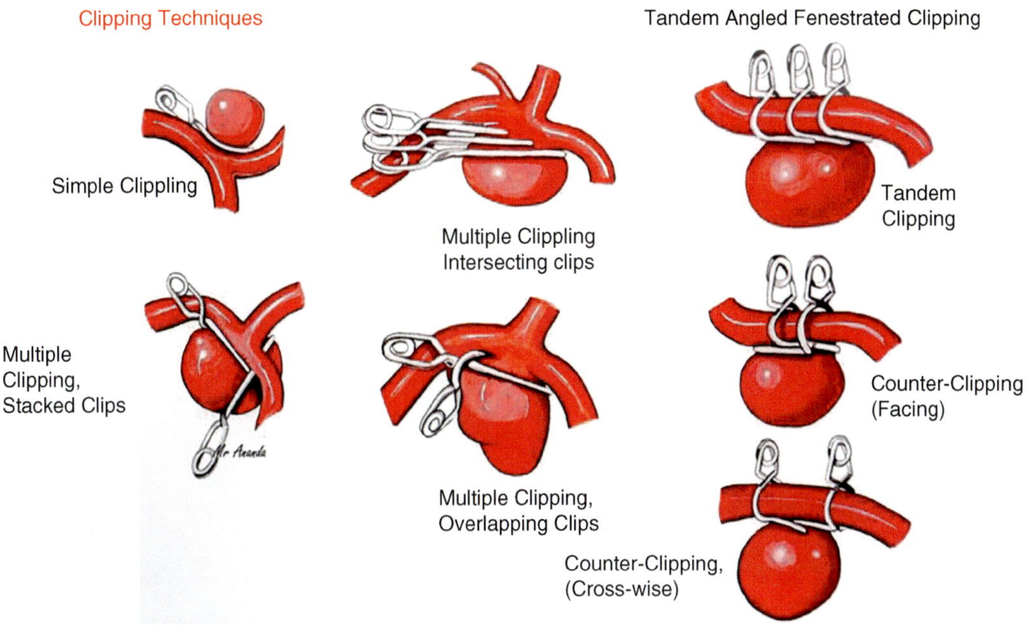

Fig. 9.5 Different clipping techniques with tandem and neck construction

ally performing the procedure [59]. This helps understand the anatomical detail, create an imaginative plan of dissection and microsurgical orientation under the microscope with handling of microsurgical instruments and virtual application of clips with their appropriate selection and anticipating the associated complications. It is also useful to mentally rehearse the steps of surgery progressively [59–61].

In contemporary neurosurgical practice, aneurysm clipping is considered at the acme of operative skill pyramid. Below we discuss some of the nuanced steps in few important aneurysm locations that are encountered most commonly in clinical practice [22, 29, 43, 62, 63].

9.7.1 Aneurysm of Anterior Communicating Artery

Anterior communicating artery (ACom) aneurysms are the most common among all the aneurysms of anterior circulation and these pose significant complexity in understanding the anatomical challenges during the surgical exposure. Unless there is vascular codominance of A1 from both sides, most neurosurgeons approach from the dominant A1 side taking advantage of proximal vascular control for meticulous dissection around and close to aneurysm. The usual sequential approach for surgical exposure in ACom aneurysm complex is from A1 (ipsilateral), A1 (contralateral), artery of Heubner, A2 ipsilateral, and A2 contralateral. Complete vivid orientation and identification of all these anatomical structures is key to successful aneurysm clipping (Fig. 9.6). In some situation, ipsilateral rectus gyrus has to be resected medial to optic tract to gain access without traction. It is utmost important to respect and preserve all the perforators to avoid any postoperative sequelae. Familiarity and anatomical orientation under the microscope ensure understanding the key structures in ACom aneurysm complex including any anatomical variations.

Choice of aneurysm clip depends upon the orientation of aneurysmal dome, site of origin, relationship to ipsilateral A2. In most cases, a bayonet shaped clip is used but other shapes may be preferred accordingly. Once all the key components of ACom complex are visualized, then aneurysm clip is carefully applied with both

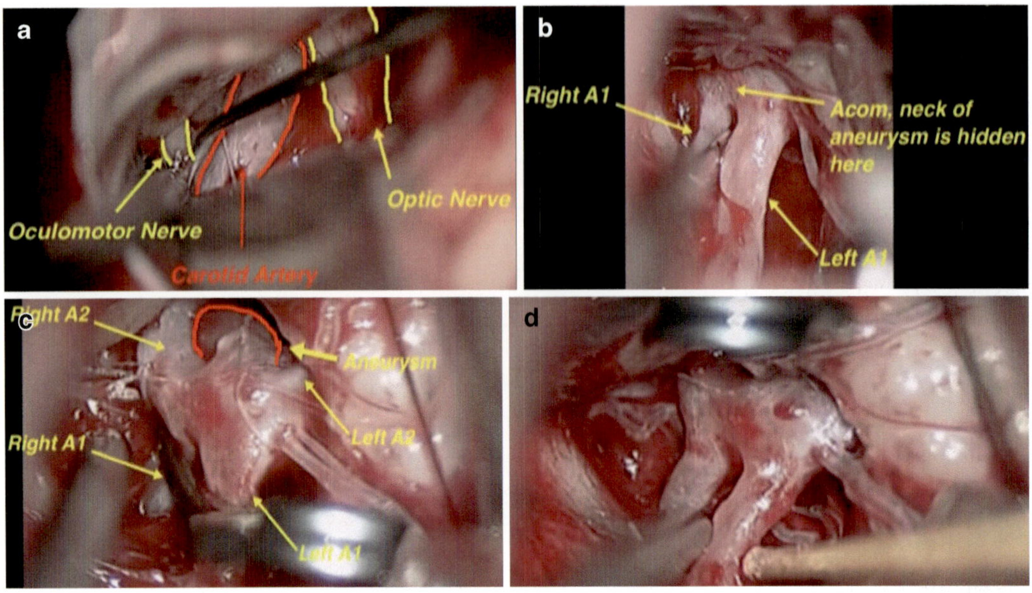

Fig. 9.6 Progressive exposure of Anterior Communicating artery from the left side (**a** and **b**) with proximal temporary clip applied on left A1 (**c**) and final clip applied (**d**) with Doppler ultrasound (yellow tip in **d**) for confirmation vascular patency

blades in constant vision to avoid compromising any vessel or perforator and at the same time achieving a perfect placement at the neck. After Initial placement, a thorough survey is conducted to confirm that all the vessels are patent, and clip is optimally obliterating the neck with no stenosis of parent artery.

9.7.2 Middle Cerebral Artery Aneurysm

Middle cerebral artery (MCA) aneurysm is the second most common aneurysm site and their relatively superficial location favors their treatment by microsurgical clipping. The key step in the surgical exposure for MCA aneurysm is splitting of the Sylvian fissure. Depending on the preference of the neurosurgeon, Sylvian fissure splitting can be started from medial to lateral (from the sphenoid wing end) or from lateral to medial (from superficial cortical location). In general, as a standard clinical practice, it is started from medial to lateral and at least 1/3 of the fissure is opened to gain adequate exposure. Presence of Sylvian (subarachnoid) hemorrhage technically facilitates the splitting as approximated arachnoid layers are set already split apart by blood clot. Relatively superficial insular or cortical M3/4 branches are identified and helps guide exposure and identification M1 and M2 in the depth of fissure. Sequential progression of surgical exposure of MCA bifurcation complex includes M1, identification of bi/trifurcation origin, M2/3 branches distally and all the adherent lenticulostriate perforators.

Before preparing for clip application, a detailed visualization and orientation is ensured of the branches in MCA bifurcation complex followed by analyzing the orientation of aneurysm with its relationship to the parent artery. The most crucial and difficult step is to identify the M2 branches as one of them may be lying under the dome of aneurysm and any uncontrolled dissection or manipulation may result in intraoperative rupture of aneurysm. Judicious use of proximal temporary clipping at M1 can be helpful to decompress the aneurysm sac while identifying the M2 branches. Once adequate exposure is achieved, the choice of aneurysm clip is made depending on the orientation of aneurysm sac and its relationship to the parent artery of origin. In general, an angled clip is required, and it is applied along the axis of the M2 branch from where the aneurysm neck is arising (Fig. 9.7). In certain situation, the aneurysm neck is wide and parent artery wall has to be reconstructed by application of tandem clips until an optimal obliteration is achieved. Finally, the patency of all the branches in vascular complex along with adequate aneurysm obliteration is confirmed with intraoperative Doppler ultrasound or ICG accordingly.

9.7.3 Posterior Communication and Anterior Choroidal Artery Aneurysm

The posterior communicating (PCom) artery is also one of the most common sites for aneurysm formation and it is within only a few millimeters in proximity of the Anterior Choroidal (Ach) artery aneurysm, thereby surgical exposure for both involves common operative steps. Surgical exposure of these aneurysms is considered less technically challenging and proximal vascular control is achieved early while exposing internal carotid artery (ICA). Some of the key nuances related to aneurysm projection/orientations are technically of

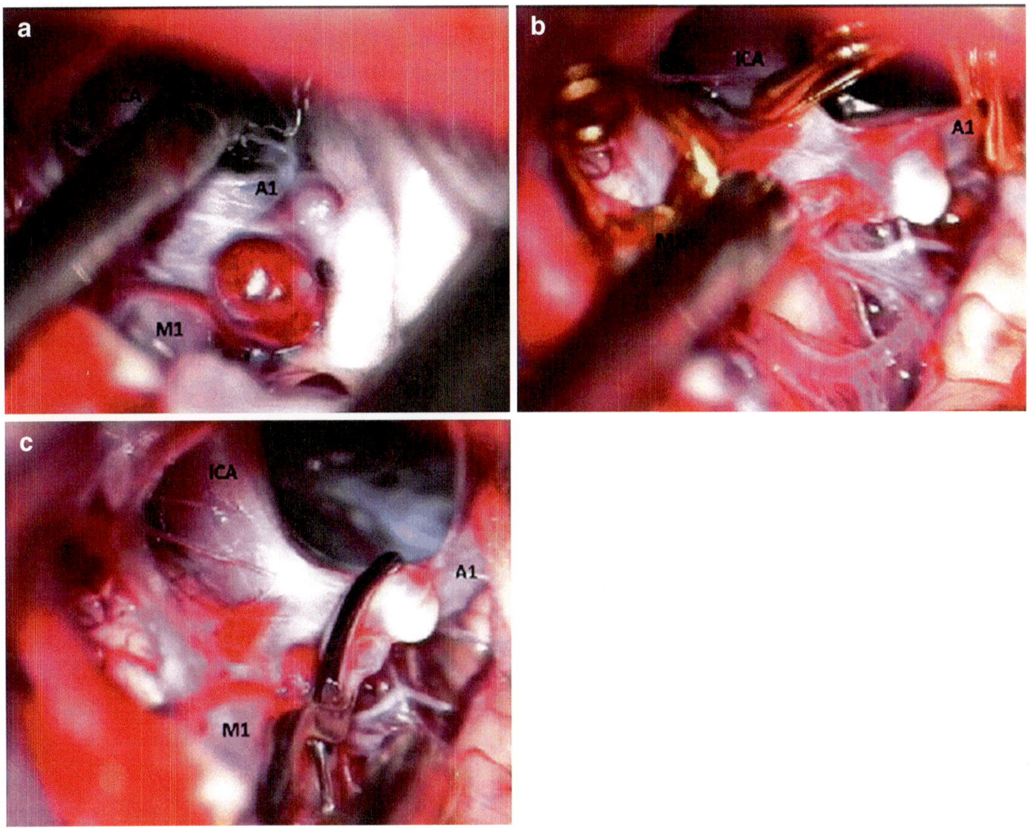

Fig. 9.7 Intraoperative images showing the key steps for aneurysm clipping. (**a**) Small aneurysm on the right carotid bifurcation; (**b**) positioning of a temporary clip on the right internal carotid artery, A1 segment of the right anterior cerebral artery, and M1 segment of the right middle cerebral artery; (**c**) aneurysm closure by miniclip application. Source: Under the free license of Creative Commons Attribution 4.0 International https://creativecommons.org/licenses/by/4.0/ available from https://www.researchgate.net/figure/Intraoperative-images-showing-the-key-steps-for-aneurysm-clipping-a-Small-aneurysm-on_fig 2_287212443

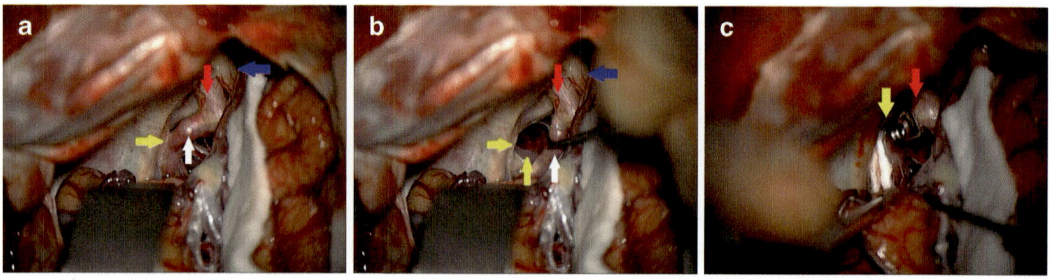

Fig. 9.8 Intraoperative image showing the optic nerve (blue arrow), proximal internal carotid artery (red arrow), and the fetal posterior communicating artery (PCOM, white arrow) indenting and displacing the cranial nerve (CN) III (yellow arrows) laterally (**a** and **b**). The clipped aneurysm and Teflon felt between the PCOM and CN III are shown (**c**). Source: Under the free license of Creative Commons Attribution 4.0 International https://creativecommons.org/licenses/by/4.0/ Available from https://www.cureus.com/articles/16585-acute-oculomotor-nerve-palsy-caused-by-compression-from-an-aberrant-posterior-communicating-artery

important concern; first, its close proximity to 3rd (oculomotor) cranial nerve and second, its potential adherent location to temporal lobe (in medial projection). The sequential surgical exposure (Fig. 9.8) includes identification of proximal ICA segment, distal ICA segment, oculomotor nerve, the adjacent artery (PCom or Ach), and all the proximal perforators arising in this anatomical complex. Another important key tenet to confirm at this point is "fetal" pattern of origin of the PCom artery, although this may have been already identified on preoperative imaging evaluation to mitigate its inadvertent compromise affecting a larger vascular territory as compared to non-fetal pattern of origin.

For clip application, it is convention to access the vascular complex from lateral to medial as it provides surgeon a good view of the origin of PCom or Ach artery and at the same time the relationship and extent of neck of aneurysm with parent artery. In case the aneurysm involves a large origin from ICA with wide neck, tandem clips are applied in succession to reconstruct the ICA wall and to ensure adequate aneurysmal obliteration. Final step involves intraoperative Doppler or ICG monitoring to confirm the obliteration of aneurysmal neck and patency of all the identified vessels in aneurysmal complex.

9.7.4 Aneurysms of the Pericallosal Artery

Aneurysms of the distal anterior cerebral artery in close proximity of origin of pericallosal or callosomarginal artery are typically smaller in size and are less frequently seen in neurosurgical practice. These aneurysms are exposed by interhemispheric approach and surgical corridor is narrow in this location. One of the important nuances is to localize the small sized aneurysm, as the absence definite anatomical landmarks makes it difficult to approximate whether exposure is proximal or distal to site of aneurysm. Neuronavigation is a useful adjunct in these cases to overcome this difficulty and routinely used in some centers as part of preoperative planning. Sequential progression in surgical exposure involves identification of ipsilateral parent artery of origin (both proximal and distal to aneurysm) and closely associated contralateral vessels. In this location, due to hemodynamic situation, the aneurysm is directed away from the approach of angle of surgical field. As these aneurysms are usually small in size, a short-blade bayonet shaped aneurysm clip is suitable in most cases. The aneurysms obliteration or vascular patency if the complex is essentially confirmed with available adjuncts in addition to thorough visual inspection under high magnification of microscope.

9.7.5 Aneurysms of Basilar Quadrification

Aneurysms in this location are mainly originating from the posterior circulation that are preferably be subjected to endovascular treatment as per current guidelines [64]. However, there is still need to have microsurgical clipping for these aneurysms when there is no feasibility to treat by endovascular procedures. In this challenging anatomical location, vascular complex includes four distal branches from basilar artery; two posterior cerebral arteries (PCA) and two superior cerebellar arteries (SCA) forming a basilar quadrification. The sequential progression of surgical exposure includes identification of proximal basilar artery, bilateral SCAs and PCA, oculomotor nerves (bilateral), and thalamo-perforator vessels. The key anatomical landmark is oculomotor nerve that is usually used by the surgeon to make progressive dissection towards the basilar tip. It is extremely important to understand all the anatomical details and variations with preoperative imaging analysis. Another crucial consideration is to carefully dissect and identify the important thalamoperforators. Both excessive manipulation of third cranial nerve or damaging/sacrificing any thalamoperforators may lead to devastating postoperative sequalae.

Once the aneurysm sac is optimally exposed (Fig. 9.9), the choice of aneurysm clip shape and number is approximated by using microdissection instruments. Usually, a straight or bayonet shaped clip is placed or alternatively fenestrated clips may be required to include P1. In patients who have a "fetal" PCom, the ipsilateral P1 can sometimes be sacrificed as a result of compensation from the anterior circulation. Tandem clip application may be necessary in most cases in basilar quadrification except when aneurysm neck is narrow where a single straight clip may be sufficient.

9.8 Confirmation of Aneurysm Obliteration

After clip application, it is extremely important to confirm the complete obliteration of the aneurysm neck without compromising the parent artery along with other normal vasculature in close proximity that may be in danger either due to being directly entangled in the blades of aneurysm clips or being affected indirectly due to kinking or compression from the clip construct. This confirmation can be accomplished by the following intraoperative techniques:

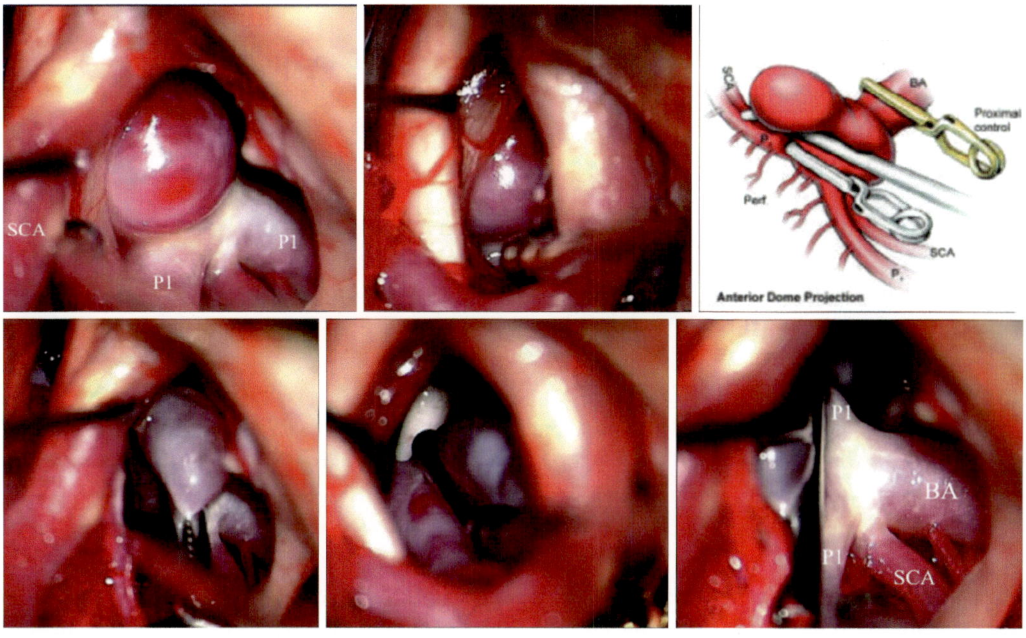

Fig. 9.9 Complex giant aneurysm of basilar artery (BA) tip with anterior dome projection, incorporating origins of posterior cerebral arteries (P1). Progressive stepwise exposure is with temporary clip at basilar artery done and obliteration by applying large straight clip

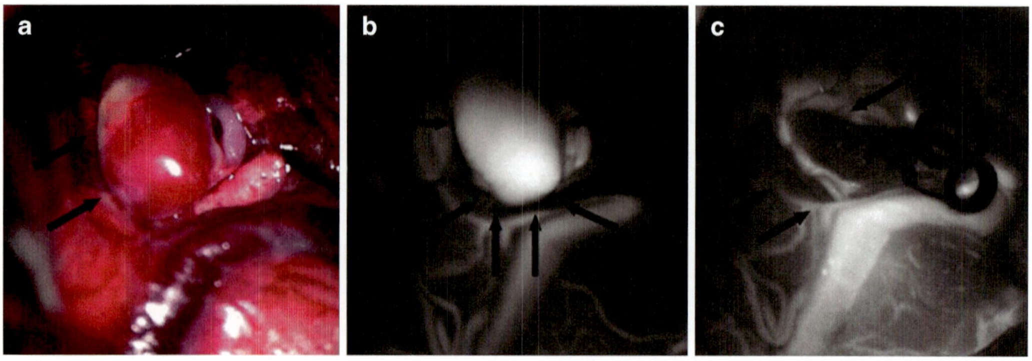

Fig. 9.10 (**a**): Intraoperative Illustration of the Middle Cerebral Artery Aneurysm (Arrows). (**b**) Video angiography showing the perfusion of the untreated aneurysm (arrows). (**c**) After clipping no perfusion of the aneurysm is detectable anymore (arrows). Source: Under the free license of Creative Commons Attribution 4.0 International https://creativecommons.org/licenses/by/4.0/ available from https://www.researchgate.net/figure/Microscope-based-indocyanine-green-video-angiography-supporting-the-microsurgical_fig 1_314227020

9.8.1 Intraoperative Doppler Ultrasound

Traditionally, a microvascular ultrasound Doppler probe is used to confirm the patency of surrounding vasculature in addition to visual confirmation under magnified view of microscope [65, 66]. A microvascular Doppler sonographic probe with a 20-MHz probe (1-mm diameter) is used before and after clip application [67]. The clip adjustment or augmentation can be done by surgeon if required. Intraoperative Doppler technique is a safe, instantaneous, effective, reliable, and cost-effective method for documenting the patency of parent vessels, arterial branches, and major perforators and the complete occlusion of cerebral aneurysms [68].

9.8.2 Indocyanine Green Video Angiography (ICG-VA)

In the late 1960s, Feindel [69] was the first to document the use of intraoperative assessment with fluorescent dye. Indocyanine Green (ICG) is a near-infrared dye that has absorption and emission peaks (805 and 835 nm, respectively) within the optical window of tissue [70]. ICG was routinely being used in ophthalmic procedures but it was only approved in 2002 by FDA for intraoperative cerebral angiography [71]. Afterwards, this technique has become very useful, safe, and essential adjunct in cerebrovascular surgery procedures including in aneurysm clipping procedures. A 0.2–0.5 mg/kg bolus of ICG dye is injected intravenously and this dye can be visualized using fluorescent operating microscope after the clip application (Fig. 9.10) [72]. If occlusion of the parent artery or its branches or residual aneurysm or neck remnant is visualized, repositioning of clip is done or additional clips may be applied in tandem as indicated [72–74].

9.8.3 Cerebral Angiography

Formal digital subtraction cerebral angiography (DSA) is the gold standard to delineate the details of morph-dimension of aneurysm as well as its branching complex both preoperatively and postoperatively [9, 32]. In complex cases, if the facility of hybrid operating suite equipped with intraoperative angiography is available, then it provides an important and unmatched tool to evaluate the effectiveness of aneurysm obliteration as well as preservation of the branches and perforators in close proximity. This also gives a superior advantage of exact matching comparison with preoperative cerebral angiography images and assessment of real-time dynamic flow [74]. Conventionally, if intraoperative cerebral angiography is not available, most neurosurgeons prefer to do postoperative DSA as standard of their practice. It also provides a baseline imaging for follow-up and dictate the planning of management in case of recurrences or progression of any neck remnants in future [75, 76].

9.9 Intraoperative Aneurysm Rupture

Premature rupture of aneurysm during the surgical exposure is one of the most dramatic and devastating complications for the operating neurosurgeon. The reported incidence of intraoperative rupture varies in the literature, from 7% to 19% [77, 78]. Premature aneurysm rupture should be anticipated at any time starting from the anesthesia induction and at any surgical step afterwards until the definitive clipping of the aneurysm is accomplished. One of the general principles of aneurysm exposure adopted to avoid encountering previously ruptured site is not to expose the dome of the aneurysm first. Similarly, sharp dissection is preferred in surgical exposure especially in close proximity of aneurysm sac and neck. In certain situations, the aneurysm dome is tamponade by or adherent to cerebral tissue, thus any uncontrolled and inadvertent traction or manipulation of the lobe can lead to aneurysm rupture with the release of tamponade. If the aneurysm is associated with surrounding intracerebral or perisylvian clot, a safe and precise exposure with gradual manipulation and suctioning of the clot may facilitate the aneurysm exposure; excessive evacuation of the clot can result in intraoperative rupture of the aneurysm and on the other hand, inadequate clot decompression may necessitate excessive retraction, which also carries its risks, as mentioned above [77, 78].

A crucial timing of rupture is usually at the time of dissection around the neck while preparing the surgical field for clip application. At this stage, proximal vascular occlusion by intermittently applying a temporary aneurysm clip is very helpful as it slackens the aneurysm dome and facilitates the circumferential dissection. Application of temporary clip is an important strategy to achieve control of bleeding if there is a sudden rupture of aneurysm [32, 79]. In certain anatomical situations, when there is no proximal vascular control available or clip application is not adequately achieved in broad neck aneurysms, a temporary flow arrest can be induced by administering intravenous adenosine. Adenosine is injected in dosage of 0.3–0.4 mg/kg body weight and a median duration of flow arrest achieved is about 60 second (range 30–90 s). Adenosine has inter-patient variability in efficacy for achieving effective hypotension and dose adjustment or repetition is considered by anesthetist if deemed necessary [80–84]. A number of other maneuvres may also be used to control intraoperative rupture, including suction decompression (Dallas technique) of the aneurysm, coagulation of the aneurysmal rent, clip application to the distal sac and severe induced hypotension complemented with barbiturate induced neuroprotection [22, 32, 57]. All these techniques are very handy and useful to mitigate the emergent intraoperative aneurysm rupture but no one technique can be helpful in all situations, therefore familiarity with all these operative armamentariums can be of significant benefit in time of real surgical challenges. Intraoperative rupture has been reported with higher rate of mortality or morbidity (31%) but interestingly there is no increase in the risk of vasospasm despite additional hemorrhagic incidents [78, 85].

9.10 Postoperative Complications

Postoperative complications after clipping of ruptured intracranial aneurysms can be categorized into generalized and anatomy-specific for individual aneurysm location [22, 88]. Generalized complications are due to the presence of blood in the subarachnoid spaces that is neurotoxic and produces complications like seizures, vasospasm, electrolyte imbalance (usually cerebral salt wasting syndrome), and hydrocephalus. The anatomy-specific complications include injury frontalis branch of facial nerve, frontal air sinus injury, and injury to optic nerve. Other possible complications include deep venous thrombosis, pulmonary embolism, strokes, infections, postoperative pain and risk of death. Late sequalae of subarachnoid hemorrhages, that may have been exacerbated by operative manipulation, are neuropsychological impairments reported as memory dysfunction, emotional instability, and performance impairment [86, 87]. Some of the important complications pertinent to surgical management of intracranial aneurysms are briefly discussed below.

9.10.1 Vasospasm

Vasospasm is one of the most common complications following subarachnoid hemorrhage with overall incidence of symptomatic vasospasm and angiographic vasospasm being 27% and 63%, respectively. Out of these, 13.6% developed delayed ischemic neurological deficits (DIND) as evident on CT scans [88, 89]. Symptomatic vasospasm is less severe in patients with better clinical grades at presentation of subarachnoid hemorrhage (WFNS Grade I-III). Similarly, the extent of subarachnoid and intraventricular hemorrhage burden has been shown to result in more severe vasospasm and delayed cerebral ischemia (DCI). In some centers, transcranial Doppler is applied as a screening tool for vasospasm in the postoperative period and can detect about 51% of cases that has proven angiographic vasospasm [89]. In regard to comparing incidence of symptomatic vasospasm in endovascular versus microsurgical clipping, there is higher vasospasm reported in patients who have undergone clipping (25%) than those who have had a coiling (15%) procedure [90, 91]. Hyponatremia and high hematocrit are associated with higher occurrences of vasospasm. In most centers, oral administration of Nimodipine is used for prevention of vasospasm. There is evidence to suggest that it reduces the risk of DCI and poor clinical outcomes following aneurysmal SAH despite significant reduction in the incidence of angiographic vasospasm [92]. Patients need to be well hydrated with normal sodium level (135–145 meq/L) and hematocrit level of 35–50%. In cases of severe vasospasm with neurological deficits, patient may be subjected to hypertensive therapy and endovascular intraarterial spasmolytic administration of vasodilators, such as calcium channel blockers [64, 91, 93].

9.10.2 Hydrocephalus

Hydrocephalus in subarachnoid hemorrhage is quite variable and reported in about 50% of cases. It can be obstructive, communicating or a combination of both. In certain cases, patients present with acute hydrocephalus and undergo urgent ventriculostomy (external ventricular drain) [94]. About one-third of all patients who develops hydrocephalus, end up requiring permanent shunting (most commonly ventriculoperitoneal shunt) [95]. Some neurosurgeons have adopted fenestration of lamina terminalis as an adjunct, during a pterional approach, to treat the hydrocephalus, but its routine use has not been recommended [96]. There is no convincing evidence to suggest significant differences in risks of hydrocephalus between patients undergoing microsurgical clipping in comparison to those treated by endovascular coiling. Similarly, the duration of temporary CSF drainage for acute hydrocephalus has not been shown to increase the need for permanent CSF shunting procedure [64, 97].

9.10.3 Seizures

In the landmark International Subarachnoid Hemorrhage Trial (ISAT) [97], the incidence of seizures in the neurosurgical arm was 3.1% while in a recent review of literature, the prevalence of early (within 7 days) and delayed postoperative seizures are 2.3% and 5.5%, respectively [98]. There are no significant differences in risks of seizure in patient who have been treated for unruptured versus ruptured intracranial aneurysms [98]. There is significant variability in the use of prophylactic anti-epileptic drugs (AED) in the neurosurgical practice but in most centers, patients who are considered at higher risk or who have suspicion of subclinical seizures are given prophylactic AED for 7 days [64, 97, 99]. Higher risk patients are those who have associated intracerebral hematomas, age < 40 years, middle cerebral artery aneurysms and patients with poor clinical status. The American Heart Association SAH guidelines state that administration of prophylactic anticonvulsants may be considered in the immediate post-hemorrhagic period, although routine long-term treatment is not recommended [64].

9.10.4 Postoperative Pain

In subarachnoid hemorrhage patients who have undergone craniotomy for microsurgical clipping, pain is related to both surgical procedure as well as from presence of brain hemorrhage itself [100–102]. Most commonly, patients are given non-narcotic analgesics like acetaminophen and complemented with narcotic analgesics as per need. But the use of narcotic analgesics is associated with nausea, vomiting, sedation, and respiratory depression. Significant controversy exists in the literature about postoperative pain management in patients after craniotomy. Intravenous tramadol has been recommended in combination with narcotic pain medications [103]. In another comparative study for use of tramadol, codeine, and morphine, use of morphine was found superior to tramadol and codeine in relieving pain, as well as being associated with less episodes of nausea and vomiting [102]. Patient-controlled analgesia (PCA) with fentanyl is getting more commonly used in clinical practice as an effective strategy in getting pain relief and it is found to be safe and efficacious in randomized controlled trial for even complex approaches like posterior fossa and skull base cerebrovascular pathologies [104]. In clinical practice, a short-acting intravenous narcotic analgesic is given in immediate postoperative period for 24–48 h and then switched to oral analgesics medications [64]. The use of scalp block in reducing need for postoperative analgesics has also been claimed effective [101].

9.10.5 Mortality

The postoperative mortality rates reported after microsurgical clipping of ruptured aneurysm are quite variable, ranging from 11% to 26% [86, 87]. The death rate after aneurysmal clipping is multifactorial depending upon patient factor as well as related to quality of postoperative management. Patient factors include pre-existing clinical comorbidities, age, coagulopathy, chronic obstructive pulmonary diseases, and strokes [86, 87, 97]. While quality of management includes experience of operating surgeon, medical care facilities and institutional capabilities to provide and handle complex clinical conditions in a multidisciplinary setting [64, 87, 97]. In comparison to clipping, mortality associated with coiling for unruptured ($\leq$ 1%) and ruptured aneurysm is on lower side (9%) [87, 97].

9.11 Post-Clipping Remnants, Growth, and Recurrences

As early as in the 1960s, Drake et al. [105] emphasized the complete obliteration of aneurysm to avoid late sequelae. Despite advancement in microsurgical clipping adjuncts, the rate of aneurysm remnants after microsurgical clipping has been reported homogenously, in the range of 1–8% with a rebleeding rate from the remnants up to 3.7% [105–108]. More recent publications have reported higher, probably related to higher detection rates [108, 109]. Independent predictors for inadequate obliteration are topographic peculiarities (location, size, morphology, flow dynamics) and intraoperative rupture of aneurysm that may have influenced the effectiveness of aneurysm clip placement and reconstructive techniques. Interestingly, other factors like timing of surgery, surgeon's experience, and presence of acute subarachnoid bleed have no influence on incomplete obliteration. Other patient-specific factors (multiple intracranial aneurysms (IA), previous SAH, family history, smoking, hypertension) that are known to influence growth of unruptured IA likewise influence growth of IA remnants. Clip remnants may be left "intentionally" to preserve the perforators or a branch arising from the neck of aneurysms and sometime due the atherosclerotic/calcified wall of aneurysm neck that may impair the ability to place clip perfectly [108].

Clip remnants exhibit growth as high as 3.5–15% and this progression is independent of the duration of follow-up [107, 108]. One independent factor that correlates with the growth of aneurysm remnants is the age of the patient, as younger patients (<45 years) show significantly higher rate of progression of aneurysmal remnants. True recurrence of aneurysm after complete obliteration is extremely rare with annual incidence of 0.02–0.52% and mostly correlated with the fragility of the neck of aneurysm, noted at the time of clip application [106]. Management of the aneurysm remnants usually involves serial imaging follow-ups and any decision to treat depends on progression and feasibility to offer re-treatment options [109]. As reoperation with microsurgical clipping is usually anticipated to have higher postoperative complications, the usual course of treatment is to offer endovascular treatment for remnants as well as for recurrences following multidisciplinary consensus with endovascular team [110].

9.12 Future Prospects, Advances, and Innovations

Since the advent of clipping procedure over 200 years ago, the technological advances both in the field of cerebrovascular surgery, better understanding of vascular angioarchitecture due to improved details from the neuroimaging, improved knowledge about the neurovascular disease and complementary revolution in endovascular treatment strategies, aneurysm treatment has completely revolutionized [17, 18]. Recently, awake craniotomy (Conscious Surgery) has been touted as a game changer in microsurgical clipping to reduce morbidity, as it avails real-time intraoperative neurological assessment of patients when operating close to eloquent cerebral tissues [111]. In addition to aneurysm repair strategies, it is expected that there will be revolutionary advancements in the non-microsurgical treatment arena in the coming decades and it includes at least two upcoming platforms. First is the use of progenitor cell or regenerative medicine technologies that aim on cells, growth factors or in combination to assist in the repair of injured endothelial wall to heal the defect [112]. A second approach is the application of next-generation genome and transcriptome sequencing that utilizes the samples of patient aneurysms for identification of potential targets that are involved in the development of aneurysm [113, 114]. These approaches provide unprecedented insight into the biological pathways involved in endothelial cell damage, remodeling, and regeneration, and they can be harnessed for potential medical treatments [112–115].

9.13 Conclusions

Microsurgical clipping for ruptured intracranial aneurysm has gone through a significant historical revolution over the past two centuries and it continues to evolve. The knowledge of aneurysm formation, natural history, and understanding of perianeurysmal environment with highly detailed neuroimaging technologies have facilitated the cerebrovascular neurosurgeons to consolidate their operative skills and perform repair of aneurysms with improved safety and high standards of quality care. Cerebrovascular surgery has advanced as a highly subspecialized field with improved surgical corridors along with efficient utilization of microscope, aneurysm clips, and other microsurgical instruments. All these improvements in microsurgical techniques, advancements in medical technology and their detailed understanding along with clinical experience of cerebrovascular diseases has significantly reduced the complications and mortality with aneurysm clipping. The future of aneurysm treatments is expected to move in the direction of non-operative domains, based on regenerative medicine and next-generation genomic technology assisting in repair of defective endothelial wall.

Acknowledgements Thanks are extended to Dr. Mohammed Ben Husien[2] (Neurosurgery consultant) and Dr. Michael Amoo[2] (Neurosurgery specialist registrar).
[2]Beaumont Hospital, Dublin, Ireland

References

1. Hunter J. The works of John Hunter: with notes. London: Longman; 1835.
2. Cooper A. A case of aneurism of the carotid artery. Med Chir Trans. 1809;1:1.
3. Drake CG. Earlier times in aneurysm surgery. Clin Neurosurg. 1985;32:41–50.
4. Halsted WS. The partial occlusion of blood vessels especially of the abdominal aorta. Bull Johns Hopkins Hosp. 1905;14:345.
5. Selverstone B, White JC. A method for gradual occlusion of the internal carotid artery in the treatment of aneurysms. Proc New England Cardiovasc Soc. 1952;9:24.
6. Cushing HI. The control of bleeding in operations for brain tumors: with the description of silver "clips" for the occlusion of vessels inaccessible to the ligature. Ann Surg. 1911 Jul;54(1):1.
7. Dandy WE. Intracranial arterial aneurysms in the carotid canal: diagnosis and treatment. Arch Surg. 1942 Sep 1;45(3):335–50.
8. Dandy WE. Intracranial arterial aneurysms. Ithaca: Comstock Pub. Co.; 1944.
9. Moniz E. L'encephalographie arterielle, son importance dans la localisation des tumeurs cerebrales. Rev Neurol (Paris). 1927;2:72.
10. Kurze T. Microtechniques in neurological surgery. Neurosurgery. 1965 Jan 1;11(CN_suppl_1):128–37.
11. Sundt TM. Surgical technique for giant intracranial aneurysms. Neurosurg Rev. 1982 Dec 1;5(4):161–8.
12. Dolenc V. Direct microsurgical repair of intracavernous vascular lesions. J Neurosurg. 1983 Jun 1;58(6):824–31.
13. Spetzler RF, Selman W, Carter LP. Elective EC-IC bypass for unclippable intracranial aneurysms. Neurol Res. 1984 Mar 1;6(1–2):64–8.
14. Drake CG, Peerless SJ, Hernesniemi J. Surgery of vertebrobasilar aneurysms: London, Ontario experience on 1,767 patients. Springer-Verlag: New York; 1996. p. 221–48.
15. Yaşargi G. A legacy of microneurosurgery: memoirs, lessons, and axioms. Neurosurgery. 1999 Nov 1;45(5):1025–92.
16. Smith RR, Zubkov YN, Tarassoli Y. The history of aneurysm surgery. In: Cerebral aneurysms. New York: Springer; 1994. p. 1–9.
17. Lai LT, O'Neill AH. History, evolution, and continuing innovations of intracranial aneurysm surgery. World Neurosurg. 2017 Jun 1;102:673–81.
18. Peschillo S, Caporlingua A, Caporlingua F, Guglielmi G, Delfini R. Historical landmarks in the management of aneurysms and arteriovenous malformations of the central nervous system. World Neurosurg. 2016 Apr 1;88:661–71.
19. Suzuki J, Ohara H. Clinicopathological study of cerebral aneurysms: origin, rupture, repair, and growth. J Neurosurg. 1978 Apr 1;48(4):505–14.
20. Ferguson GG. Physical factors in the initiation, growth, and rupture of human intracranial saccular aneurysms. J Neurosurg. 1972 Dec 1;37(6):666–77.
21. Tateshima S, Murayama Y, Villablanca JP, Morino T, Nomura K, Tanishita K, Viñuela F. In vitro measurement of fluid-induced wall shear stress in unruptured cerebral aneurysms harbouring blebs. Stroke. 2003 Jan 1;34(1):187–92.
22. Yasargil MG. Microneurosurgery. Thierne. 1984;1:169–85.
23. Mower WR, Baraff LJ, Sneyd J. Stress distributions in vascular aneurysms: factors affecting risk of aneurysm rupture. J Surg Res. 1993 Aug 1;55(2):155–61.
24. Ruiz DS, Yilmaz H, Dehdashti AR, Alimenti A, De Tribolet N, Rüfenacht DA. The perianeurysmal environment: influence on saccular aneurysm shape and rupture. Am J Neuroradiol. 2006 Mar 1;27(3):504–12.
25. Kassell NF, Drake CG. Timing of aneurysm surgery. Neurosurgery. 1982 Apr 1;10(4):514–9.
26. Whitfield PC, Kirkpatrick P. Timing of surgery for aneurysmal subarachnoid haemorrhage. Cochrane Database Syst Rev. 2001;2:CD001697.
27. de Gans K, Nieuwkamp DJ, Rinkel GJ, Algra A. Timing of aneurysm surgery in subarachnoid hemorrhage: a systematic review of the literature. Neurosurgery. 2002 Feb 1;50(2):336–42.
28. Dorhout Mees SM, Molyneux AJ, Kerr RS, Algra A, Rinkel GJ. Timing of aneurysm treatment after subarachnoid hemorrhage: relationship with delayed cerebral ischemia and poor outcome. Stroke. 2012 Aug;43(8):2126–9.
29. Yaşargil MG. Microneurosurgery: principles, applications, and training. In: Practical handbook of neurosurgery. Vienna: Springer; 2009. p. 3–30.
30. Lougheed WM, Marshall BM. The diploscope in intracranial aneurysm surgery: results in 40 patients. Canadian journal of surgery. 1969 Jan;12(1):75.
31. Dandy WE. Intracranial aneurysm of the internal carotid artery: cured by operation. Ann Surg. 1938 May;107(5):654.
32. Yasargil MG, Vise WM, Bader DC. Technical adjuncts in neurosurgery. Surg Neurol. 1977 Nov;8(5):331–6.
33. Sugita K, Hirota T, Iguchi I, Mizutani T. Comparative study of the pressure of various aneurysm clips. J Neurosurg. 1976 Jun 1;44(6):723–7.
34. Louw DF, Asfora WT, Sutherland GR. A brief history of aneurysm clips. Neurosurg Focus. 2001 Aug 1;11(2):1–4.
35. McFadden JT. Magnetic resonance imaging and aneurysm clips: a review. J Neurosurg. 2012 Jul 1;117(1):1–1.
36. Chaddad-Neto F, Doria-Netto HL, Campos-Filho JM, Ribas ES, Ribas GC, Oliveira ED. Head positioning for anterior circulation aneurysms microsurgery. Arq Neuropsiquiatr. 2014 Nov;72(11):832–40.
37. Chaddad-Neto F, et al. The pterional craniotomy: tips and tricks. Arq Neuropsiquiatr. 2012;70:727–32.
38. Yaşargil MG, Reichman MV, Kubik S. Preservation of the frontotemporal branch of the facial nerve using the interfascial temporalis flap for pterional craniotomy: technical article. J Neurosurg. 1987 Sep 1;67(3):463–6.

39. Rhoton AL. Microsurgical anatomy of common aneurysm site. Clin Neurosurg. 1979;26:248–306.
40. Yasargil MG. Microsurgical pterional approach to the aneurysms of the basilar bifurcation. Surg Neurol. 1976;6:83–91.
41. Hernesniemi J, Ishii K, Niemelä M, Kivipelto L, Fujiki M, Shen H. Subtemporal approach to basilar bifurcation aneurysms: advanced technique and clinical experience. In: New trends of surgery for stroke and its perioperative management. Vienna: Springer; 2005. p. 31–8.
42. Rhoton AL Jr. The far-lateral approach and its transcondylar, supracondylar, and paracondylar extensions. Neurosurgery. 2000 Sep 1;47(suppl_3):S195–\\.
43. Welch BG, de Oliveira SR, White JA, Batjer HH. Technical principles of aneurysm clipping. In: Intracranial aneurysms. London: Academic Press; 2018 Jan 1. p. 207–32.
44. Samson D, Batjer HH, Gary B, Mootz L, Krippner WJ Jr, Meyer YJ, Allen BC. A clinical study of the parameters and effects of temporary arterial occlusion in the management of intracranial aneurysms. Neurosurgery. 1994 Jan 1;34(1):22–9.
45. Taylor CL, Selman WR, Kiefer SP, Ratcheson RA. Temporary vessel occlusion during intracranial aneurysm repair. Neurosurgery. 1996;39:893–905.
46. Lavine SD, Masri LS, Levy ML, Giannotta SL. Temporary occlusion of the middle cerebral artery in intracranial aneurysm surgery: time limitation and advantage of brain protection. J Neurosurg. 1997;87:817–24.
47. Tanabe J, Ishikawa T, Moroi J. Safe time duration for temporary middle cerebral artery occlusion in aneurysm surgery based on motor-evoked potential monitoring. Surg Neurol Int. 2017;8:79.
48. Malinova V, Schatlo B, Voit M, Suntheim P, Rohde V, Mielke D. The impact of temporary clipping during aneurysm surgery on the incidence of delayed cerebral ischemia after aneurysmal subarachnoid hemorrhage. J Neurosurg. 2017 Sep 15;129(1):84–90.
49. Greenberg IM. Self-retaining retractor and handrest system for neurosurgery. Neurosurgery. 1981 Feb 1;8(2):205–8.
50. Chaichana KL, Vivas-Buitrago T, Jackson C, Ehresman J, Olivi A, Bettegowda C, Quinones-Hinojosa A. The radiographic effects of surgical approach and use of retractors on the brain after anterior cranial fossa meningioma resection. World Neurosurg. 2018 Apr 1;112:e505–13.
51. Rosenørn J. Self-retaining brain retractor pressure during intracranial procedures. Acta Neurochir. 1987 Mar 1;85(1–2):17–22.
52. Bennett MH, Albin MS, Bunegin L, Dujovny MA, Hellstrom HA, Jannetta PJ. Evoked potential changes during brain retraction in dogs. Stroke. 1977 Jul;8(4):487–92.
53. Kashimura H, Ogasawara K, Kubo Y, Kakino S, Sasoh M, Takahashi H, Suzuki K, Ogawa A. Brain retraction technique using gelatin sponge in the subtemporal approach. Neurol Med Chir. 2008;48(3):143–6.
54. Spetzler RF, Sanai N. The quiet revolution: retractorless surgery for complex vascular and skull base lesions. J Neurosurg. 2012 Feb 1;116(2):291–300.
55. Sun H, Safavi-Abbasi S, Spetzler RF. Retractorless surgery for intracranial aneurysms. J Neurosurg Sci. 2016 Mar;60(1):54.
56. Kalani MY, Wanebo JE, Martirosyan NL, Nakaji P, Zabramski JM, Spetzler RF. A raised bar for aneurysm surgery in the endovascular era. J Neurosurg. 2017 May 1;126(5):1731–9.
57. Batjer HH, Samson DS. Retrograde suction decompression of giant paraclinoidal aneurysms. J Neurosurg. 1990 Aug 1;73(2):305–6.
58. Flores BC, White JA, Batjer HH, Samson DS. The 25th anniversary of the retrograde suction decompression technique (Dallas technique) for the surgical management of paraclinoid aneurysms: historical background, systematic review, and pooled analysis of the literature. J neurosurgery. 2018 Apr 1;1(aop):1–5.
59. Kimura T, Morita A, Nishimura K, Aiyama H, Itoh H, Fukaya S, Sora S, Ochiai C. Simulation of and training for cerebral aneurysm clipping with 3-dimensional models. Neurosurgery. 2009 Oct 1;65(4):719–26.
60. Tenjin H, Okano Y. Training model for cerebral aneurysm clipping. Interdiscip Neurosurg. 2017 Dec 1;10:114–8.
61. Spicer MA, van Velsen M, Caffrey JP, Apuzzo ML. Virtual reality neurosurgery: a simulator blueprint. Neurosurgery. 2004 Apr 1;54(4):783–98.
62. Caplan J, Naval N, Huang J, Tamargo RJ. Aneurysm surgery. In: Neurocritical care management of the neurosurgical patient. Philadelphia: Elsevier; 2017 Mar 30. p. 95–104.
63. Savardekar AR, Patra DP, Narayan V, Bollam P, Guthikonda B, Nanda A. Internal carotid artery bifurcation aneurysms: microsurgical strategies and operative nuances for different aneurysmal directions. Oper Neurosurg. 2018 Oct 1;15(4):386–94.
64. Connolly ES Jr, Rabinstein AA, Carhuapoma JR, Derdeyn CP, Dion J, Higashida RT, Hoh BL, Kirkness CJ, Naidech AM, Ogilvy CS, Patel AB. Guidelines for the management of aneurysmal subarachnoid hemorrhage: a guideline for healthcare professionals from the American Heart Association/American Stroke Association. Stroke. 2012 Jun;43(6):1711–37.
65. Bailes JE, Tantuwaya LS, Fukushima T, Schurman GW, Davis D, Bailes JE. Intraoperative microvascular Doppler sonography in aneurysm surgery. Neurosurgery. 1997 May 1;40(5):965–72.
66. Gilsbach JM. Intraoperative Doppler Sonography in Neurosurgery. New York: Springer-Verlag; 1983.
67. Bailes JE, Tantuwaya LS, Fukushima T, Schurman GW, Davis D, Bailes JE. Intraoperative microvascular Doppler sonography in aneurysm surgery. Neurosurgery. 1997 May 1;40(5):965–72.
68. Stendel R, Pietilä T, Al Hassan AA, Schilling A, Brock M. Intraoperative microvascular Doppler ultrasonography in cerebral aneurysm surgery. J Neurol Neurosurg Psychiatry. 2000 Jan 1;68(1):29–35.

69. Feindel W, Garretson H, Yamamoto YL, Perot P, Rumin N. Blood flow patterns in the cerebral vessels and cortex in man studied by intracarotid injection of radioisotopes and Coomassie blue dye. J Neurosurg. 1965 Jul 1;23(1):12–22.
70. Kuroiwa T, Kajimoto Y, Ohta T. Development and clinical application of near-infrared surgical microscope: preliminary report. Minim Invasive Neurosurg. 2001 Dec;44(04):240–2.
71. Raabe A, Beck J, Gerlach R, Zimmermann M, Seifert V. Near-infrared indocyanine green video angiography: a new method for intraoperative assessment of vascular flow. Neurosurgery. 2003 Jan 1;52(1):132–9.
72. Dashti R, Laakso A, Niemelä M, Porras M, Celik Ö, Navratil O, Romani R, Hernesniemi J. Application of microscope integrated indocyanine green video-angiography during microneurosurgical treatment of intracranial aneurysms: a review. In: Surgical Management of Cerebrovascular Disease. Vienna: Springer; 2010. p. 107–9.
73. Fischer G, Stadie A, Oertel JM. Near-infrared indocyanine green videoangiography versus microvascular Doppler sonography in aneurysm surgery. Acta Neurochir. 2010 Sep 1;152(9):1519–25.
74. Sharma M, Ambekar S, Ahmed O, Nixon M, Sharma A, Nanda A, Guthikonda B. The utility and limitations of intraoperative near-infrared indocyanine green videoangiography in aneurysm surgery. World Neurosurg. 2014 Nov 1;82(5):e607–13.
75. Macdonald RL, Wallace MC, Kestle JR. Role of angiography following aneurysm surgery. J Neurosurg. 1993 Dec 1;79(6):826–32.
76. Scheer N, Ghaznawi R, van Walderveen MA, Koot RW, Willems PW. Evaluation of the yield of post-clipping angiography and nationwide current practice. Acta Neurochir. 2019 Apr 1;161(4):783–90.
77. Batjer H, Samson D. Intraoperative aneurysmal rupture: incidence, outcome, and suggestions for surgical management. Neurosurgery. 1986 Jun 1;18(6):701–7.
78. Schramm J, Cedzich CC. Outcome and management of intraoperative aneurysm rupture. Surg Neurol. 1993 Jul 1;40(1):26–30.
79. Giannotta SL, Oppenheimer JH, Levy ML, Zelman V. Management of intraoperative rupture of aneurysm without hypotension. Neurosurgery. 1991 Apr 1;28(4):531–6.
80. Owall A, Gordon E, Lagerkranser M, Lindquist C, Rudehill A, Sollevi A. Clinical experience with adenosine for controlled hypotension during cerebral aneurysm surgery. Anesth Analg. 1987 Mar;66(3):229–34.
81. Nussbaum ES, Sebring LA, Ostanny I, Nelson WB. Transient cardiac standstill induced by adenosine in the management of intraoperative aneurysmal rupture: technical case report. Neurosurgery. 2000 Jul 1;47(1):240–3.
82. Bendok BR, Gupta DK, Rahme RJ, Eddleman CS, Adel JG, Sherma AK, Surdell DL, Bebawy JF, Koht A, Batjer HH. Adenosine for temporary flow arrest during intracranial aneurysm surgery: a single-center retrospective review. Neurosurgery. 2011 Oct 1;69(4):815–21.
83. Intarakhao P, Thiarawat P, Jahromi BR, Kozyrev DA, Teo MK, Choque-Velasquez J, Luostarinen T, Hernesniemi J. Adenosine-induced cardiac arrest as an alternative to temporary clipping during intracranial aneurysm surgery. J Neurosurg. 2017 Oct 27;129(3):684–90.
84. Meling TR, Lave A. What are the options for cardiac standstill during aneurysm surgery? A systematic review. Neurosurg Rev. 2019 Dec 1;42(4):843–52.
85. Elijovich L, Higashida RT, Lawton MT, Duckwiler G, Giannotta S, Johnston SC. Predictors and outcomes of intraprocedural rupture in patients treated for ruptured intracranial aneurysms: the CARAT study. Stroke. 2008 May 1;39(5):1501–6.
86. Bekelis K, Missios S, MacKenzie TA, Desai A, Fischer A, Labropoulos N, Roberts DW. Predicting inpatient complications from cerebral aneurysm clipping: the Nationwide inpatient sample 2005–2009. J Neurosurg. 2014 Mar 1;120(3):591–8.
87. Molyneux AJ, Kerr RS, Birks J, Ramzi N, Yarnold J, Sneade M, Rischmiller J. ISAT collaborators. Risk of recurrent subarachnoid haemorrhage, death, or dependence and standardised mortality ratios after clipping or coiling of an intracranial aneurysm in the international subarachnoid aneurysm trial (ISAT): long-term follow-up. Lancet Neurol. 2009 May 1;8(5):427–33.
88. Fisher CM, Roberson GH, Ojemann RG. Cerebral vasospasm with ruptured saccular aneurysm—the clinical manifestations. Neurosurgery. 1977 Nov 1;1(3):245–8.
89. Kolias AG, Sen J, Belli A. Pathogenesis of cerebral vasospasm following aneurysmal subarachnoid hemorrhage: putative mechanisms and novel approaches. J Neurosci Res. 2009 Jan;87(1):1–1.
90. Dehdashti AR, Mermillod B, Rufenacht DA, Reverdin A, de Tribolet N. Does treatment modality of intracranial ruptured aneurysms influence the incidence of cerebral vasospasm and clinical outcome? Cerebrovasc Dis. 2004;17(1):53–60.
91. Hofmann E, Marbacher S, Jakob SM, Takala J, Remonda L, Fandino J. Incidence of vasospasm, outcome, and quality of life after endovascular and surgical treatment of ruptured intracranial aneurysms: results of a single-center prospective study in Switzerland. ISRN Vasc Med. 2011 Aug;15:201.
92. Bederson JB, Connolly ES Jr, Batjer HH, Dacey RG, Dion JE, Diringer MN, et al. Guidelines for the management of aneurysmal subarachnoid hemorrhage: a statement for healthcare professionals from a special writing group of the stroke council. Am Heart Assoc Stroke. 2009;40(3):994–1025.
93. Wagner M, Steinbeis P, Güresir E, Hattingen E, de Rochemont RD, Weidauer S, Berkefeld J. Beyond delayed cerebral vasospasm: infarct patterns in patients with subarachnoid hemorrhage. Clin Neuroradiol. 2013 Jun 1;23(2):87–95.
94. van Gijn J, Hijdra A, Wijdicks EF, Vermeulen M, van Crevel H. Acute hydrocephalus after aneurysmal subarachnoid hemorrhage. J Neurosurg. 1985 Sep 1;63(3):355–62.

95. Dehdashti AR, Rilliet B, Rufenacht DA, de Tribolet N. Shunt-dependent hydrocephalus after rupture of intracranial aneurysms: a prospective study of the influence of treatment modality. J Neurosurg. 2004 Sep 1;101(3):402–7.
96. Tomasello F, d'Avella D, de Divitiis O. Does lamina terminalis fenestration reduce the incidence of chronic hydrocephalus after subarachnoid hemorrhage? Neurosurgery. 1999 Oct 1;45(4):827–32.
97. Molyneux AJ, Kerr RS, Yu LM, Clarke M, Sneade M, Yarnold JA, Sandercock P. International subarachnoid aneurysm trial (ISAT) collaborative group. International subarachnoid aneurysm trial (ISAT) of neurosurgical clipping versus endovascular coiling in 2143 patients with ruptured intracranial aneurysms: a randomised comparison of effects on survival, dependency, seizures, rebleeding, subgroups, and aneurysm occlusion. Lancet. 2005 Sep 3;366(9488):809–17.
98. Raper DM, Starke RM, Komotar RJ, Allan R, Connolly ES Jr. Seizures after aneurysmal subarachnoid hemorrhage: a systematic review of outcomes. World Neurosurg. 2013 May 1;79(5–6):682–90.
99. Dewan MC, Mocco J. Current practice regarding seizure prophylaxis in aneurysmal subarachnoid hemorrhage across academic centers. J Neurointervent Surg. 2015 Feb 1;7(2):146–9.
100. Gottschalk A, Berkow LC, Stevens RD, Mirski M, Thompson RE, White ED, Weingart JD, Long DM, Yaster M. Prospective evaluation of pain and analgesic use following major elective intracranial surgery. J Neurosurg. 2007 Feb 1;106(2):210–6.
101. Hwang JY, Bang JS, Oh CW, Joo JD, Park SJ, Do SH, Yoo YJ, Ryu JH. Effect of scalp blocks with levobupivacaine on recovery profiles after craniotomy for aneurysm clipping: a randomized, double-blind, and controlled study. World Neurosurg. 2015 Jan 1;83(1):108–13.
102. Sudheer PS, Logan SW, Terblanche C, Ateleanu B, Hall JE. Comparison of the analgesic efficacy and respiratory effects of morphine, tramadol and codeine after craniotomy. Anaesthesia. 2007 Jun;62(6):555–60.
103. Rahimi SY, Alleyne CH, Vernier E, Witcher MR, Vender JR. Postoperative pain management with tramadol after craniotomy: evaluation and cost analysis. J Neurosurg. 2010 Feb 1;112(2):268–72.
104. Morad A, Winters B, Stevens R, White E, Weingart J, Yaster M, Gottschalk A. The efficacy of intravenous patient-controlled analgesia after intracranial surgery of the posterior fossa: a prospective, randomized controlled trial. Anesth Analg. 2012 Feb 1;114(2):416–23.
105. Drake CG, Vanderlinden RG. The late consequences of incomplete surgical treatment of cerebral aneurysms. J Neurosurg. 1967 Sep 1;27(3):226–38.
106. Ebina K, Suzuki M, Andoh A, Saitoh K, Iwabuchi T. Recurrence of cerebral aneurysm after initial neck clipping. Neurosurgery. 1982 Dec 1;11(6):764–8.
107. Feuerberg I, Lindquist C, Lindqvist M, Steiner L. Natural history of postoperative aneurysm rests. J Neurosurg. 1987 Jan 1;66(1):30–4.
108. Sindou M, Acevedo JC, Turjman F. Aneurysmal remnants after microsurgical clipping: classification and results from a prospective angiographic study (in a consecutive series of 305 operated intracranial aneurysms). Acta Neurochir. 1998 Nov 1;140(11):1153–9.
109. Burkhardt JK, Chua MH, Weiss M, Do AS, Winkler EA, Lawton MT. Risk of aneurysm residual regrowth, recurrence, and de novo aneurysm formation after microsurgical clip occlusion based on follow-up with catheter angiography. World Neurosurg. 2017 Oct 1;106:74–84.
110. Moon JU, Koh JS, Kim TS, Kim GK, Rhee BA, Lim YJ. Treatment of remnant aneurysms previously treated with endovascular coiling or surgical clipping. J Korean Soc Intravasc Neurosurg. 2007;2(2):41–7.
111. Abdulrauf SI, Vuong P, Patel R, Sampath R, Ashour AM, Germany LM, Lebovitz J, Brunson C, Nijjar Y, Dryden JK, Khan MQ. "Awake" clipping of cerebral aneurysms: report of initial series. J Neurosurg. 2017 Aug 1;127(2):311–8.
112. Adibi A, Sen A, Mitha AP. Cell therapy for intracranial aneurysms: a review. World Neurosurg. 2016 Feb 1;86:390–8.
113. Yasuno K, Bilguvar K, Bijlenga P, Low SK, Krischek B, Auburger G, Simon M, Krex D, Arlier Z, Nayak N, Ruigrok YM. Genome-wide association study of intracranial aneurysm identifies three new risk loci. Nat Genet. 2010 May;42(5):420.
114. Farlow JL, Lin H, Sauerbeck L, Lai D, Koller DL, Pugh E, Hetrick K, Ling H, Kleinloog R, Van Der Vlies P, Deelen P. Lessons learned from whole exome sequencing in multiplex families affected by a complex genetic disorder, intracranial aneurysm. PLoS One. 2015;10(3):e0121104.
115. Liu D, Han L, Wu X, Yang X, Zhang Q, Jiang F. Genome-wide microRNA changes in human intracranial aneurysms. BMC Neurol. 2014 Dec 1;14(1):188.

Complications and Critical Care Management of Aneurysmal Subarachnoid Hemorrhage

10

Adel E. Ahmed Ganaw,
Sohel Mohamed Gamal Ahmed, Moad Ehfeda,
and Sirajeddin Belkhair

10.1 Introduction

Aneurysmal subarachnoid hemorrhage (aSAH) is a devastating neurovascular disease which is associated with high morbidity and mortality. It can have profound impact on the brain and other organs. Although the management strategies improved significantly in the last 30 years, the 30-day mortality and before admission death remain high, around 35% and 15%, respectively. Mortality and morbidity outcomes following aSAH largely depends on the severity of initial insult and the complications that might follow the insult. SAH patients are normally managed by multiciliary team including neurosurgeons, intensivists, interventional neuroradiologist, and anesthesiologists in an intensive care unit (ICU). Their course in the ICU ranges from a few days to a few weeks and repeatedly accompanied by neurological and non-neurological complications. Neurological complications include re-bleeding, delayed cerebral ischemia, hydrocephalus, brain edema, and seizures while non-neurological complications are cardiac complications, electrolyte disturbances, fever, hyperglycemia, anemia, and deep venous thrombosis. Treating clinicians must grasp the pathophysiology, recognition, risk factors, and therapeutic options of these complications [1, 2].

A. E. A. Ganaw (✉) · S. M. G. Ahmed · M. Ehfeda
Anesthesia, Perioperative Medicine and Critical Care Department, Hamad General Hospital, Hamad Medical Corporation, Doha, Qatar
e-mail: aganaw@hamad.qa; SAhmed65@hamad.qa; MEhfeda@hamad.qa

S. Belkhair
Neurosurgery Department, Hamad General Hospital, Hamad Medical Corporation, Doha, Qatar

Neurosurgery Department, Weill Cornell Medical College, Ar-Rayyan, Qatar

Neurosurgery Department, Michigan State University, East Lansing, MI, USA
e-mail: SBelkhair@hamad.qa

10.2 Complications Associated with SAH

Complications of subarachnoid hemorrhage can be divided into neurological and non-neurological complications.

10.2.1 Neurological Complications

Re-bleeding, cerebral vasospasm, hydrocephalus, and seizures are the most important neurological complications of aSAH. The high rates of mortality and morbidity after aneurysmal subarachnoid hemorrhage are mainly due to neurological complications.

A. E. A. Ganaw et al. (eds.), *Management of Subarachnoid Hemorrhage*,
https://doi.org/10.1007/978-3-030-81333-8_10

10.2.1.1 Re-bleeding

Re-bleeding following aSAH is one of the most devastating neurological complications of SAH. It is associated with very high mortality and morbidity, especially if it occurs in the first 12 h after the initial insult, the mortality rate may reach 50–70%. In the first 24 h, the risk of re-bleeding ranges between 4 and 13%. Early securing of ruptured aneurysm by either clipping or coiling significantly reduces the risk of re-bleeding. Rebleeding occurs more frequently within the first 6 hours after initial bleed. Some factors associated with rebleeding are non-modifiable, making it impossible to completely eliminate this complication [1–3].

Risk Factors of Re-bleeding

No doubt, knowing the risk factors of re-bleeding is very important for prioritizing the surgical management strategies and improving the outcome of SAH patients. The following are the most important risk factors:

Amount of Subarachnoid Blood on Initial Non-contrast CT Head

The modified Fisher grade of 3 or 4 is one of the strongest predictors of re-bleeding within first 24 h post-ictus. It is independent of patient's clinical status as evaluated by the World Federation of Neurosurgery score at admission. The amount of the blood measured by mFisher scale on initial CT scan is an indicator of the defect size and stability of the damaged aneurysm wall, regardless of the patient's neurological status [3].

Poor Neurological Status on Admission

There is a significant association between rate of re-bleeding and poor Hunt–Hess grade which have been reported in large number of studies. Guo L et al. reported that the incidence of re-bleeding was low in patients with good Hunt–Hess grades (I–III) in comparison with those with poor Hunt–Hess grades (IV–V) [3].

Aneurysmal Factors (Size, Location, Total Number)

Aneurysm larger than 10 mm is independent risk factor of re-bleeding. Guo et al. found that when the aneurysm is larger than 10 mm, bleeding was 1.624-fold higher compared to an aneurysm less than 10 mm [3].

Furthermore, posterior cerebral circulation aneurysms are at higher rate of re-bleeding than anterior cerebral circulation aneurysms.

Total number of aneurysms in angiography of patients who present with one ruptured aneurysm is strongly associated with re-bleeding. Although there is no clear explanation of this association, it may be due to high fragility of cerebral blood vessels causing multiple aneurysms and increased risk of re-bleeding of ruptured aneurysms [4].

High Blood Pressure (More than 160 mmHg)

Systolic blood pressure (SBP) more than 160 mmHg is independent risk factor of re-bleeding. It is presumed that the fibrin cloth formed over the ruptured aneurysm during the early stages of SAH is very fragile, therefore the significant increase of transmural pressure may lead to rupture of the fibrin clot and re-bleeding [3, 5].

Patient Age

Age is considered as independent risk factor of re-bleeding and poor outcome. Lanzino et al. reported that the rate of re-bleeding was significantly high in patients older than 70 years, it reached up to 16.4%, while the rate of re-bleeding in the youngest age group was only 4.5% [6].

Angiography within 6 h After Initial SAH

Digital subtraction angiography (DSA) within 6 h of ictus has been considered to be a risk factor for re-bleeding. The incidence of the re-bleeding when angiography performed within 6 h of initial insult may reach 3.3%. Re-bleeding may result from sudden increase in intra-atrial pressure during contrast injection. In one study, internal aneurysmal pressure was measured during cerebral angiography, contrast injection was found to lead to a sudden increase in intra-aneurysmal pressure of 5–23 mmHg in the absence of fluctuations in blood pressure [7, 8].

Sentinel Headache Preceding SAH

Sentinel headache (SH) is an intense secondary headache, sudden onset, persistent at least for 1-h, preceding SAH by days or weeks. It is an indicator of blood leak from fragile aneurysms. Beck et al. reported that the history of SH was associated with a significant increase in incidence of re-bleeding in unsecured aneurysm [4].

Longer Interval from Ictus to Admission

Delay in admission, blood pressure control, and securing of aneurysm are strongly associated with re-bleeding. Park et al. revealed that immediate intervention (median time from admission to start of aneurysm repair 3 h) was associated with significant decrease in re-bleeding risk and clinical outcome [9].

Ventriculostomy Before Aneurysmal Treatment

Insertion of external CSF drainage may cause sudden changes in transmural pressure over the already ruptured and weak aneurysm wall increasing risk of re-bleeding [9–11].

Coagulopathy

Coagulopathy may interfere with hemostasis and cloth formation leading to increased risk of re-bleeding.

Pathophysiology of Re-bleeding

There are many theories have been suggested based on experimental studies. Change of transmural pressure gradient theory (TMPG) is the most important theory. The aneurysm's transmural pressure gradient (TMPG) is equal to the pressure within the aneurysm (arterial blood pressure) minus the pressure outside/around the aneurysm (ICP), i.e. TMP = MAP-ICP. Sudden increase in arterial pressure or decrease ICP leads to an increase of TMPG and aneurysmal rupture. Therefore the balance between intra-atrial and external pressure on the arterial wall is mandatory to maintain integrity of the initial clot after the initial aneurysmal rupture [12].

Diagnosis

Diagnosis of re-bleeding based on new clinical manifestations and new radiological changes. The clinical manifestations range from a mild increase of headache to coma. Most patients with re-bleeding complain of an abrupt increase in headache intensity along with deterioration in GCS score. However, some patients present with loss of consciousness after a convulsion or appearance of new neurological deficit. Brain (CT) scans are indicated in all patients with new neurological manifestations and compared with admission CT study to confirm the re-bleeding. Sometimes diagnosis of re-bleeding is challenging if it occurs in pre-hospital stage, before the initial CT scan has not been done and patients has not properly assessed by emergency physicians [13].

Prevention of Re-bleeding

Early Obliteration of the Aneurysm

Early securing of the aneurysm is the treatment of choice to prevent re-bleeding. The American Stroke Association (ASA) and the European Stroke Organisation (ESO) recommend securing the aneurysm as soon as feasibly possible, preferably within 72 hours. The adoption of these recommendations in clinical practice varies among neurosurgical centers. While some centers consider aSAH as an emergency and advocate securing the aneurysm as soon as diagnosed, others prefer to intervene during the daytime only. Obviously, early obliteration of the aneurysm avoids the possible administration of antifibrinolytic medications which may increase the risk of delayed cerebral ischemia and thrombosis. Phillips et al. reported securing of ruptured aneurysm within first 24 h (ultra-early) post-ictal was associated with improved clinical outcome compared with securing the aneurysm after 24 h (Table 10.1) [5, 10, 14].

Blood Pressure Control

Although there is no strong evidence to determine blood pressure extreme, there is general settlement that the acute hypertension in aSAH patients with unsecured aneurysm should be

Table 10.1 Medical measures recommended by AHA/ASA to prevent re-bleeding of aSAH [10] (Courtesy from Dr Adel E. Ahmed Ganaw)

AHA/ASA guidelines 2012	Level of evidence
1. Between the time of aSAH symptom onset and aneurysm obliteration, blood pressure should be controlled with a titratable agent to balance the risk of stroke, hypertension-related re-bleeding, and maintenance of cerebral perfusion pressure	Class I; Level of evidence B
2. The magnitude of blood pressure control to reduce the risk of re-bleeding has not been established, but a decrease in systolic blood pressure to <160 mmHg is reasonable	Class IIa; Level of evidence C
3. For patients with an unavoidable delay in obliteration of aneurysm, a significant risk of re-bleeding, and no compelling medical contraindications, short-term (<72 h) therapy with tranexamic acid or aminocaproic acid is reasonable to reduce the risk of early aneurysm re-bleeding	Class IIa; Level of evidence B

controlled till the aneurysm secured to avoid re-bleeding. However, post securing the aneurysm by clipping or coiling, tight blood pressure may increase the risk of cerebral ischemia. It looks acceptable but without strong evidence to suspend all antihypertensive medications that the patients were taking, and treat hypertension only when it is extremely high. It is extremely hard to set limits for blood pressure extreme, because extreme varies between patients and it is affected by many factors such as previous blood pressure, cardiac disease, patient age, and other factors. The management of high blood pressure in acute setting (before securing the aneurysm) after aSAH is still debatable due to the lack of evidence from randomized controlled trial. Data from observational studies propose that aggressive management of blood pressure reduces the risk of re-bleeding, however, at the expense of an increase in secondary ischemia. Expert opinion suggests starting with short active intravenous titratable antihypertensive medications when systolic blood pressure more than 160 mmHg. Nicardipine is short-acting calcium channel blocker, used for smooth control of blood pressure**.** Nicardipine infusion should start with 2.5–5 mg/h, with increase 2.5 mg/h every 15 min. The infusion should not exceed 15 mg/h. Clevidipine, a very short-acting calcium channel blocker, is another option for acute control of hypertension, but data for aSAH are lacking at this time. Labetalol is non-selective beta blocker, commonly used for blood pressure control with intracranial hemorrhage as it has no effect on ICP (Table 10.1) [5, 10].

Short Course of Antifibrinolytic Medications

In patients who are at high risk of rebleeding and whom the delay in securing the aneurysm is unavoidable, short-course therapy with tranexamic acid or aminocaproic acid (start at diagnosis; continued till aneurysm secured or up to 72 h post ictus, whichever is earlier) is advisable provided there is no medical contraindication to decrease the risk of early re-bleeding [14]. Antifibrinolytic therapy should be stopped at least 2 h before coiling of the aneurysm. Continue administration of antifibrinolytic therapy for more than 72 h exposes patients to side effects of therapy when jeopardy of re-bleeding is significantly decreased and should be avoided. DVT is the most important side effect of prolonged course of antifibrinolytic therapy especially in patients who have other DVT risk factors, therefore they should have close screening for DVT. All antifibrinolytic therapies have not been approved by US Food and Drug Administration (FDA) for prevention of re-bleeding (Table 10.1) [2, 5, 10, 15].

10.2.1.2 Vasospasm, Delayed Cerebral Ischemia (DCI)

Cerebral ischemia is considered the worst subacute complications of aSAH, affecting almost a third of patients surviving the initial insult. It usually occurs between the 4th and 10th day after the initial hemorrhage. The most common clinical features of cerebral ischemia are focal neurological deficits such as aphasia, hemiparesis or a drop in level of consciousness. Occasionally, cerebral ischemia is reversible but may progress to cerebral infarction leading to severe neurological deficits and even death. Cerebral ischemia and neurological deficits are usually associated with angiographic narrowing of cerebral blood vessels. However, both cerebral ischemia and angiographic narrowing may occur independently of each other [2, 16].

Furthermore, there is no direct association between the severity of angiographic vasospasm and clinical manifestations of cerebral ischemia. Some aSAH patients develop DCI despite moderate vasospasm, while others who have significant angiographic vasospasm are might stay asymptomatic. Several factors other than vasospasm, such as impairment of collateral circulation, variations in tolerance cerebral ischemia and genetic susceptibility, contribute to DCI and cerebral infarction acquirement. Therefore, vasospasm refers to the luminal narrowing of large cerebral blood arteries following aSAH confirmed by either radiographic images such as CT angiography, MRA, DSA or ultrasonography (TCD). This narrowing may impair cerebral perfusion and oxygen delivery, causing cerebral infarction or ischemia. Generally, cerebral vasospasm starts on the third day after aneurysm rupture, though early vasospasm has been reported. The most significant degree of vasospasm occurs between the 5th and 14th day after initial insult and resolves spontaneously after 21 days [2, 16].

Delayed cerebral ischemia (DCI) refers to a drop in the GCS by 2 points either on the total score or on one of its components (Eye, motor on either side, verbal) or occurrence of focal neurological deficit such as hemiparesis, aphasia, hemianopia, and apraxia and worsening headache. This should continue at least for an hour, it is not apparent straightaway after aneurysm securing and cannot be explained by other causes, for instance, medications, seizures, metabolic derangement, sepsis, re-bleeding, and hydrocephalus [16].

These clinical manifestations may resolve spontaneously or after treatment. However, it may lead to cerebral infarction.

Cerebral infarction refers to the presence of cerebral infarction on radiological investigations (brain CT scan or MRI) within 6 weeks post-ictus, or on the last CT scan or MRI made prior to death within 6 weeks or confirmed at autopsy and not reported on CT scan or MRI within first 48 h post early securing of a cerebral aneurysm, as well as not related to other reasons such as surgical clipping or coiling [2, 16].

Risk Factors

The pathophysiology of cerebral vasospasm and delayed cerebral ischemia is exceptionally complicated, not yet fully understood. Therefore, recognizing risk factors and markers of cerebral vasospasm and delayed cerebral ischemia is essential for better understanding, prediction and timely effective management. Many factors have been investigated for possible correlation with cerebral vasospasm, such as age, hypertension, diabetes mellitus, smoking, gender, and heart disease [17].

Age

There are contradicting data regarding the association of a patient's age with cerebral vasospasm. Generally, younger age is considered as a predictor of symptomatic cerebral vasospasm. Furthermore, vasospasm in young SAH patients is usually more severe and necessitate more aggressive interventions than vasospasm in elderly patients. Stiffens of the cerebral blood vessels in the elderly population may explain low vasospasm risk in elderly patients. However, the elderly are more susceptible to cerebral infarction as their brains have less tolerance for vascular narrowing [17, 18].

Gender

Although female gender is relatively considered as risk factor for aSAH, most studies showed no association between gender and occurrence or severity of cerebral vasospasm [19].

Cigarette Smoking

There are conflicting data regarding the correlation of cigarette smoking with cerebral vasospasm and DCI. Some studies reported a strong association between cigarette smoking and severe cerebral vasospasm and DCI, while nine studies found no association. Smoking may cause arteriopathy and make patients less tolerant of cerebral ischemia [17].

Diabetes Mellitus

Dumont et al. showed that longstanding preexisting diabetes mellitus in aSAH patients is an independent risk factor for developing symptomatic vasospasm, despite adequate glycemic control. The possible explanation is that the presence of endothelial and muscularis dysfunction of vessels' wall due to longstanding microvascular disease. Moreover, hypoglycemia is considered by some researchers as a risk factor for cerebral vasospasm and DCI [20].

Initial Loss of Consciousness

Hop et al. reported that the length of initial unconsciousness following aneurysm rupture was a strong predictor of cerebral vasospasm and DCI [21].

Hypertension

Most studies found no correlation between cerebral vasospasm and pre-existing hypertension. However, longstanding hypertension may cause arteriopathy. Therefore, cerebral vasospasm in hypertensive patients is poorly tolerated and associated with poor outcome [17].

Severity of aSAH Clot on CT Scan

The amount of subarachnoid blood detected by the initial CT scan following aneurysm rupture is the most potent predictor of vasospasm occurrence. However, few studies could not find a significant association between cerebral vasospasm and radiological grading of SAH. Fisher et al. reported a strong association between thick cisternal clot and cerebral vasospasm. Fisher scale and recently developed modified Fisher scales are most commonly used by clinicians as a significant predictor for vasospasm. Several techniques (lumbar drain, intracisternal and intrathecal lysis) to reduce the amount of subarachnoid blood or to facilitate clearance of blood clot from basal cisterns, have been investigated with variable outcomes [17, 19].

Electrolyte Disturbance

Clinical studies showed a significant correlation between cerebral vasospasm incidence and some electrolyte disturbance, especially sodium and magnesium. Van den Bergh et al. proposed that hypomagnesemia following rupture of cerebral aneurysm is a risk factor for cerebral vasospasm and DCI. Administration of magnesium might be worthy to reduce the risk of cerebral vasospasm. Furthermore, most studies found no association between serum potassium, urea nitrogen, liver enzymes, lactate dehydrogenase, and creatine phosphokinase and development of cerebral vasospasm [2, 22].

Myocardial Dysfunction

Myocardial dysfunction occurs in almost half of patients with aSAH. It ranges from mild elevation in cardiac biomarkers, electrocardiogram (ECG) changes to recognizable clinical and echocardiographic abnormalities. Numerous studies reported that elevation of cardiac troponin I, brain natriuretic peptide (BNP), creatine kinase MB, left ventricular hypertrophy (LVH) on ECG, severe left ventricular dysfunction (Ejection fraction less than 40%), and regional wall motion abnormalities on the echocardiography were associated with severe cerebral vasospasm, DCI, and poor outcome [2, 17].

Diagnosis of DCI

Close neurological monitoring of SAH patients is crucial for early diagnosis and treatment of reversible causes of neurological deterioration. The neurological insult can be caused by DCI, hypoxia, sepsis, seizures, hypoxia, metabolic disturbance, re-bleeding, and hydrocephalus. Hence, frequent neurological evaluations, availability of urgent neuro-imaging and EEG are standards in treatment of aSAH. Neurological monitoring approach to early detection of DCI contains three components: clinical, radiological, and physiological monitoring [2].

Clinical Monitoring

Frequent neurological examinations is crucial for detecting new neurological deficits caused by DCI or cerebral infarction. Any worsening change in neurological examination should trigger for further investigations and interventions that may vary according to the patient's clinical condition. Unfortunately, clinical examinations alone are not enough to detect all ischemic events, especially in poor obtunded, sedated, and mechanically ventilated patients. Shimonda et al. found that MRI detected cerebral infarction in 23% of patients with aSAH which were not recognized clinically. Furthermore, Schmidt et al. reported that the brain CT scan identified asymptomatic infarction in 20% of patients with aSAH. It was mostly reported in comatose patients. Therefore, supplementary radiological investigations or physiological monitoring or both should be regularly performed for SAH patients during the high-risk period (5–14 day post-ictus) even in the absence of clinical evidence of DCI [2].

Radiological Monitoring

Radiological imaging including digital subtraction angiography (DSA), Computed tomogram angiography (CTA), Computed tomogram perfusion (CTP), and MR angiogram should be considered to diagnose, assess the severity, location, and complications of cerebral vasospasm and DCI [2].

Digital Subtraction Angiography (DSA)

DSA is considered the gold standard for the diagnosis of cerebral arterial narrowing. It is accurate and permits immediate intervention by balloon angioplasty and or intra-arterial injection of vasodilators. However, it is a slightly invasive technique, requires general anesthesia, has a limited role in assessment sufficiency of perfusion to gather cerebral metabolic demands and is associated with slightly increased risk of cerebral ischemia and stroke [2].

Computed Tomogram Angiography (CTA)

CTA is a noninvasive investigation to diagnose vasospasm in patients with aSAH. It directly visualizes arterial narrowing caused by cerebral vasospasm. Compared with DSA, it requires less human resources and is easily accessible and can be performed immediately after a non-contrast brain CT scan. Numerous studies compared CTA with DSA and reported the tendency of CTA to overestimate the degree of stenosis. CTA has a specificity of 96% and a sensitivity of 64% in evaluating the severity and location of cerebral vasospasm. It could be used as a screening tool to limit using DSA in the emergency setting when immediate management decisions are required and in unstable patients to undergo DSA [2].

Computed Tomogram Perfusion (CTP)

CTP assesses brain perfusion hemodynamics, is noninvasive, can be performed repeatedly, and can easily be incorporated into the standard CT/CTA protocol that is classically performed for aSAH patients with suspected vasospasm. CTP uses standard CT equipment and requires only dedicated post-processing software to generate perfusion maps of the brain within 5 min of data acquisition. Unlike TCD, CTP can assess blood flow throughout the whole territory perfused by a cerebral artery. Quantitative CTP maps have been validated by comparison with xenon CT20 and positron-emission tomography (PET) studies [21]. CTP plays a role in the early management of adult patients with acute stroke and other cerebrovascular disorders [22–24] because it affords insight into the relative areas of cerebral infarction and the associated ischemic penumbra. However, experience with CTP in vasospasm following SAH is limited. To date, only one small series has been reported [25], and there has been no systematic comparison with DSA or TCD results [23].

CTP affords some brain perfusion measurements, which could improve the predictive value of multi-modality CT (non-contrast + CTA + CTP) for assessment and diagnosis of DCI. CTP finding of delayed mean transit time (MTT) >6.4 s in conjunction with arterial narrowing on CTA was more accurate in predicting the need for endovascular intervention for vasospasm. However, all published CTP studies are small (less than 100 patients), and CTP does not currently evaluate the posterior fossa well. There were too few MR perfusion reports to consider this as a proper DCI monitoring tool at this time [2, 20, 23].

Physiological Monitoring

Transcranial Doppler ultrasonography (TCD), electroencephalography (EEG), brain tissue oxygen monitoring, cerebral microdialysis, cerebral blood flow thermal diffusion (TD-CBF) monitoring, and near-infrared spectroscopy are physiological monitoring modalities for cerebral vasospasm and DCI [2].

Transcranial Doppler (TCD)

Transcranial Doppler is an ideal surveillance tool to detect cerebral vasospasm in symptomatic patients with aSAH and patients with poor neurological status when clinical suspicion of cerebral aneurysm is unreliable. Cerebral vasospasm in patients with SAH is a dynamic phenomenon that may worsen or improve over time. Thus, bedside TCD is considered as the most appropriate tool for monitoring of cerebral vasospasm in comparison with DSA, CTA or CTP which they cannot be used daily for monitoring patients with SAH, as they are invasive tools, requiring administration of contrast and transferring of critically ill patients to angiography suits. Besides, in contrast to TCD, they are static tools and give snapshot information on the disease process. The AHA/ASA guidelines on the management of aneurysmal subarachnoid hemorrhage (2012) recommend using TCD as a reliable noninvasive tool to monitor the development of cerebral vasospasm in patients with aSAH (Class II a, Level) [23].

TCD probe (2 MHz) is fixed in a headset or applied manually in the region of acoustic windows. Acoustic windows are regions of the skull, either thin bone or foramina where ultrasound waves can be transmitted to the cerebral circulation. There are four acoustic windows (transtemporal, transorbital, suboccipital, and submandibular windows) (Fig. 10.1) [23].

The calculated flow velocity is directly proportional in milliliters per minute to the amount of blood flowing through the artery and inversely proportional to the square of the vessel's diameter. Vasospasm narrows the diameter of blood vessels and increases flow velocity by assuming continuous flow. Low (<120 cm/s) or very high (>200 cm/s) middle cerebral artery flow velocity reliably indicates the presence or absence of clinically significant cerebral vasospasm. The intermediate velocities (120–199 cm/s) are unreliable and inconclusive for determining significant angiographic cerebral vasospasm [24].

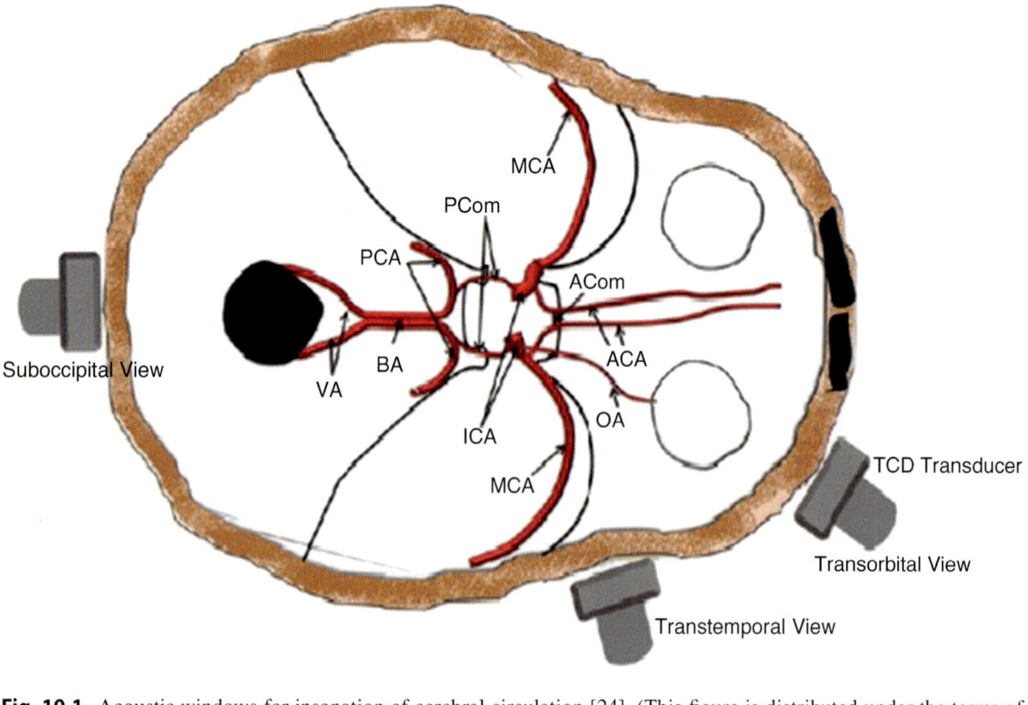

Fig. 10.1 Acoustic windows for insonation of cerebral circulation [24]. (This figure is distributed under the terms of the Creative Commons 4.0 License)

Table 10.2 Grading of the severity of MCA vasospasm using LR [24] (This table is distributed under the terms of the Creative Commons 4.0 License)

Degree of MCA vasospasm	MCA MFV (cm/s)	LR
Mild	120–149	3–6
Moderate	150–199	3–6
Sever	>200	>6

TCD is used to calculate the Lindegaard ratio (LR), which is the ratio between mean flow velocity of the middle cerebral artery (MCA MFV) and mean flow velocity of the ipsilateral extracranial proximal internal carotid artery (ICA MFV). LR plays a vital role in grading vasospasm as well as in distinguishing between hyperemia and vasospasm (Table 10.2). In patients with hyperemia, the mean blood flow velocity increases in both ICA and MCA; therefore, LR is less than 3. While in cerebral vasospasm, mean blood flow velocity in MCA is much higher than that of ICA, and subsequently, LR is greater than 6 [24].

TCD has several significant limitations. It helps in recognition vasospasm with only 67% specificity in comparison with DSA. Vasopressor may affect the measurements of TCD, resulting in false-positive vasospasm. Sensitivity and specificity of TCD may vary significantly, depending on the skills and capability of the operative. Furthermore, about 15% of patients do not have a temporal acoustic window that permits accurate TCD measurements. TCD is not reliable in detecting anterior cerebral artery (ACA) and posterior cerebral artery (PCA) vasospasm [24].

Prevention of Delayed Cerebral Ischemia

Although DCI prevention has been studied extensively for the last few decades, most studies have been disappointing and currently only limited treatment choices are available to reduce the risk of delayed cerebral ischemia (Table 10.3) [1].

Nimodipine

Nimodipine is a dihydropyridine L-type calcium channel blocker is the only medication recommended for aSAH by the American Heart Association (AHA), Neurocritical Care Society (NCS), and European guidelines. It seems to improve the long-term outcome in patients with poor-grade aSAH. British aneurysm nimodipine trial reported that oral nimodipine 60 mg four hourly for 21 days was well tolerated, reduced the risk of cerebral infarction, death and improved neurological outcome in patients with subarachnoid hemorrhage. Currently, this regimen is recommended and widely used. Nimodipine dose may be divided to 30 mg two hourly or reduced to 30 mg four hourly if associated with hypotension. Adequate cerebral perfusion (systolic blood pressure 130–150 mmHg) takes priority over nimodipine. Nimodipine should be suspended if perfusion pressure cannot be maintained. Intravenous nimodipine is not superior to an oral formulation. It is associated with hemodynamic instability, particularly in hypovolemic or cardiac patients. It may be considered an instance of enteral malabsorption. The mechanisms by which nimodipine improves the outcome are not entirely understood. It might increase the endogenous fibrinolytic activity in patients with SAH and prevent ischemic events in these patients. Also, the reduction of the calcium influx by nimodipine after cerebral ischemia may have a neuroprotection effect in SAH patients [25, 26].

Avoidance Hyponatremia and Hypovolemia

Cerebral Salt Wasting Syndrome (CSWS) and Syndrome of Inappropriate Antidiuretic Hormone (SIADH) are common medical complications following aSAH. They are the leading cause of hypovolemia and hyponatremia, and consequently, DCI. Wijdicks et al. reported that hyponatremia correction secondary to SIADH with fluid restriction was dangerous and increased cerebral infarction risk. Maintaining euvolemia and normal serum sodium with isotonic crystalloid is currently recommended to prevent DCI. Fludrocortisone (200–400μg/day) reduces the incidence of hyponatremia. Hypertonic saline 3% may be considered to correct symptomatic hyponatremia [27, 28].

Table 10.3 Evidence review of drugs used in aneurysmal subarachnoid hemorrhage [27]

Medication	Type of the medications	Suggested mechanism of action	Status	Guidelines
Nimodipine	Calcium channel blocker (L-type)	Reduces angiographic vasospasm, neuroprotective, augment fibrinolytic activity and decreases cortical spread of ischemia	Meta-analysis of clinical trials reported that oral nimodipine decreased the risk of DCI and poor outcome	Class 1, level A, Nimodipine should be administered orally to prevent DCI
Clazosentan	Endothelin A receptor antagonist	Reduction of angiographic vasospasm	4 RCTs and a meta-analysis Clazosentan reduced angiographic vasospasm without a significant effect on outcome. Hypotension and pulmonary complications effect of Clazosentan could have counteracted its favorable effects	Not addressed. Nonetheless, after the publication of the CONSCIOUS trials and following meta-analysis, clazosentan infusion will not be recommended for patients with SAH, as a class I, level A
Fasudil	Rho-kinase inhibitor	Decreases smooth muscle contraction and inhibits TNF-induced IL-6 release from C6 glioma cells	8 RCTs, reported that Fasudil significantly decreased the incidence of angiographic vasospasm and cerebral infarction and improved the odds ratio for good recovery in comparison with placebo or nimodipine and other medications	Not addressed. Fasudil is approved for use in Japan and China but not in Europe or USA
Statins	Inhibit HMG-CoA reductase	Preserve endothelial function, anti-inflammatory, antioxidant, antithrombotic effect. Neuroprotective. Vascular protection	7 RCTs of statins in patients with SAH. An additional study showing no benefit of higher dose of simvastatin (80 mg versus 40 mg). Systematic review reported that statin had no effect of poor outcome	Statin considered only if aSAH patient was receiving statin at time of the insult. (class I, level A)
Magnesium	Antagonism of calcium channels on vascular smooth muscle	Vasodilation, increased endothelial cell prostacyclin. Endothelial protection Protect the BBB. Decrease cerebral edema Anticonvulsant (NMDA antagonist)	Seven RCTs, Meta-analysis reported no effect of magnesium on poor outcome	Class I, level A magnesium is not recommended for prevention of DCI

Table 10.3 (continued)

Medication	Type of the medications	Suggested mechanism of action	Status	Guidelines
Dantrolene	Inhibits ryanodine receptors	Decreases intracellular calcium release in smooth muscle and may be neuroprotective	One small dose-escalation study, Dantrolene in a dose of 2.5 mg/kg was associated with reduced cerebral blood flow velocities measured by transcranial Doppler	Not addressed. Remains experimental
Intrathecal thrombolytics (i.e., urokinase and recombinant tissue plasminogen activator)	Fibrinolytic agents	The rapid clearance of subarachnoid clot could reduce angiographic vasospasm and complications, such as cortical spreading ischemia and microthrombosis	5 RCTs and a meta-analysis, thrombolysis was associated with significant reductions in angiographic vasospasm, delayed neurological deficits, hydrocephalus, and poor outcome	Not addressed Further studies are required
Antiplatelet drugs (Acetylsalicylic acid, OKY-046 (Cataclot), selective thromboxane synthetase inhibitor, Dipyridamole, Ticlopidine	Acetylsalicylic acid. OKY-046 (Cataclot)—direct drug action L-type calcium channel antagonist. Endothelin A receptor antagonist. Rho-kinase inhibitor inhibit HMG-CoA reductase. Antagonism of calcium channels on vascular smooth muscle, inhibits ryanodine receptors Fibrinolytic agents Inhibition of platelet aggregation	Inhibition of platelet aggregation	7 RCTs and a meta-analysis found trends toward reduction in poor outcome but also toward increased intracranial hemorrhage. Only ticlopidine was associated with statistically significant fewer occurrences of a poor outcome (only one small RCT)	Not addressed Further trials are needed. According to the meta-analysis results, treatment with antiplatelet agents to prevent DCI or poor outcome cannot be recommended
Albumin	Multiple	Neuroprotection	Open-label dose-escalation trial reported improvement in the outcome	Not addressed. Remains experimental
Erythropoietin	Multiple	Prevent loss of autoregulation • Reduce angiographic vasospasm • Inhibits apoptosis and stimulates neurogenesis and angiogenesis	2 RCTs, one negative study and one showing that patients who received erythropoietin had fewer cerebral infarcts, shorter duration of autoregulatory dysfunction, and better clinical outcome	Not addressed. Remains experimental

(continued)

Table 10.3 (continued)

Medication	Type of the medications	Suggested mechanism of action	Status	Guidelines
Cilostazol	Phosphodiesterase 3 inhibitors	Vasodilatation, antithrombotic, anti-smooth muscle proliferation, inotropic and chronotropic effects	One small (109 patients) randomized, single-blind study, Cilostazol significantly reduced angiographic vasospasm, DCI, and cerebral infarction but had no effect on outcome	Not addressed. Remains experimental

CONSCIOUS Clazosentan to Overcome Neurological Ischemia and Infarction Occurring After Subarachnoid Hemorrhage, *IL-6* interleukin-6, *RCT* randomized controlled trial, *STASH* simvastatin in aneurysmal subarachnoid hemorrhage, *BBB* blood–brain barrier. (This table from Creative Commons Attribution 4.0 International License (http://creativecommons.org/licenses/by/4.0/) [1]

Induced Hypertension

Induced hypertension is an effective technique to reverse the neurological symptoms of DCI. Vasopressor is considered as the first-line therapy for augmentation of blood pressure. Vasopressors such as Norepinephrine, dopamine, and phenylephrine have been shown to significantly improve CBF and or cerebral oxygenation, leading to clinical improvement of neurological deficits in almost 70% of SAH patients. Norepinephrine is considered as vasopressor of choice due to its agonist effect on alpha and beta receptors, reliable hemodynamic response, and relatively low incidence of tachycardia. Arginine vasopressin is also effective and may be considered rescue therapy for refractory DCI patients when multiple vasopressors are needed to achieve targeted CPP. Isotonic saline bolus (15 mL/kg/over 1 h) at the institution of therapy improves cerebral blood flow (CBF). The initial systolic blood pressure target depends on baseline blood pressure; it usually ranges between 140 and 180 mmHg. In symptomatic good grade patients, the blood pressure should be titrated to clinical response and gradually increased. The absence of the response for 30 min should trigger increasing the blood pressure target; the goal is resolving the symptoms. Systolic blood pressure of 220 mmHg or MAP of 140 mmHg is the highest target used by most centers. In poor-grade patients, clinical examinations are not reliable. The treating physician should rely on accessible neuromonitoring such as ICP, continuous EEG and brain tissue oxygen monitoring ($PbtO_2$) and titrate blood pressure to optimize CPP. CPP of 120 mmHg is the highest target used by neuro centers. Induced hypertension is safe in patients with an unsecured, unruptured cerebral aneurysm. However, induced hypertension may lead to cardiac complication, such as heart failure or myocardial ischemia. De-escalation of the induced hypertension should be gradual and should be started after obtaining a stable neurological condition for at least 24–48 h [28, 29].

Rescue Therapy for Medically-Refractory DCI (Tier One Interventions)

Haemoglobin Optimization

Anemia in aSAH patients is not uncommon. It is observed in more than half of patients with aSAH and is usually associated with poor outcome. In poor-grade patients, anemia with hemoglobin less than 10 g/dL is associated with brain anoxia and increased metabolic distress. Transfusion of packed red blood cells in aSAH patients with a baseline hemoglobin level of 8 g/dL is associated with improved oxygen delivery and increases brain tissue oxygen tension. Neurocritical care society guidelines recommend packed red blood cell transfusion trigger of 8 g/dL in patients with aSAH without DCI and transfusion trigger of 9–10 g/dL as rescue therapy in aSAH patients with refractory DCI unresponsive to induced hypertension [26].

Endovascular Therapy

Endovascular intervention should be considered when DCI is refractory to hemodynamic optimization or for patients with multiple medical comorbidities, in whom medical therapy can cause medical complications such as myocardial infarction, heart failure, and fluid overload. Endovascular therapy can be carried out through either mechanical dilatation via percutaneous transluminal balloon angioplasty (PTCA) or intra-arterial infusion of vasodilators [28].

Mechanical Dilatation

Mechanical dilatation of spastic arteries via PTCA is usually considered to dilate spastic proximal vessels such as the internal carotid artery, vertebral or basilar artery, M1 and sometimes M2 segments of the MCA, and A1 and P1 segments of the anterior and posterior cerebral artery, respectively. It is a successful procedure with more than a 90% success rate, primarily if performed within less than 2 h after neurological deterioration. Although, because of recurrence of arterial vasospasm, repeating the intervention may be required. The rate of serious complications from mechanical dilatation such as a cerebral artery rupture, thrombosis, embolism, and arterial dissection may occur in up to 5% of patients [28].

Intra-arterial Vasodilators

Several case series have reported intra-arterial vasodilators' success in reversing cerebral vasospasm assessed by cerebral angiography, TCD, cerebral oxygenation, and angiographic cerebral circulation time. Although no single vasodilator has been tested objectively in a clinical trial against a control group, many vasodilators such as papaverine, nicardipine, verapamil, nimodipine, milrinone, and fasudil have used intra-arterial effectively to treat the vasospasm. Verapamil (20–40 mg) and nicardipine (10–20 mg) are the most commonly used agents. They are typically infused over 1 h. Intra-arterial vasodilator is usually administered with balloon angioplasty to treat diffuse and distal vasospasm. It has numerous pros over PTCA; better distal penetration with a more diffusing effect and a better safety profile. The most important limitations of intra-arterial vasodilators are recurrent vasospasm due to short-term effects of these agents, jeopardy of hypotension due to systemic effect, and cerebral vasodilatation may increase the ICP [28, 30].

10.2.1.3 Hydrocephalus

Hydrocephalus is considered as one of the common serious neurological complications of SAH which affects 20–30% of aSAH patients. It may cause significant neurological deterioration; long hospital stay and increase the mortality. Therefore, early diagnosis and treatment is vital and may improve patient's outcome [31].

Hydrocephalus is defined as "an active distention of the ventricular system of the brain resulting from inadequate passage of CSF from its point of production within cerebral ventricles to its point of absorption into systemic circulation" [32].

Pathophysiology

Acute hydrocephalus occurs in 20% of the patients in first 72 h post-ictus. A sub-acute develops between 4th and 14th day after the hemorrhage and affects only 2–3% of patients. While chronic hydrocephalus develops 2 weeks after initial hemorrhage, it affects 10–20% of patients. The pathophysiology of hydrocephalus after SAH is still unclear and poorly understood. However, altered CSF dynamics in acute and chronic hydrocephalus have been extensively investigated [31, 33]. There are two forms of post-SAH hydrocephalus:

Communicating Hydrocephalus

Subarachnoid hemorrhage leads to fibrosis of leptomeninges as well as deposition of blood and blood products in arachnoid granulation of the superior sagittal sinus causing impairment of CSF absorption and circulation. For instance, rupture of anterior cerebral aneurysm causes fibrosis of leptomeninges and arachnoid granulation and considered as common cause of acute and chronic communicating hydrocephalus. In communicating hydrocephalus, the CT scan shows all four ventricles are evenly dilated. However, this analysis can be misleading if obstruction occurs in fourth ventricle outflow (foramina of Luschka and Magendie), which might be falsely interpreted radiologically as being communicating as all ventricles are evenly dilated [31].

Noncommunicating Hydrocephalus

Subarachnoid hemorrhage may lead to obstruction of CSF pathways causing noncommunicating or obstructive hydrocephalus. For example, rupture of posterior cerebral aneurysm can lead to intraventricular hemorrhage which may obstruct fourth ventricle outflow (foramina of Luschka and Magendie) and lead to obstructive hydrocephalus [34].

Diagnosis

Clinical diagnosis of the acute hydrocephalus in aSAH can be challenging. Most of SAH patients complain of headache, vomiting, disturbance of consciousness, and nausea as result of presence of blood in subarachnoid space, therefore treating physicians cannot rely on symptoms to diagnose hydrocephalus. Hence the diagnosis of hydrocephalus relays mainly on radiographic finding, specifically CT scan [31].

CT Scan

CT scan is the quickest and the most efficient investigation to detect hydrocephalus. Numerous ventricular measurements based on CT scan studies have been tried to establish diagnosis of hydrocephalus. Presently, bicaudate index (BCI) and relative bicaudate index (RBCI) are considered as markers of choice to make a diagnosis. In 1980s Gijn et al. suggested that hydrocephalus should be diagnosed once the BCI was more than the age-corrected 95th percentile to limit effect of aging on the ventricular size (Table 10.2). The BCI is the width of the frontal horns of the caudate nuclei divided by corresponding diameter of the brain at the same level (Fig. 10.2), While RBCI calculated by dividing BCI by the upper limit of normal for that age (Table 10.4). Diagnosis of hydrocephalus is highly suspected if RBCI more than1. For example, if a 73 year old patient had BCI of 0.24, the RBCI was calculated by dividing BCI by the upper limit for age 73

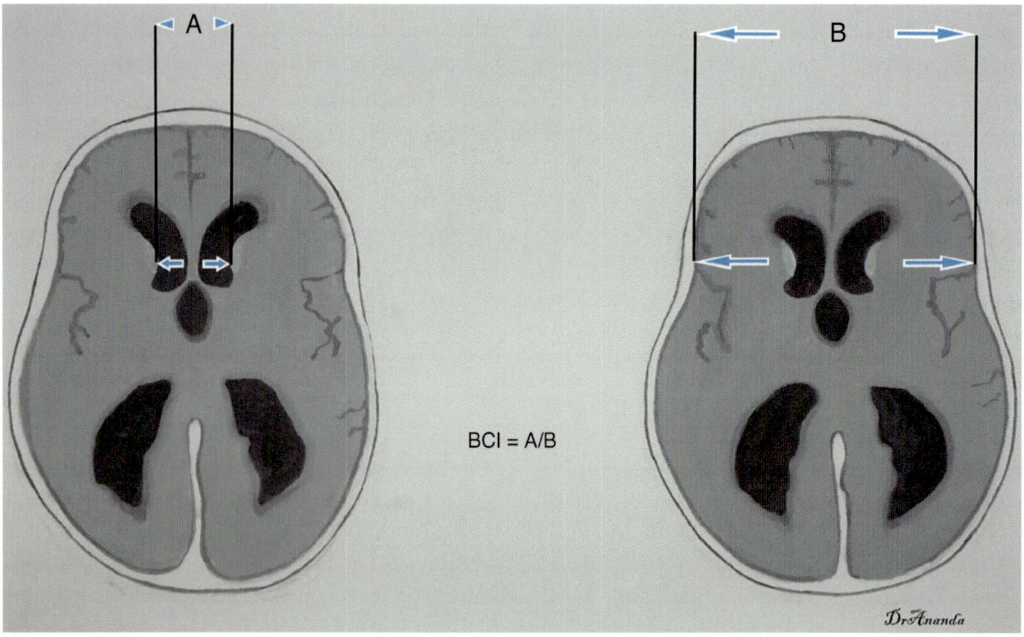

Fig. 10.2 CT brain to explain how to calculate BCI, (A) is the distance between caudate nuclei, while B is the width of brain at same level. BCI is A/B. (Courtesy from Dr. Adel E. Ahmed Ganaw)

Table 10.4 Upper 95% confidence value for BCI stratified by age as suggested by van Gijn et al. [35]

Patient age in years	Upper 95% confidence value
Less than 30	0.16
30–49	0.18
50–59	0.19
60–79	0.21
80–100	0.25

which is 0.21, which gives 1.14, so diagnosis of hydrocephalus is approved [31, 35].

Magnatic Resonance Imaging (MRI)

MRI provides more details than CT scan on the extent of damaging effect of hydrocephalus on periventricular brain parenchyma and gives more details on the morphology of the aqueduct and dynamic of CSF and consequently determine if it is stenosed or completely blocked. Therefore, MRI may help treating clinician to determine the cause and pathophysiology of hydrocephalus. However, MRI is an expensive, time consuming, sedation is required which may affect conscious level and interfere with neurological assessment [36].

Clinical Predictor of Shunt-Dependent Hydrocephalus

Shunt-dependent hydrocephalus is one of the devastating neurological complications of aSAH. It represent 4.3–48% of complications. The pathophysiology of shunt-dependent hydrocephalus is not well understood. It is different from acute hydrocephalus. Meningeal inflammation leads to arachnoid inflammation and adhesion, which impair and prevent CSF absorption at the arachnoid villi and basal cisterns causing shunt-dependent hydrocephalus. Prediction of occurrence of shunt-dependent hydrocephalus and timely diversion of CSF are very important to reduce parenchymal damage. The following are the independent risk factors for shunt-dependent hydrocephalus;

1. Poor High Hunt and Hess Scale score.
2. Intraventricular hemorrhage.
3. Age older than 60 years.
4. Ruptured Posterior circulation aneurysm.
5. Re-bleeding [37, 38].

Table 10.5 AHA/ASA guidelines for management of hydrocephalus following aneurysmal subarachnoid hemorrhage [10] (Courtesy from Dr. Adel E. Ahmed Ganaw)

AHA/ASA guidelines 2012	Level of evidence
1. aSAH-associated acute symptomatic hydrocephalus should be managed by cerebrospinal fluid diversion (EVD or lumbar drainage, depending on the clinical scenario)	Class I; Level of evidence B
2. aSAH-associated chronic symptomatic hydrocephalus should be treated with permanent cerebrospinal fluid diversion	Class I; Level of evidence C
3. Weaning EVD over >24 h does not appear to be effective in reducing the need for ventricular shunting	Class III; Level of evidence B
4. Routine fenestration of the lamina terminalis is not useful for reducing the rate of shunt-dependent hydrocephalus and therefore should not be routinely performed	Class III; Level of evidence B

Management of Hydrocephalus

External Ventricular Drain (EVD)

EVD insertion is considered a treatment choice for management of acute hydrocephalus regardless the cause of the hydrocephalus. It is associated of rapid improvement of neurological status. According to AHA/ASA guidelines (Table 10.5), EVD should be considered for aSAH patients who presented with symptomatic hydrocephalus (decrease in GCS, drowsiness and or confusion). EVD placement should be established in operating theater or at bedside (critical care or emergency department) using established sterile, anatomical land-mark approach. If EVD placed before securing of the aneurysm, the drainage pressure should be kept at 20 mmHg to avoid over drainage of CSF and re-bleeding. Once the aneurysm secured, the drainage pressure should be decreased to 5–10 mmHg to drain sufficient bloody CSF [39].

Most of the neurocritical care centers in the USA prefer continues EVD draining with gradual weaning over intermittent draining and rapid weaning. However, rapid weaning of EVD may improve recruitment and utilization of blocked CSF resorption pathways in the arachnoid granulations. Therefore, may decrease duration of EVD placement, risk of infection, and staying in critical care. The Barrow RCT propose that rapid weaning of EVD may reduce hospital and critical care staying without harmful effect on frequency of delayed cerebral ischemia or other adverse effects [40].

EVD drainage pressure can be gradually increased by 5 mmHg daily up to 20 mmHg and monitor amount of drained CSF, ICP, and neurological status. The neurosurgeon/intensivist can clamp EVD for 24–48 h if EVD draining CSF less than 5 mL/h. They de-clamp the EVD only if the ICP is persistent at 20 mmHg or greater for 5 min or enormous spikes in ICP are noticed. EVD removed if there is no increase in ICP or change in neurological status, it is recommended by some neurosurgeons to have baseline CT head prior to start weaning EVD and do follow-up CT after clamping the drain [39].

Nevertheless, in spite simplicity and frequent insertion of EVD, there are concerns regarding number of serious complications such as infection, bleeding, and malposition. Infection rate of EVD ranges between 3 and 32%. Therefore, NCS recommends prophylactic antibiotics before insertion, use of antimicrobial-impregnated catheter, avoidance of routine CSF sampling and obtaining of CSF for analysis only when clinically indicated, as well as removal of EVD as early as clinical situation allows. Bleeding is another important complication of EVD insertion. The incidence of bleeding varies widely in the literatures, rates have been reported to be as high as 41% or as low as 0%. NCS recommends correction of coagulopathy before EVD insertion unless it is dire emergencies necessitating prompt ventricular drainage. NCS advises using Kocher's point as entry point in the skull, and direct the EVD vertical to the skull or pointing the contralateral medical canthus in normal ventricular anatomy to afford the uppermost possibility of optimum EVD position. Advancement of EVD catheter more than 6.5 cm from skull surface should be avoided. Moreover, NCS suggests the use of image guidance if it is available for patients with small ventricle or distorted ventricular anatomy [40, 41].

Lumbar Drain

Lumbar drain is safe and simple bedside intervention for patients with persistent communicating hydrocephalus after intraventricular hemorrhage (IVH), to avoid frequent replacement of EVD, which is associated with the risk of ventriculitis, bleeding, subdural hematoma, repeated damage to brain tissue and repeated exposure to anesthesia. Moreover, lumbar drain extends duration of extracorporal CSF drainage with less side effects than EVD, therefore increasing the chance of arachnoid recovery and re-start reabsorption of CSF, which may avoid ventriculoperitoneal shunt insertion. Small retrospective studies stated that, serial lumbar drainage of communicating hydrocephalus in patients with a SAH is safe. If obstructive hydrocephalus, supratentorial mass, intraparenchymal hematoma are suspected, the risk of downward herniation is high and lumbar drain must be avoided. Obviously, lumbar drain should be avoided in coagulopathic patients [42].

Ventriculoperitoneal Shunt (VPS)

About 25% of patients may fail to be weaned from EVD after aSAH and would require cerebrospinal fluid diversion to treat hydrocephalus, also sometimes after successful weaning and removal of the EVD, some patients developed delayed hydrocephalus which is slowly developed up to 6 months after discharge. It is shunt-dependent hydrocephalus and treated with ventriculoperitoneal shunt. Regrettably, complications associated with VPS placement are quite common, and frequent shunt revision might be needed throughout a patient's life. The most common complications are shunt malfunction secondary to shunt obstruction, infection, pseudocyst formation, and bowel perforation. Recently, several interventions have been introduced to reduce the rate of VPS complications, for example, better-quality sterile techniques, using antibiotic impregnated catheters, programmable valves. However, VPS malfunctions still a major issue which frequently causing frequent and costive hospital re-admission. Fenestration of the Lamina terminals has been proposed to decrease the occurrence of delayed hydrocephalus, however, a meta-analysis of non-randomized studies, failed to show meaningful decrease in the incidence of shunt-dependent hydrocephalus in patients who had undergone fenestration of the lamina terminalis [10, 42].

10.2.1.4 Seizures

Seizure like movement is common after initial aneurysm rupture. It occurs in 26% of aSAH patients. However, it is still unclear whether it is real seizure or represents post-ictus posturing. Clinical seizures are rare, it occurs only in 1–7% of SAH patients. It is usually representing re-bleeding in patients with unsecured aneurysms. The majority of seizures manifest before medical care are accessed. The seizures incidence decrease dramatically after intervention. A systemic review reported that the incidence of post-intervention seizures during staying in the hospital was only 2.3% (early seizures), while the incidence of late seizures (after discharge from the hospital) was only 5.5% with average latency of 7.45 months. Claassen et al. reported that 11% of aSAH patients had at least one seizure in first year which may be secondary to gliosis and development of meningocerebral cicatrix [43, 44].

Furthermore, the incidence of late epilepsy post-SAH ranges between 3 and 35%. Nevertheless, it seems to be declining over the years which may be explained by improvements in the managing of aSAH patients. ISAT trial reported that late epilepsy was developed only in 4% of SAH patients after 1 year of follow-up [45]. There are several risk factors that associate with development seizures in aSAH patients such as aneurysm in middle cerebral artery, thick subarachnoid clot, surgical repair of cerebral aneurysm in patients who are older than 65 years, history of seizure disorder, intracerebral hematoma, re-bleeding, cerebral infarction, and poor neurological grade [2, 5, 46, 47].

Management

There is a debate about anticonvulsant prophylaxis, best anticonvulsant medications, and duration of anticonvulsant treatment in SAH patients. This was enlightened by the lack of randomized clinical trials or high-quality researches comprehending this issue. A Cochrane review 2013 neither support nor rebut the primary and secondary prevention treatment of seizures in aSAH. Furthermore, the prophylactic administration of anticonvulsant in aSAH diverges significantly among clinicians from different countries [48].

Although multidisciplinary Consensus Conference of the Neurocritical Care Society (NCS) and American heart association/ American stroke association (AHA/ASA) published very important clinical recommendations (Table 10.6) none of these societies support or rebut one or another approach in managing seizures in SAH patients grounded on strong evidence [2, 10, 49]. Initially, it is essential to highlight that there is no general agreement on the primary or secondary anticonvulsant prophylaxis in SAH patients. Actually, recent studies reported routine use of anticonvulsants especially phenytoin in SAH was associated with worsening of the cognitive function, and increased in hospital complications. Hence, the decision of starting anticonvulsant prophylaxis still empirical than evidence-based [5, 46, 50].

NCS and AHA/ASA support consideration of routine short course of anticonvulsant prophylaxis in immediate post-hemorrhagic period. However, AHA/ASA recommend consideration of routine long-term anticonvulsant therapy for patients who have risk factors for delayed seizures such as MCA aneurysm, refractory hypertension, cerebral infarction, history of seizures, and intracerebral hematoma [10].

Table 10.6 Management of seizures after SAH according to the Neurocritical Care Society (NCS) recommendations and the AHA/ASA guideline [46]

NCS recommendations 2011	AHA/ASA guidelines 2012
1. Routine use of anticonvulsant prophylaxis with phenytoin is not recommended after SAH (low-quality evidence—Strong recommendation)	
2. Routine use of other anticonvulsants for prophylaxis may be considered (very low-quality evidence—weak recommendation)	1. The use of prophylactic anticonvulsants may be considered in the immediate post-hemorrhagic period (Class IIb; Level of evidence B)
3. If anticonvulsant prophylaxis is used, a short course (3–7 days) is recommended (low-quality evidence—weak recommendation)	
4. In patients who suffer a seizure after presentation, anticonvulsants should be continued for a duration defined by local practice (low-quality evidence—weak recommendation)	2. The routine long-term use of anticonvulsants is not recommended (Class III; Level of evidence B), but may be considered for patients with known risk factors for delayed seizure disorder, such as prior seizure, intracerebral hematoma, intractable hypertension, infarction, or aneurysm at the middle cerebral artery (Class IIb; Level of evidence B)
5. Continuous EEG monitoring should be considered in patients with poor-grade SAH who fail to improve or who have neurological deterioration of undetermined etiology (low-quality evidence—Strong recommendation)	

10.2.2 Non-neurological Complications Associated with SAH

The high morbidity and mortality associated with SAH is not only due to neurological complications, non-neurological complications also play a major role in increasing mortality and morbidity rates. More than 80% will develop serious non-neurological complications which may increase the risk for secondary brain injury (Fig. 10.3) [51–53].

10.2.2.1 Cardiac Complications

Cardiac manifestations occur in about 50% of patients with aSAH; it ranges from mild elevation in cardiac enzymes and electrocardiogram (ECG) changes to obvious clinical and echocardiographic pathology. Cardiac damage markers are associated with an increased mortality and poor outcome and DCI [52].

Pathophysiology

Mild Myocardial Injury

Mild myocardial injury occurs in 20–68% of patients with SAH. The severity of neurological injury as scored by the Hunt–Hess scale is independent predictor of myocardial injury. Mild increase in serum cardiac troponin I is considered as main manifestation of mild myocardia injury. Troponin I does not reach threshold of myocardial infarction.

It is a specific and sensitive indicator of myocardial injury; thus, trend of serial troponin level should be monitored especially in patients with past history of cardiovascular disease. In addition, serum troponin is a strong predictor for cardiac, pulmonary, and neurological complication such as left ventricular dysfunction, requirement of vasopressor, pulmonary edema, DCI particularly in patients present with poor WFNS grades [52].

Cardiomyopathy

Neurogenic stunned myocardium (NSM) is the severest form of myocardial injury following

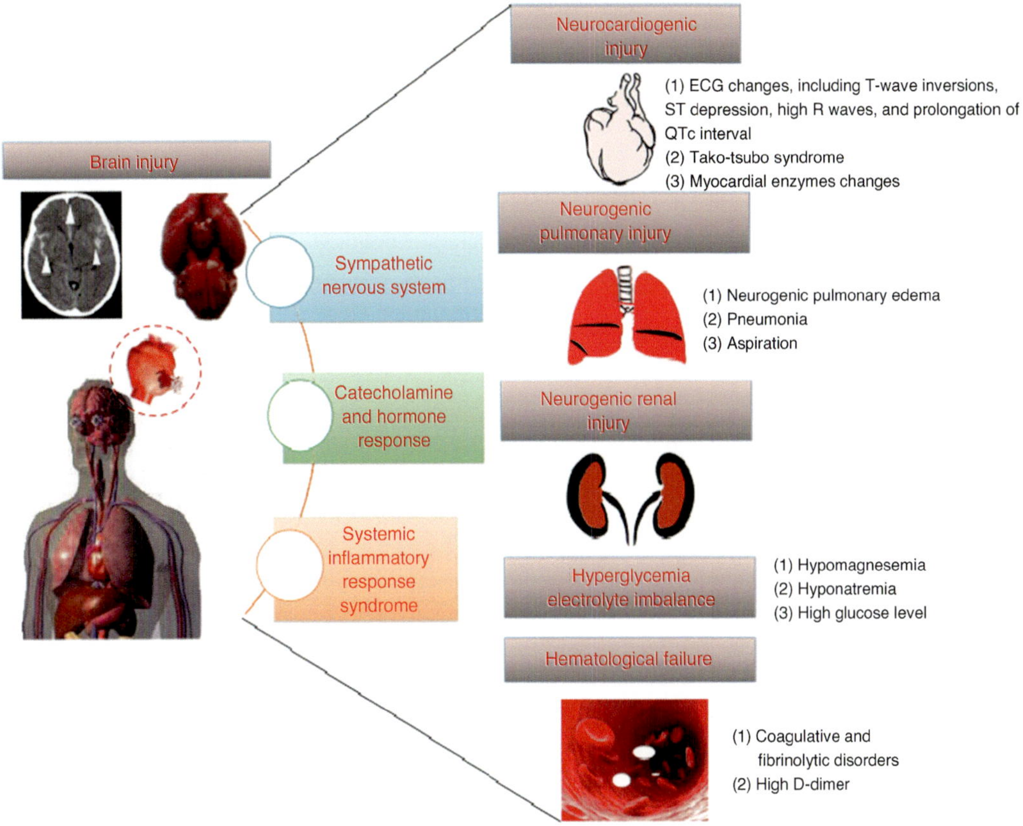

Fig. 10.3 Non-CNS complications of aSAH [53]. (This Figure distributed under the Creative Commons Attribution License)

SAH. The incidence of NSM ranges between 20 and 30% of SAH patients. The increase of sympathetic tone after acute insult leads to transient calcium overload with reduction in response of myocardial filaments to calcium, eventually leading to myocardial depression. The theoretical role of oxygen-derived free radicals also has been described in the pathophysiology of NSM. Furthermore, the specific histopathological feature of NSM is charecterized by subendocardial band necrosis. Predictors of left ventricular dysfunction are CK-MB, female gender, and poor neurological grade.

Clinically, NSM is characterised by severe yet reversible impairment of the left ventricle (LV) function. Echocardiography shows a decrease of LV contractility and regional wall motion abnormality. Although, NSM is reversible, full recovery of myocardial function may take several weeks. The impairment of left ventricular function may severely compromise the cardiac output, causing cardiogenic shock which may decrease cerebral blood flow (CBF) and worsen cerebral vasospasm and DCI. Thus, cardiac output monitoring and optimization of myocardial function is extremely important in patients with SAH. Inodilators such as dobutamine and milrinone may be considered to optimize myocardial function. However, the inodilators may cause peripheral vasodilatation, leading to decrease in mean arterial blood pressure and cerebral perfusion; therefore, advanced cardiac output monitoring should be used to titrate the Inodilators. In critical cases where cardiac output severely

Table 10.7 ECG changes after subarachnoid hemorrhage [56]

ECG abnormality	Recorded incidence (%)
ST-segment alterations	15–51
T wave changes	12–92
Prominent U waves	4–47
QT prolongation	11–66
Conduction abnormalities	7.5
Sinus bradycardia	16
Sinus tachycardia	8.5

reduced and refractory to inodilators, intra-aortic balloon pump should be considered [52].

Arrhythmia

ECG changes are commonly observed in SAH patients, particularly in the first 3 days post-ictus, nearly 50–100% of SAH patients show different forms of arrhythmia such as ST segments changes, T wave changes, QTc prolongation, and Prominent U wave (Table 10.7). Malignant arrhythmias such as ventricular tachycardia (VT), torsade de pointe, and asystole are observed only in 4–8% of SAH patients [52]. These arrhythmias are commonly observed in patients with severe neurological insults, nevertheless they are not independent predictors of mortality. Sakr et al. reported that repolarization abnormalities are the commonest form of ECG changes in patients with acute subarachnoid hemorrhage, ST depression was associated with Hunt–Hess grading scale, WFNS score, and Acute Physiology and Chronic Health Evaluation II score (APACHE II score), but was not associated with cerebral vasospasm or increase in ICP. In addition, it was commonly observed in patients who had poor outcome. However, ECG changes were not independently predictor of poor outcome [54, 55].

Severity of neurological injury, elderly, and history of arrhythmia are predictors for development of arrhythmia in SAH patients. Pathophysiology of ECG changes following SAH is poorly understood, SAH may damage paraventricular nuclei of hypothalamus, leading to activation of sympathetic outflow through the rostral ventrolateral medulla, and induce arrhythmia, ECG changes and myocardial necrosis. Furthermore, electrolyte disturbance especially hypokalemia may contribute in development ECG changes [57].

Management of arrhythmia following SAH depends on type of arrhythmia, clinical significance, and patient condition. Treating physician should correct electrolyte and metabolic abnormalities. Optimization of the oxygenation is extremely important to prevent malignant arrhythmia. Treatment of tachyarrhythmia with beta-blockers should be balanced against hypotension and decrease of CBF [10].

10.2.2.2 Electrolyte Disturbances

Electrolyte disturbances are commonly observed in patients with aneurysmal subarachnoid hemorrhage which can have an impact on the prognosis of these groups of patients. They include hyponatremia, hypernatremia, hypokalemia, hypocalcemia, and hypomagnesaemia. Hyponatremia is commonest electrolyte disturbance following SAH.

10.2.2.3 Hyponatremia

Hyponatremia is defined as serum sodium concentration less than 135mml/L. Clinically significant hyponatremia is defined as serum sodium concentration less than 131 mmol/L. Hyponatremia is considered as the commonest electrolyte disturbance associated with aneurysmal SAH. The incidence of hyponatremia ranges between 30 and 56%, frequently reported following rupture of anterior communicating artery (AComA). It was reported in 52.4% of SAH patients with AComA; most probably secondary to disturbance of blood supply to the hypothalamus which is supplied by branch from AComA [58–60].

The most common cause of hyponatremia following SAH is the syndrome of inappropriate anti-diuretic hormone secretion (SIADH); hypothalamic ischemic insults following aSAH secondary to cerebral vasospasm leads to excessive secretion of antidiuretic hormone which increases water reabsorption in distal convoluted tubules of the kidney, causing fluid retention, increase blood volume and dilutional hyponatremia [61]. The second important cause of hyponatremia is cerebral salt wasting syndrome (CSW), increase urinary excretion of sodium and urine output due to abnormal release of atrial and brain natriuretic hormone, leading to decrease of extracellular and circulating blood volume which leading to increase secretion of antidiuretic hormone (ADH), aldosterone and renin and decrease release of atrial/brain natriuretic peptide to restore plasma volume.

Kao et al. stated that SIADH was responsible on 34.5% of severe hyponatremia. While, CSW was responsible on only 23% of hyponatremia in SAH patients. Noteworthy, the inclusion criteria were a serum sodium less than 130 mmol/L. Thus, the patients included in this trial had more significant hyponatremia than in the comparative studies [62, 63].

Irrespective of the pathophysiology, hyponatremia is an independent jeopardy of high mortality and morbidity. Hyponatremia in aSAH is associated with long hospital stay, cerebral vasospasm, and poor outcome; hyponatremia shifts water from extracellular compartment to intracellular compartment leading to worsening of brain edema and ICP in SAH patients. Furthermore, hyponatremia increases jeopardy of seizures and neurological injury. Therefore, prompt diagnosis and appropriate management are extremely important to improve the outcome [59, 64, 65]. However, the proper treatment of hyponatremic SAH patients requires resolving the diagnostic and therapeutic dilemma of determining whether to restrict water in patients with SIADH or administer sodium and water in patients with CSWS [63].

Clinically it is very difficult to differentiate between SIADH and CSW syndrom due to significant overlapping clinical findings between both syndrome: both syndromes follow brain insults, have normal thyroid, adrenal and kidney function. Furthermore, in both syndromes, patients have hyponatremia, hypouricemic and concentrated urine, elevated urinary sodium >40 mmol/L, and high fractional excretion of urate (FE urate). Status of the extracellular volume (ECV) is the only clinical difference between both syndromes; patients are hypervolemic or euvolemic in SIADH and hypovolemic in CSWS (Table 10.8). However, accurate assessment of ECV clinically is extremely difficult [63].

Table 10.8 Difference between SIADH and CSWS (This table is distributed under the terms of the Creative Commons Attribution License (http://creativecommons.org/licenses/by/3.0) [66]

	SIADH	CSWS
Plasma volume	↑ or ↔	↓↓
Water balance	↑ or ↔	Negative
Signs and symptoms of dehydration	Absent	Present
Central venous pressure	↑ or ↔	↓↓
Salt balance	Variable	Negative
Hematocrit	↔	↑ or ↔
Serum osmolality	↓↓	↓↓
Urine sodium	↑	↑↑
Urine volume	↓or ↔	↑↑
Plasma BUN/creatinine	↓↓	↑ or ↔
Treatment	Fluid restriction, hypertonic saline, furosemide, Democycline	Normal saline, hypertonic saline, Fludrecortisone

Determination FE urate is very useful to distinguish between SIADH and CSW syndrome, normal FE urate ranges between 4 and 11%, increased to more than 11% in both syndromes, correction hyponatremia will normalize FE urate (4–11%) in patients with SIADH, but it persists more than 11% after correction the hyponatremia in patients with CSWS (Fig. 10.4). This algorithm eradicates the requirement of volume status assessment, terminate the need of determination of urine sodium concentration, plasma renin, aldosterone, blood urea nitrogen to creatinine ratio, and atrial / brain natriuretic peptide. The main limitation of this algorithm that it is not reliable in patients with reduced glomerular filtration rate (GFR) as FE urate may exceed the normal value [63].

Another important cause of hyponatremia such as acute cortisol insufficiency, diuretics, and fluid therapy should be considered during assess-

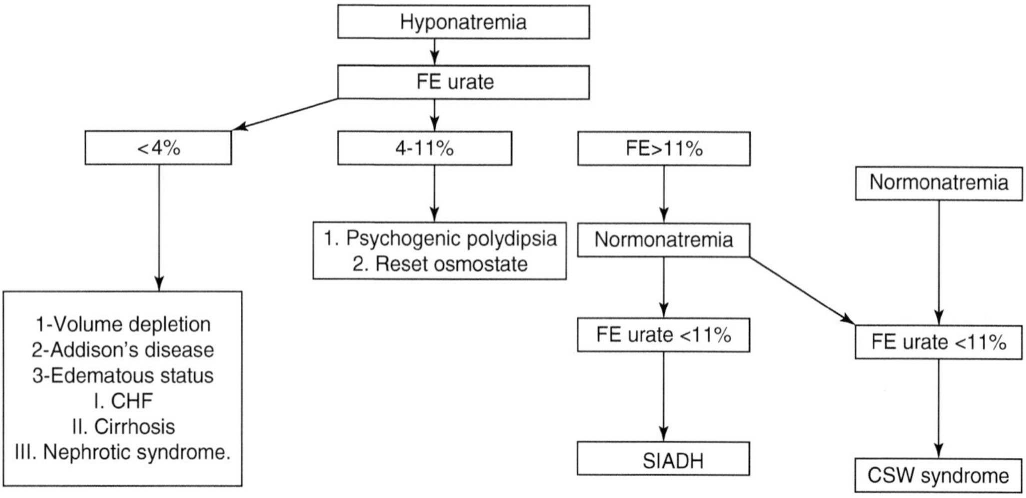

Fig. 10.4 Algorithm for determining cause of hyponatremia, using FE urate. (This figure distributed under the terms and conditions of the Creative Commons Attribution license (http://creativecommons.org/licenses/by/4.0/) [63])

ment and management of hyponatremia. Klose et al. and Parenti et al. reported that the incidence of cortisol deficiency in SAH patients ranges between 7.1 and 12% at presentation [67, 68].

Treatment of Hyponatremia

Determination of the etiology of hyponatremia by proper clinical assessment, biochemical hormonal, and urinary investigations is mandatory to guarantee well-timed and effective management of hyponatremia.

All subarachnoid hemorrhage patients should be closely monitored for signs and symptoms of cerebral vasospasm, DCI, as well as daily fluid and electrolyte balance for at least 2–3 weeks post-insult in neurosurgery high-dependent unit, which may help treating doctors in early detection and immediate management of hyponatremia or other electrolyte disturbances. Bedside sodium and fluid balance assessment is best economical and valuable approach for avoiding hyponatremia in patients with SAH. Sodium level should be immediately checked if there are fluctuations in the mental status, significant changes of the fluid balance due to polyuria [59].

Generally, patients with SAH should be maintained on balanced crystalloid or sodium chloride-based fluids (i.e., 0.9% normal saline) at rate 3 L/day, infusion rate should be adjusted for oral intake, glucose containing solution and hypotonic fluid should be avoided to prevent cerebral edema due to fluid shifts across a damaged blood–brain barrier.

Neurocritical care society recommend that fluid restriction to treat hyponatremia should be avoided to prevent cerebral vasospasm. However, large volume of free water intake should be avoided. Furthermore, AHA recommend isotonic solution to treat hypovolemia (Class IIa, Level B evidence), and that avoiding of large volumes of hypotonic solutions in patients with SAH. Balanced solutions in the early SAH period may prevent electrolyte imbalance associated with saline-based intravenous fluids, such as hyperchloremia, hyperosmolality, and extreme positive fluid balances [49, 59].

Fluid restriction to less than 500 mL/day is considered as treatment of choice of SIADH. Unfortunately, it is not feasible in patients with SAH due to risk of cerebral vasospasm and DCI. In addition, most of these patients are unconscious on enteral feeding, subsequently daily fluid intake ranges between 1 and 2 L. Administration of hypertonic saline (2–3%) or albumin may be considered when fluid restriction is required. However, it may increase risk of pulmonary edema, especially in patients with impaired cardiac function. Hypertonic saline may rapidly correct hyponatremia resulting in central myelinolysis. Therefore, sodium level should be checked four hourly if patient is receiving hypertonic saline [59].

Fludrocortisone may be considered to treat hyponatremia due to CSWS, but there is no strong evidence support its effectiveness and it is associated with fluid overload [59].

Conivaptan (Vasopressin receptor antagonists) have been investigated in small studies, it increases rapidly sodium level rapidly. Therefore, it is not recommended to treat hyponatremia [69].

Steroids may be considered to treat acute cortisol deficiency; however, the beneficial effect of steroid is indeterminate. Further studies are required to support using steroid in patients with SAH especially steroid may increase risk of hyperglycemia which associated with poor outcome [70].

10.2.2.4 Hyperglycemia

Hyperglycemia is a serious medical complication of aSAH. It is usually recognized during initial assessment of SAH patients. It affects one third of aSAH patients. Admission hyperglycemia is associated with poor clinical grade of SAH. Hyperglycemia is associated with vasospasm, long stay in critical care, and poor outcome. Blood glucose of 220 mg/dL is associated with amplified infection jeopardy. However, continuous insulin infusion for tight glucose control (80–110 mg/dL) may place patients at danger of hypoglycemia, vasospasm, cerebral infarction, and poor outcome even if sever hypoglycemia does not happen. Schlenk et al. reported that tight glucose control with insulin infusion induced cerebral hypoglycemia and cerebral metabolic stress in SAH patients despite absence of systemic hypoglycemia. Pasternak et al., reported that targeting glucose between 80 and 140 mg/dL was associated with improved outcomes [2, 71–73].

10.2.2.5 Fever

Fever is one of the common medical complications of aSAH which affects 41–72% of aSAH patients. It is commonly reported in patients who present with intraventricular hemorrhage (IVH) and poor Hunt–Hess grade which considered as strongest predictors of fever in aSAH patients. It is most likely secondary to the inflammatory response to extravasated blood in subarachnoid space. However, infectious causes must be excluded. Fever is associated with cerebral infarction poor outcome of aSAH patients. There are neither randomized controlled trials on the role of cooling in SAH patients nor studies that have proofed that treatment of fever has beneficial effect on outcome of aSAH patients. There are pharmacological and non-pharmacological techniques to treat fever in SAH patients. Paracetamol is commonly used to treat fever in aSAH patients. However, it is not very effective, it is normalizing the temperature only in minority of patients. NSAID such as Ibuprofen has been used to treat fever in SAH, also it has limited effect in management of fever in aSAH patients. Moreover, it may interfere with normal blood clotting. Non-pharmacological techniques include evaporative cooling, ice packs, and cooling blanket. Aggressive cooling may cause shivering which leads to increase oxygen consumption, carbon dioxide production, marked increase in resting energy expenditure and reduction in in brain oxygen tension. Several measures have been introduced to reduce shivering. This includes counter warming of extremities as well as medications such as magnesium, buspirone, meperidine, propofol and other sedatives [2, 13, 74–76].

10.2.2.6 Anemia

Anemia is a common medical complication of aSAH. It affects about 50% of SAH and develops within 3–4 days after SAH. Generally, hemoglobin concentrations drops 3 g/dL following aSAH. Normally, cerebral oxygen delivery exceeds metabolic demands. This affords oxygen store, hence any drop in cerebral blood flow and oxygen delivery compensated by increase in oxygen extraction.

Cerebral oxygen delivery is determined by-product of cerebral blood flow and arterial oxygen contents which is directly associated with hemoglobin concentration. Therefore, CBF rises significantly in anemic patients to maintain oxygen delivery. This compensation mechanism exhausts in severely anemic patients and the oxygen delivery significantly compromised leading to worsening in the outcome. Although, optimal hemoglobin concentration in SAH patients remains uncertain, anemia correction improves outcome in SAH patients. Dhar et al. stated that raising hemoglobin concentration from 8 to 10 was associated with improvement in cerebral oxygen delivery. There are no evidences that address beneficial role of higher hemoglobin (more than 10 g/dL) on cerebral oxygen delivery. Generally, blood transfusion is associated with serious complication such as immunosuppression, infection, fever, volume overload, pneumonia, and electrolyte disturbance. Hence, the risk of blood transfusion must be considered in aSAH patients. Current guidance recommends to keep hemoglobin concentration between 8 and 10 g/dL [2, 77–79].

10.2.2.7 Deep Venous Thrombosis (DVT)

Deep venous thrombosis is a serious medical complication of aSAH. Significant medical comorbidities, surgical interventions, prolonged mechanical ventilation as well as immobilization in the critical care department render aSAH patients exceptionally vulnerable to DVTs. The rate of DVTs in aSAH patients ranges between 1.5 and 18%. Early mobilization and DVT prophylaxis are the most important intervention to prevent and reduce the incidence of DVTs [80].

There are two types of DVT prophylaxis in a SAH, mechanical DVT prophylaxis such as pneumatic stocking and sequential compression devices, and pharmacological DVT prophylaxis which include heparin (unfractionated and low molecular weight heparin LMWH). Collen et al. (Meta-analysis) reported that intermittent pneumatic compression (IPC), unfractionated heparin, and LMWH were equally effective in prevention DVTs. Moreover, there was an increase in the rate of ICH with LMWH with no overall influence on the outcome. Therefore, mechanical prophylaxis is safest DVT prophylaxis approach, especially before securing the aneurysm and when the risk of re-bleeding is high [2].

Lacut et al. stated that a combination of stockings and IPC was superior to stocking alone in prevention of DVT in stroke patients. The starting time of pharmacological prophylaxis in SAH patients is controversial, but ideally should be started after securing the aneurysm and continued till the patients pass the risk of developing DVTs [2, 5, 81].

10.2.2.8 Heparin-Induced Thrombocytopenia (HIT)

SAH patients are at high risk of developing HIT due to number of angiographic procedures performed and frequent exposure to unfractionated heparin. It occurs in 5% of SAH patients. HIT is associated with high rates of thrombotic complication, DCI, high mortality, and poor outcomes. It is vital to recognize this complication to prevent further exposure to heparin and to use another DVT prophylaxis [10].

10.3 Conclusion

Complications of aneurysmal subarachnoid hemorrhages are significant determinants in the prognosis of patients who have suffered a ruptured aneurysm. At the early phase, re-bleeding constitutes the most severe complication and necessitates immediate intervention. Cerebrospinal fluid diversion, usually in the form of an extraventricular drain (EVD), should be considered if acute hydrocephalus develops. Delayed cerebral ischemia (DCI) and Vasospasm commonly evolve from day three to the end of the third week. Cases at high risk of developing DCI should be followed closely with bedside transcranial Doppler ultrasonography. Clinically suspected cases of DCI require immediate perfusion-weighted imaging. Because of the recurrence risk of the re-bleeding from recurrence of the aneurysm, all patients should be followed up.

Medical complications after ruptured cerebral aneurysm, such as cardiomyopathy, arrhythmias, electrolyte disturbances, etc., are potentially preventable but may add to patients' total mortality rate if not addressed and it may lead to an unwarranted increase in an intensive care unit (ICU) and hospital stay.

References

1. de Oliveira Manoel AL, Goffi A, Marotta TR, Schweizer TA, Abrahamson S, Macdonald RL. The critical care management of poor-grade subarachnoid haemorrhage. Crit Care. 2016;20:21.
2. Diringer MN, Bleck TP, Claude Hemphill J 3rd, Menon D, Shutter L, Vespa P, et al. Critical care management of patients following aneurysmal subarachnoid hemorrhage: recommendations from the Neurocritical Care Society's Multidisciplinary Consensus Conference. Neurocrit Care. 2011;15(2):211–40.
3. Guo LM, Zhou HY, Xu JW, Wang Y, Qiu YM, Jiang JY. Risk factors related to aneurysmal rebleeding. World Neurosurg. 2011;76(3–4):292–8; discussion 53–4.
4. Beck J, Raabe A, Szelenyi A, Berkefeld J, Gerlach R, Setzer M, et al. Sentinel headache and the risk of rebleeding after aneurysmal subarachnoid hemorrhage. Stroke. 2006;37(11):2733–7.
5. Steiner T, Juvela S, Unterberg A, Jung C, Forsting M, Rinkel G, et al. European Stroke Organization guidelines for the management of intracranial aneurysms and subarachnoid haemorrhage. Cerebrovasc Dis. 2013;35(2):93–112.
6. Lanzino G, Kassell NF, Germanson TP, Kongable GL, Truskowski LL, Torner JC, et al. Age and outcome after aneurysmal subarachnoid hemorrhage: why do older patients fare worse? J Neurosurg. 1996;85(3):410–8.
7. Lim YC, Kim CH, Kim YB, Joo JY, Shin YS, Chung J. Incidence and risk factors for rebleeding during cerebral angiography for ruptured intracranial aneurysms. Yonsei Med J. 2015;56(2):403–9.
8. Sampei T, Yasui N, Mizuno M, Nakajima S, Ishikawa T, Hadeishi H, et al. Contrast medium extravasation during cerebral angiography for ruptured intracranial aneurysm—clinical analysis of 26 cases. Neurol Med Chir (Tokyo). 1990;30(13):1011–5.
9. van Donkelaar CE, Bakker NA, Veeger NJ, Uyttenboogaart M, Metzemaekers JD, Luijckx GJ, et al. Predictive factors for rebleeding after aneurysmal subarachnoid hemorrhage: rebleeding aneurysmal subarachnoid hemorrhage study. Stroke. 2015;46(8):2100–6.
10. Connolly ES Jr, Rabinstein AA, Carhuapoma JR, Derdeyn CP, Dion J, Higashida RT, et al. Guidelines for the management of aneurysmal subarachnoid hemorrhage: a guideline for healthcare professionals from the American Heart Association/American Stroke Association. Stroke. 2012;43(6):1711–37.
11. Naidech AM, Janjua N, Kreiter KT, Ostapkovich ND, Fitzsimmons BF, Parra A, et al. Predictors and impact of aneurysm rebleeding after subarachnoid hemorrhage. Arch Neurol. 2005;62(3):410–6.
12. Priebe HJ. Aneurysmal subarachnoid haemorrhage and the anaesthetist. Br J Anaesth. 2007;99(1):102–18.
13. Dippel DW, van Breda EJ, van Gemert HM, van der Worp HB, Meijer RJ, Kappelle LJ, et al. Effect of paracetamol (acetaminophen) on body temperature in acute ischemic stroke: a double-blind, randomized phase II clinical trial. Stroke. 2001;32(7):1607–12.
14. Phillips TJ, Dowling RJ, Yan B, Laidlaw JD, Mitchell PJ. Does treatment of ruptured intracranial aneurysms within 24 hours improve clinical outcome? Stroke. 2011;42(7):1936–45.
15. Starke RM, Kim GH, Fernandez A, Komotar RJ, Hickman ZL, Otten ML, et al. Impact of a protocol for acute antifibrinolytic therapy on aneurysm rebleeding after subarachnoid hemorrhage. Stroke. 2008;39(9):2617–21.
16. Vergouwen MD, Vermeulen M, van Gijn J, Rinkel GJ, Wijdicks EF, Muizelaar JP, et al. Definition of delayed cerebral ischemia after aneurysmal subarachnoid hemorrhage as an outcome event in clinical trials and observational studies: proposal of a multidisciplinary research group. Stroke. 2010;41(10):2391–5.
17. Inagawa T, Yahara K, Ohbayashi N. Risk factors associated with cerebral vasospasm following aneurysmal subarachnoid hemorrhage. Neurol Med Chir (Tokyo). 2014;54(6):465–73.
18. Kale SP, Edgell RC, Alshekhlee A, Borhani Haghighi A, Sweeny J, Felton J, et al. Age-associated vasospasm in aneurysmal subarachnoid hemorrhage. J Stroke Cerebrovasc Dis. 2013;22(1):22–7.
19. Kongable GL, Lanzino G, Germanson TP, Truskowski LL, Alves WM, Torner JC, et al. Gender-related differences in aneurysmal subarachnoid hemorrhage. J Neurosurg. 1996;84(1):43–8.
20. Dumont T, Rughani A, Silver J, Tranmer BI. Diabetes mellitus increases risk of vasospasm following aneurysmal subarachnoid hemorrhage independent of glycemic control. Neurocrit Care. 2009;11(2):183–9.
21. Hop JW, Rinkel GJ, Algra A, van Gijn J. Initial loss of consciousness and risk of delayed cerebral ischemia after aneurysmal subarachnoid hemorrhage. Stroke. 1999;30(11):2268–71.
22. van den Bergh WM, Algra A, van der Sprenkel JW, Tulleken CA, Rinkel GJ. Hypomagnesemia after aneurysmal subarachnoid hemorrhage. Neurosurgery. 2003;52(2):276–81; discussion 81–2.
23. Wintermark M, Ko NU, Smith WS, Liu S, Higashida RT, Dillon WP. Vasospasm after subarachnoid hemorrhage: utility of perfusion CT and CT angiography on diagnosis and management. AJNR Am J Neuroradiol. 2006;27(1):26–34.
24. Samagh N, Bhagat H, Jangra K. Monitoring cerebral vasospasm: how much can we rely on tran-

scranial Doppler. J Anaesthesiol Clin Pharmacol. 2019;35(1):12–8.
25. Vergouwen MD, Vermeulen M, de Haan RJ, Levi M, Roos YB. Dihydropyridine calcium antagonists increase fibrinolytic activity: a systematic review. J Cereb Blood Flow Metab. 2007;27(7):1293–308.
26. de Oliveira Manoel AL, Goffi A, Zampieri FG, Turkel-Parrella D, Duggal A, Marotta TR, et al. The critical care management of spontaneous intracranial hemorrhage: a contemporary review. Crit Care. 2016;20:272.
27. Wijdicks EF, Vermeulen M, Hijdra A, van Gijn J. Hyponatremia and cerebral infarction in patients with ruptured intracranial aneurysms: is fluid restriction harmful? Ann Neurol. 1985;17(2):137–40.
28. Francoeur CL, Mayer SA. Management of delayed cerebral ischemia after subarachnoid hemorrhage. Crit Care. 2016;20(1):277.
29. Reynolds MR, Buckley RT, Indrakanti SS, Turkmani AH, Oh G, Crobeddu E, et al. The safety of vasopressor-induced hypertension in subarachnoid hemorrhage patients with coexisting unruptured, unprotected intracranial aneurysms. J Neurosurg. 2015;123(4):862–71.
30. Albanese E, Russo A, Quiroga M, Willis RN Jr, Mericle RA, Ulm AJ. Ultrahigh-dose intraarterial infusion of verapamil through an indwelling microcatheter for medically refractory severe vasospasm: initial experience. Clinical article. J Neurosurg. 2010;113(4):913–22.
31. van Gijn J, Hijdra A, Wijdicks EF, Vermeulen M, van Crevel H. Acute hydrocephalus after aneurysmal subarachnoid hemorrhage. J Neurosurg. 1985;63(3):355–62.
32. Rekate HL. The definition and classification of hydrocephalus: a personal recommendation to stimulate debate. Cerebrospinal Fluid Res. 2008;5:2.
33. Vale FL, Bradley EL, Fisher WS 3rd. The relationship of subarachnoid hemorrhage and the need for postoperative shunting. J Neurosurg. 1997;86(3):462–6.
34. Graff-Radford NR, Torner J, Adams HP Jr, Kassell NF. Factors associated with hydrocephalus after subarachnoid hemorrhage. A report of the Cooperative Aneurysm Study. Arch Neurol. 1989;46(7):744–52.
35. van Gijn J, Hijdra A, Wijdicks EF, Vermeulen M, van Crevel H. Acute hydrocephalus after aneurysmal subarachnoid hemorrhage. J Neurosurg. 1985;63(3):355–62.
36. Kartal MG, Algin O. Evaluation of hydrocephalus and other cerebrospinal fluid disorders with MRI: an update. Insights Imaging. 2014;5(4):531–41.
37. O'Kelly CJ, Kulkarni AV, Austin PC, Urbach D, Wallace MC. Shunt-dependent hydrocephalus after aneurysmal subarachnoid hemorrhage: incidence, predictors, and revision rates. Clinical article. J Neurosurg. 2009;111(5):1029–35.
38. de Oliveira JG, Beck J, Setzer M, Gerlach R, Vatter H, Seifert V, et al. Risk of shunt-dependent hydrocephalus after occlusion of ruptured intracranial aneurysms by surgical clipping or endovascular coiling: a single-institution series and meta-analysis. Neurosurgery. 2007;61(5):924–33; discussion 33–4.
39. Akinduro OO, Vivas-Buitrago TG, Haranhalli N, Ganaha S, Mbabuike N, Turnbull MT, et al. Predictors of ventriculoperitoneal shunting following subarachnoid hemorrhage treated with external ventricular drainage. Neurocrit Care. 2020;32(3):755–64.
40. Chung DY, Mayer SA, Rordorf GA. External ventricular drains after subarachnoid hemorrhage: is less more? Neurocrit Care. 2018;28(2):157–61.
41. Fried HI, Nathan BR, Rowe AS, Zabramski JM, Andaluz N, Bhimraj A, et al. The insertion and management of external ventricular drains: an evidence-based consensus statement: a statement for healthcare professionals from the Neurocritical Care Society. Neurocrit Care. 2016;24(1):61–81.
42. Huttner HB, Nagel S, Tognoni E, Kohrmann M, Juttler E, Orakcioglu B, et al. Intracerebral hemorrhage with severe ventricular involvement: lumbar drainage for communicating hydrocephalus. Stroke. 2007;38(1):183–7.
43. Claassen J, Peery S, Kreiter KT, Hirsch LJ, Du EY, Connolly ES, et al. Predictors and clinical impact of epilepsy after subarachnoid hemorrhage. Neurology. 2003;60(2):208–14.
44. Kvam DA, Loftus CM, Copeland B, Quest DO. Seizures during the immediate postoperative period. Neurosurgery. 1983;12(1):14–7.
45. Scott RB, Eccles F, Molyneux AJ, Kerr RS, Rothwell PM, Carpenter K. Improved cognitive outcomes with endovascular coiling of ruptured intracranial aneurysms: neuropsychological outcomes from the International Subarachnoid Aneurysm Trial (ISAT). Stroke. 2010;41(8):1743–7.
46. Miguel Bertelli Ramos MJT, Figueiredo EG. Seizures and epilepsy following subarachnoid hemorrhage: a review on incidence, risk factors, outcome and treatment. Arquivos Brasileiros de Neurocirurgia. 2018;37(3):206–12.
47. Al-Khindi T, Macdonald RL, Schweizer TA. Cognitive and functional outcome after aneurysmal subarachnoid hemorrhage. Stroke. 2010;41(8):e519–36.
48. Marigold R, Gunther A, Tiwari D, Kwan J. Antiepileptic drugs for the primary and secondary prevention of seizures after subarachnoid haemorrhage. Cochrane Database Syst Rev. 2013;(6):CD008710.
49. Lehmann L, Bendel S, Uehlinger DE, Takala J, Schafer M, Reinert M, et al. Randomized, double-blind trial of the effect of fluid composition on electrolyte, acid-base, and fluid homeostasis in patients early after subarachnoid hemorrhage. Neurocrit Care. 2013;18(1):5–12.
50. Rosengart AJ, Huo JD, Tolentino J, Novakovic RL, Frank JI, Goldenberg FD, et al. Outcome in patients with subarachnoid hemorrhage treated with antiepileptic drugs. J Neurosurg. 2007;107(2):253–60.
51. Wartenberg KE, Schmidt JM, Claassen J, Temes RE, Frontera JA, Ostapkovich N, et al. Impact of medical complications on outcome after subarachnoid hemorrhage. Crit Care Med. 2006;34(3):617–23; quiz 24.

52. Behrouz R, Sullebarger JT, Malek AR. Cardiac manifestations of subarachnoid hemorrhage. Expert Rev Cardiovasc Ther. 2011;9(3):303–7.
53. Chen S, Li Q, Wu H, Krafft PR, Wang Z, Zhang JH. The harmful effects of subarachnoid hemorrhage on extracerebral organs. Biomed Res Int. 2014;2014:858496.
54. Zaroff JG, Rordorf GA, Newell JB, Ogilvy CS, Levinson JR. Cardiac outcome in patients with subarachnoid hemorrhage and electrocardiographic abnormalities. Neurosurgery. 1999;44(1):34–9; discussion 9–40.
55. Sakr YL, Lim N, Amaral AC, Ghosn I, Carvalho FB, Renard M, et al. Relation of ECG changes to neurological outcome in patients with aneurysmal subarachnoid hemorrhage. Int J Cardiol. 2004;96(3):369–73.
56. Wartenberg KE, Mayer SA. Medical complications after subarachnoid hemorrhage: new strategies for prevention and management. Curr Opin Crit Care. 2006;12(2):78–84.
57. Chen Z, Venkat P, Seyfried D, Chopp M, Yan T, Chen J. Brain-heart interaction: cardiac complications after stroke. Circ Res. 2017;121(4):451–68.
58. Maimaitili A, Maimaitili M, Rexidan A, Lu J, Ajimu K, Cheng X, et al. Pituitary hormone level changes and hypxonatremia in aneurysmal subarachnoid hemorrhage. Exp Ther Med. 2013;5(6):1657–62.
59. Marupudi NI, Mittal S. Diagnosis and management of hyponatremia in patients with aneurysmal subarachnoid hemorrhage. J Clin Med. 2015;4(4):756–67.
60. Rahman M, Friedman WA. Hyponatremia in neurosurgical patients: clinical guidelines development. Neurosurgery. 2009;65(5):925–35; discussion 35–6.
61. Benvenga S. What is the pathogenesis of hyponatremia after subarachnoid hemorrhage? Nat Clin Pract Endocrinol Metab. 2006;2(11):608–9.
62. Kao L, Al-Lawati Z, Vavao J, Steinberg GK, Katznelson L. Prevalence and clinical demographics of cerebral salt wasting in patients with aneurysmal subarachnoid hemorrhage. Pituitary. 2009;12(4):347–51.
63. Maesaka JK, Imbriano L, Mattana J, Gallagher D, Bade N, Sharif S. Differentiating SIADH from cerebral/renal salt wasting: failure of the volume approach and need for a new approach to hyponatremia. J Clin Med. 2014;3(4):1373–85.
64. Mount DB. The brain in hyponatremia: both culprit and victim. Semin Nephrol. 2009;29(3):196–215.
65. Corona G, Giuliani C, Parenti G, Norello D, Verbalis JG, Forti G, et al. Moderate hyponatremia is associated with increased risk of mortality: evidence from a meta-analysis. PLoS One. 2013;8(12):e80451.
66. Ahmed AE, Ganaw AMT, Mohamed AO, Khair B. Aneurysmal subarachnoid hemorrhage. ICU book. Intechopen; 2017. p. 73–99.
67. Klose M, Brennum J, Poulsgaard L, Kosteljanetz M, Wagner A, Feldt-Rasmussen U. Hypopituitarism is uncommon after aneurysmal subarachnoid haemorrhage. Clin Endocrinol. 2010;73(1):95–101.
68. Parenti G, Cecchi PC, Ragghianti B, Schwarz A, Ammannati F, Mennonna P, et al. Evaluation of the anterior pituitary function in the acute phase after spontaneous subarachnoid hemorrhage. J Endocrinol Investig. 2011;34(5):361–5.
69. Wright WL, Asbury WH, Gilmore JL, Samuels OB. Conivaptan for hyponatremia in the neurocritical care unit. Neurocrit Care. 2009;11(1):6–13.
70. Weant KA, Sasaki-Adams D, Dziedzic K, Ewend M. Acute relative adrenal insufficiency after aneurysmal subarachnoid hemorrhage. Neurosurgery. 2008;63(4):645–9; discussion 9–50.
71. Pasternak JJ, McGregor DG, Schroeder DR, Lanier WL, Shi Q, Hindman BJ, et al. Hyperglycemia in patients undergoing cerebral aneurysm surgery: its association with long-term gross neurologic and neuropsychological function. Mayo Clin Proc. 2008;83(4):406–17.
72. Schlenk F, Graetz D, Nagel A, Schmidt M, Sarrafzadeh AS. Insulin-related decrease in cerebral glucose despite normoglycemia in aneurysmal subarachnoid hemorrhage. Crit Care. 2008;12(1):R9.
73. Naidech AM, Levasseur K, Liebling S, Garg RK, Shapiro M, Ault ML, et al. Moderate hypoglycemia is associated with vasospasm, cerebral infarction, and 3-month disability after subarachnoid hemorrhage. Neurocrit Care. 2010;12(2):181–7.
74. Naidech AM, Bendok BR, Bernstein RA, Alberts MJ, Batjer HH, Watts CM, et al. Fever burden and functional recovery after subarachnoid hemorrhage. Neurosurgery. 2008;63(2):212–7; discussion 7–8.
75. Oddo M, Frangos S, Milby A, Chen I, Maloney-Wilensky E, Murtrie EM, et al. Induced normothermia attenuates cerebral metabolic distress in patients with aneurysmal subarachnoid hemorrhage and refractory fever. Stroke. 2009;40(5):1913–6.
76. Aiyagari V, Diringer MN. Fever control and its impact on outcomes: what is the evidence? J Neurol Sci. 2007;261(1–2):39–46.
77. Dhar R, Zazulia AR, Videen TO, Zipfel GJ, Derdeyn CP, Diringer MN. Red blood cell transfusion increases cerebral oxygen delivery in anemic patients with subarachnoid hemorrhage. Stroke. 2009;40(9):3039–44.
78. Naidech AM, Drescher J, Ault ML, Shaibani A, Batjer HH, Alberts MJ. Higher hemoglobin is associated with less cerebral infarction, poor outcome, and death after subarachnoid hemorrhage. Neurosurgery. 2006;59(4):775–9; discussion 9–80.
79. Levine J, Kofke A, Cen L, Chen Z, Faerber J, Elliott JP, et al. Red blood cell transfusion is associated with infection and extracerebral complications after subarachnoid hemorrhage. Neurosurgery. 2010;66(2):312–8; discussion 8.
80. Mack WJ, Ducruet AF, Hickman ZL, Kalyvas JT, Cleveland JR, Mocco J, et al. Doppler ultrasonography screening of poor-grade subarachnoid hemorrhage patients increases the diagnosis of deep venous thrombosis. Neurol Res. 2008;30(9):889–92.
81. Lacut K, Bressollette L, Le Gal G, Etienne E, De Tinteniac A, Renault A, et al. Prevention of venous thrombosis in patients with acute intracerebral hemorrhage. Neurology. 2005;65(6):865–9.

Headache in Subarachnoid Hemorrhage

11

Hassan Abdallah Mitwally
and Sohel Mohamed Gamal Ahmed

11.1 Introduction

Headache is the chief complaint of patients who develop ruptured aneurysmal subarachnoid hemorrhage (SAH) and is the most common reason for visiting the emergency department for these patients [1]. Headache secondary to aneurysmal SAH usually starts as thunderclap which is severe in nature and sudden in onset [2]; patients describe the headache as the worst headache have ever experienced.

Headache post-aneurysmal SAH reaches its maximum intensity in minutes after a spontaneous bleed, and it may last for days or even weeks. Patients who develop cerebral vasospasms have higher pain score than patients without vasospasm [3]. In general, the pain severity correlates non-linearly with Hunt and Hess grade and correlates linearly with Hijdra score [4]. For more details please refer to Chap. 6. SAH in younger age and patients with high Hijdra score tend to be associated with severe headache [4].

H. A. Mitwally (✉)
Pharmacy Department, Al-Wakra Hospital, Hamad Medical Corporation, Doha, Qatar
e-mail: hmitwally@hamad.qa

S. M. G. Ahmed
Anesthesia Department, ICU and Perioperative Medicine, Hamad General Hospital, Hamad Medical Corporation, Doha, Qatar
e-mail: SAhmed65@hamad.qa

SAH headache may be associated with one or more sign and symptom. Nausea and or vomiting was reported in around 70% of patients, loss of consciousness was reported in around half of the patients. Other signs and symptoms associated with SAH headache, as photophobia, neck rigidity, and focal neurological deficit [5].

11.2 Pathophysiology of Headache in Aneurysmal SAH

The exact etiology behind SAH headache is not entirely understood. Many theories have been postulated over the three last decades. The most held up mechanism proposes that the headache is primarily due to the chemical irritation of the blood products on the brain meninges. Once the aneurysm ruptures, the blood extravasates from the blood vessels to the subarachnoid space causing a sharp rise in intracranial pressure (ICP) which leads to the feeling of sudden intolerable pain. The presence of blood in the subarachnoid space causes chemical irritation and subsequent inflammation that thought to contribute to the pathophysiology of pain [6, 7].

Vasospasm is associated with increasing intensity of headache secondary to decrease in cerebral perfusion which considered as one of the most important mechanisms of severe headache in SAH patients [8]. The decrease in brain perfusion

A. E. A. Ganaw et al. (eds.), *Management of Subarachnoid Hemorrhage*,
https://doi.org/10.1007/978-3-030-81333-8_11

is due to the endothelial damage that interferes with the nitric oxide production leading to vasoconstriction. Additionally, the excessive release of endothelin the potent vasoconstrictor plays a role in the induction of vasospasm and subsequently a decrease in cerebral perfusion [9, 10].

Another postulated factor is hyperalgesia caused by central sensitization by *N*-methyl-D-aspartate (NMDA) receptors. After SAH, activation of NMDA receptors facilitates pain transmission in the central nervous system, which can lead to hyperalgesia [11].

11.3 Pain Severity Evaluation in SAH

Pain should be routinely assessed as part of intensive care unit patient daily care [12]. Routine pain assessment was associated with a decrease in intensive care unit days, mechanical ventilator days, and a decrease in consumption of opioids and sedative agents in critically ill patients [13].

There is no specific tool or scale recommended to evaluate the severity of SAH headache. However self-reporting scales are the best method to assess pain in awake patients [12]. Among SAH patients whom could verbalized, 0–10 Numerical Rating Score (NRS) either verbally or visually should be used to assess the pain severity. In which 0 reflects no pain and 10 reflects the worst pain the patient could experience.

It is always difficult to assess pain in nonverbalized patients. The society of critical care medicine (SCCM) recommends two validated tools to assess pain in non-verbalized patients with a condition that they should have an intact motor function. The Critical-Care Pain Observation Tool (CPOT) and the Behavioral Pain Scale in intubated (BPS) are the most validated tools to evaluate pain in Medical, Surgical, and traumatic non-verbalizing patients critically ill patients [12, 14, 15]. Additionally, CPOT and BPS were studied in neurosurgical patients with different brain injuries; SAH, traumatic brain injury, tumor, intracranial hemorrhage, and ischemic stroke [16–19]. A COPT score cutoff of 3 or more and BPS more than 5 associated with a significant pain (Tables 11.1, and 11.2, respectively). Although nothing of these tools were extensively studied in SAH patient, clinicians may consider using these tools to monitor pain in nonverbalizing SAH patients.

11.4 Management of Headache in SAH

SAH-induced headache is difficult to be controlled and usually needs a combination between opioids and non-opioids analgesia for better pain control [4, 20]. Many clinicians still believe that pain management is still suboptimum in most of the centers. The complexity of SAH headache management came from the severity of headache and the worry of giving high drug doses that may mask the neurological deterioration of these patients. In fact, the available evidence for managing headache post-SAH is lacking, and the majority of the available evidence especially for opioids derived from post craniotomy pain control studies.

11.4.1 Pharmacological

11.4.1.1 Opioids

According to the World and Health Organization guidelines for pain management, opioids are considered a cornerstone for treating moderate to severe pain [21]. The cutoffs of moderate and severe pain were not mentioned clearly in the guidelines; some studies define the cutoffs of moderate and severe pain based on the numerical rating score (NRS) to be 4–6/10 and ≥7/10, respectively [22–24].

Morphine, codeine, and tramadol are the most studied opioids for post-craniotomy pain management [25]. Morphine is an opioid with high affinity for mu receptors and is considered one of the most effective opioids. Cumulative evidence has shown that morphine has better pain control when compared to codeine [26, 27]. The fear of masking the neurological deterioration post-craniotomy secondary to excessive sedation was usually associated with the use of potent opioids like morphine

Table 11.1 Critical-Care Pain Observation Tool (CPOT)

Indicator	Description	Score	
Facial expression	No muscular tension observed	Relaxed, neutral	0
	Presence of frowning, brow lowering, orbit tightening, and levator contraction	Tense	1
	All of the above facial movements plus eyelids tightly closed	Grimacing	2
Body movement	Does not move at all (does not necessarily mean absence of pain)	Absence of movement	0
	Slow, cautious movements; touching or rubbing the pain site; seeking attention through movements	Protection	1
	Pulling tube, trying to sit up, moving limbs/thrashing, not following commands, striking at staff, trying to climb out of bed	Restlessness	2
Muscle tension Evaluation by passive flexion and extension of upper extremities	No resistance to passive movements	Relaxed	0
	Resistance to passive movements	Tense, rigid	1
	Strong resistance to passive movements, inability to complete them	Very tense or rigid	2
Compliance with the ventilator (intubated patients)	Alarms not activated, easy ventilation	Tolerating ventilator or movement	0
	Alarms stop spontaneously	Coughing but tolerating	1
	Asynchrony: Blocking ventilation, alarms often activated	Fighting ventilator	2
Or vocalization (extubated patients)	Talking in normal tone or no sound	Talking in normal tone or no sound	0
	Sighing, moaning	Sighing, moaning	1
	Crying out, sobbing	Crying out, sobbing	2
Total, range			0–8

A CPOT score ≥3 indicates significant pain

Table 11.2 Behavioral Pain Scale (BPS)

Indicator	Description	Score
Facial expression	Relaxed	1
	Partly tightened (e.g., brow lowering)	2
	Fully tightened (e.g., eyelid closing)	3
	Grimacing	4
Upper limbs	No movement	1
	Partly bent	2
	Fully bent with finger flexion	3
	Permanently retracted	4
Compliance with ventilation	Tolerating movement	1
	Coughing but tolerating ventilation most of the time	2
	Fighting ventilator	3
	Unable to control ventilation	4

A BPS score >5 indicates significant pain

or fentanyl; however, trials showed no difference between morphine and codeine with regard to sedation, respiratory depression or cardiovascular outcomes [27, 28]. Tramadol is a weak mu-opioid receptor agonist. Intravenous tramadol may be as effective as morphine in controlling pain post-craniotomy; however, it showed more incidences of nausea and vomiting [29–31]. Vomiting is a significant concern in SAH patients as it may cause a sharp increase in ICP, which may worsen the neurological injury. Dihydrocodeine, another opioid frequently used in neurosurgical cases and incorporated in some hospital protocol [32], although it is reported to be inadequate in pain control [33]. Dihydrocodeine should be avoided in patients with severely impaired renal (Creatine clearance <10 mL/min) or hepatic functions.

Fentanyl could be considered a reasonable alternative to morphine as it also has a high affinity to mu receptors, quick onset of action, and accepted safety profile. Administration of opioids through a patient-controlled analgesia could be considered for conscious patients and may offer more patient convenience [34]. Fentanyl is may be preferred than morphine for patient-controlled analgesia, as morphine may be associated with more sedative effect when compared to fentanyl [35]. These findings may mask the neurological deterioration in SAH patients, especially in hepatic, renal impairment, and elderly patients. Moreover, continuous infusion of fentanyl is favorable than morphine In intubated patients, as morphine has two active metabolites; morphine-3-glucuronide and morphine-6-glucuronide [36], which upon accumulation might cause seizures, respiratory depression, and excessive sedation, especially in patients with renal impairment [37, 38].

Remifentanil is a short-acting mu-receptor opioid agonist. Because of its unique metabolism and clearance, remifentanil represents a new pharmacokinetic opioid class. Remifentanil context half-life (defined as; time required by continuous infusion drug plasma concentration to reach to 50% after being at steady state) was significantly less when compared to fentanyl [39]. Although being short acting is an advantage in various types of brain injuries as it allows early neurological assessment [40], it may be a disadvantage as it may lead to tolerance and hyperalgesia which subsequently increase opioids requirements; especially in patients who require prolonged remifentanil infusion [41]. Beside increasing tolerance possibility, remifentanil had conflicting efficacy data as analgesic when compared to other opioids or opioid sparing drugs which considered main concern in this context [39, 40, 42].

In general, using the least effective doses for opioids based on a valid pain assessment scores should be considered to avoid adverse drug reactions associated with opioids; as over sedation, hypotension, constipations, nausea, and vomiting. For opioids doses range; please refer to (Table 11.3) [43].

11.4.1.2 Non-opioids Therapy

Paracetamol

Intravenous Paracetamol is considered a safe analgesic with a degree of opioids sparing effect; it is found to decrease the opioids consumption postoperatively [44]. Paracetamol could be regarded as only as add on therapy to opioids as paracetamol monotherapy showed to be inferior to the combination of paracetamol and opioids [45, 46].

Table 11.3 Opioids dose ranges

Drug	Route	Dose range
Morphine[a]	Patient-controlled analgesia	– 0.5–2 mg – Lock time: 5–10 min – Maximum 30 mg in 4-h period
	Intermittent IV boluses	1–4 mg every 1–4 h as needed, up to 10 mg every 4 h as needed.
	Oral	10–20 mg every 4–6 h
Fentanyl	Continuous IV infusion	0.7–7μg/kg/h
	Patient-controlled analgesia	– 5–20μg – Lock time 5–10 min – Maximum 300μg within 4-h period
	Intermittent IV boluses	– Loading 25–100μg – Maintenance 25–50μg every 30–60 min
Remifentanil	Continuous IV infusion	0.05–0.25μg/kg/min
Dihydrocodeine	Oral	30 mg every 4–6 h

IV intravenous

[a]Avoid giving morphine as continues infusion in SAH. Morphine patient-controlled analgesia may be associated with more sedation when compared to fentanyl. Avoid morphine in renal, hepatic insufficiency, and elderly patients

Non-steroidal Anti-inflammatory Drugs (NSAIDs)

Besides its analgesic property, NSAIDs showed some beneficial outcome on ameliorating inflammatory response after aneurysmal SAH secondary to its anti-inflammatory effect [47]. Additionally, NSAIDs has an opioid sparing effect with no effect on neurological assessment. The use of NSAIDs post-aneurysmal SAH is limited because of its platelets inhibitory effect and suspicion of impacting homeostasis [48], especially in non-secured aneurysm, when risk of rebleeding is very high. Other side effects include interstitial nephritis, gastritis, gastro-intestinal bleeding, and cardiovascular complications [49, 50].

Dexmedetomidine

Dexmedetomidine is a selective α-2 agonist with sedation and analgesia properties, the mechanism of dexmedetomidine analgesic effect was thought to be through hyperpolarization of noradrenergic neurons, which suppresses neuronal firing in the locus coeruleus [51]. Dexmedetomidine showed a decrease in both pain scores and opioids requirements post-craniotomy [52–54]. Its light sedation property makes dexmedetomidine a desirable option for SAH intubated patients. Start by 0.2μg/kg/h and titrate up to 0.7μg/kg/h, doses up to 1.4μg/kg/h were used in clinical trials in mechanically intubated patients [55]. Monitoring for bradycardia and hypotension is vital while the patient is on dexmedetomidine [51]. Dose reduction needs to be considered in elderly and hepatic impairment patients [43].

Pregabalin

Although Pregabalin is a structural derivative of the inhibitory neurotransmitter GABA, it does not bind to GABA. Pregabalin reduces the release of neurotransmitters as glutamate and substance P by its presynaptic binding to α-2-delta subunit of the voltage-gated calcium channels within the central nervous system. This reduce in excitatory neurotransmitters may be the reason for anticonvulsant and analgesic effect of pregabalin [56].

A recent small well-designed randomized control trial evaluated the effect of pregabalin on perioperative headache in patients with aneurysmal subarachnoid hemorrhage. The use of pregabalin 75 mg twice daily perioperatively was associated with significant decrease in opioid and anesthetic requirements without increase in sedation [57]. Although larger trials need to be conducted to confirm these findings, pregabalin could be consider as an adjunctive therapy in controlling perioperative headache in SAH patients. Pregabalin in general in well tolerated, although it is renally eliminated and dose should be adjusted based on the patient creatinine clearance to avoid drug accumulation which may affect neurological status.

Gabapentin

Gabapentin is structurally related to (Gamma-Aminobutyric Acid) GABA, it has a high affinity towards voltage-gated calcium channels located pre-synaptically, and may modulate the release of excitatory neurotransmitters [58]. Gabapentin showed to decrease opioids consumption in post-craniotomy patient, although it causes more sedation and delay in extubation [59]. Limited evidence supporting the use of gabapentin in treating aneurysmal SAH headache, gabapentin showed to decrease the requirements of opioids in a small retrospective study [60]. The mechanism of action is that aneurysmal SAH headache may be neuropathic, as the meninges are innervated by the anterior and posterior ethmoidal nerves, the tentorial nerve (a branch of the ophthalmic nerve), and the maxillary division of the trigeminal nerve [60].

Ketamine

Some evidence suggested that ketamine may decrease ICP, opioids requirements, and delayed cerebral ischemia (DCI)-associated cerebral infarctions [61]. Prospective clinical trials need to be conducted before generalizing the use of ketamine in SAH patients.

Magnesium

Magnesium could be used as adjunctive therapy to opioids and non-opioids pain medications to decrease the intensity of pain or decrease the need for opioids. Patients with high magnesium levels (magnesium >1.0 mmol/L) had a lower pain scores when compared to patients with normal magnesium levels (magnesium <1.0 mmol/L). Additionally, these patients required lower opioids doses than required by normal magnesium level patients [62]. Case reports showed a significant pain improvement for patients with Reversible Cerebral Vasoconstriction Syndrome (RCVS) treated with intravenous magnesium sulphate the primary pathology was aneurysmal SAH and acute infarction of the bilateral parieto-occipital lobes [8].

The mechanism behind the suspected benefit of magnesium is that it may act as a neuroprotectant by decreasing the ischemic depolarization of brain cells. That helps to reduce the cerebral lesion volume presented during aneurysmal SAH acute phase [63].

Corticosteroids

Corticosteroids, especially dexamethasone, are potent anti-inflammatory drugs. As discussed in the mechanism of aneurysmal SAH, the presence of blood in the subarachnoid space irritates the meninges and cause production of inflammatory cytokines. A meta-analysis was conducted including eight clinical trials to evaluate the effect of dexamethasone in delayed cerebral ischemia and showed non-significant results [64]. Further studies need to be undertaken to assess the impact of corticosteroids in headache post-aneurysmal SAH. Till the availability of more evidence, routine use of corticosteroids in preventing delayed cerebral ischemia and subsequent headache is not recommended, especially that corticosteroids cause hyperglycemia which was proven to be associated with poor outcomes [65].

11.4.2 Non-pharmacological Options

11.4.2.1 Scalp Block

Both the trigeminal and spinal nerves provide sensory innervation of the scalp and forehead. The trigeminal nerve is the largest cranial nerve and is the principal source of sensory innervation of the head and face, including the meninges [66]. The trigeminal nerve has an ophthalmic, maxillary, and mandibular division, all of which contribute branches that innervate part of the forehead and scalp (Fig. 11.1). The greater occipital nerve arises from the posterior ramus of the second cervical nerve (C2) root and innervates the significant portion of the posterior scalp. It originates in the posterior neck, lateral to the atlantoaxial joint and deep into the inferior oblique muscle [67].

Scalp block, which entitles infiltration of local anesthesia at various spots of the scalp, has been

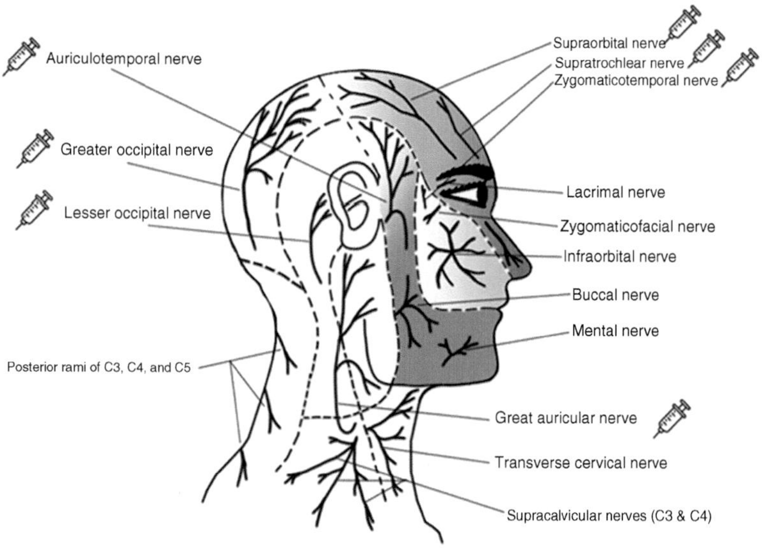

Fig. 11.1 Scalp innervation with syringes pointing out to nerves need to be blocked. (Drawing courtesy of Dr. Mohammed Bahari, London, UK)

extensively described in the literature. Scalp blocks are mainly used for neurosurgical procedures such as the sole anesthetic for awake craniotomies [68] and/or postoperative pain management of craniotomies in adults and children [69]. It has also been used to diagnose postoperative headache of unknown origin [70].

Irrespective of the etiology behind headache associated with SAH, the afferent pathway is through the meningeal branches of the various branches of the trigeminal nerve and roots of C2 and C3 nerves. Hence, scalp block has the potential to block any nociceptive stimulus from the meninges. In a series of 10 cases, Venkatesulu and colleagues utilized scalp block in the management of SAH-induced headache. Scalp block was administered if the patient's Visual Analog Scale (VAS) for pain is >7, after administration of adequate systemic analgesics, or when the patient exhibits intolerance to analgesics. Scalp blocks were performed using an anatomic method without ultrasound guidance, with 2–3 mL of 0.25% bupivacaine administered per nerve. Scalp block resulted in an average 62% reduction in VAS at 1 h after administration. Only one patient required rescue analgesia, and then only a single dose of intravenous tramadol, 48 h after block administration. All the patients were followed up for 48 h, after stopping the intravenous paracetamol, and none required further analgesia [71].

As the authors noted, scalp block might potentially mask SAH-related complications such as vasospasm and/or rebleeding, so its risks and benefits require further evaluation. Furthermore, its influence on the incidence of vasospasm or rebleeding rates also needs to be studied.

11.5 Conclusion and Recommendations

Management of SAH headache is complex, combining both opioids and non-opioids is important to control the pain and decrease opioids requirements (Table 11.4). The use of pain assessment

Table 11.4 Management of headache post-subarachnoid hemorrhage

Drug		Initial regimen or pain score ≥6	Pain score <6
Opioids	Intubated[a]	Fentanyl/Remifentanil[b] as continuous infusion	
	Non-intubated	Fentanyl: patient-controlled analgesia for awake and intermittent boluses for non-awake patients	Oral morphine/dihydrocodeine[c] (use the least effective dose)
±			
Dexmedetomidine		For intubated patients[d]	
+			
Paracetamol		1 g intravenous every 6 h	1 g orally every 6 h
±			
Pregabalin		75 mg orally twice daily[e] perioperatively	
+			
Magnesium sulfate		2–4 g daily (to keep magnesium level >1.0 mmol/L)	
+			
Laxatives/prokinetics		To avoid straining and to maintain at least one bowel motion every 24–48 h	
+			
Blood pressure control (*discussed in Chap. 10*)		• Maintain SBP <140 mmHg (in secured aneurysm up to 160 mmHg, especially if there is vasospasm) • Nimodipine 60 mg oral every 4 h for 21 days	

SBP systolic blood pressure

[a]Use behavioral assessment tools in intubated patient or patient unable to self-report [e.g. critical care pain observation tool (CPOT), or behavioral pain scale (BPS)] to assure adequate pain control

[b]Avoid prolonged use of remifentanil (risk of tolerance and hyperalgesia)

[c]Avoid using morphine or dihydrocodeine in severely impaired renal or hepatic patients

[d]May be continued after extubation to decrease the opioids consumption with monitoring for heart rate, blood pressure, and conscious level

[e]Pregabalin needs to be adjusted in renal impairment patients (Creatinine clearance <60 mL/min)

scores helps in evaluating the degree of pain and titrating medications to ensure adequate pain control with the least effect doses.

11.6 Research Gaps and Future Directions

Till now the evidence behind the best strategy to manage SAH-induced headache is lacking. Clinical trials need to be conducted to compare different opioids and non-opioids evaluating both efficacy and safety outcomes.

References

1. Wartenberg KE, Mayer SA. Medical complications after subarachnoid hemorrhage. Neurosurg Clin N Am. 2010;21(2):325–38. https://doi.org/10.1016/j.nec.2009.10.012.
2. Dodick DW. Thunderclap headache. J Neurol Neurosurg Psychiatry. 2002;72(1):6–11. https://doi.org/10.1136/JNNP.72.1.6.
3. Swope R, Glover K, Gokun Y, Fraser JF, Cook AM. Evaluation of headache severity after aneurysmal subarachnoid hemorrhage. Interdiscip Neurosurg. 2014;1(4):119–22. https://doi.org/10.1016/J.INAT.2014.07.003.
4. Glisic EK, Gardiner L, Josti L, et al. Inadequacy of headache management after subarachnoid hemorrhage. Am J Crit Care. 2016;25(2):136–43. https://doi.org/10.4037/ajcc2016486.
5. Cross DT, Tirschwell DL, Clark MA, et al. Mortality rates after subarachnoid hemorrhage: variations according to hospital case volume in 18 states. J Neurosurg. 2003;99(5):810–7. https://doi.org/10.3171/jns.2003.99.5.0810.
6. Gaetani P, Tartara F, Pignatti P, Tancioni F, Rodriguez Y, Baena R, De Benedetti F. Cisternal CSF levels of cytokines after subarachnoid hemorrhage. Neurol Res. 1998;20(4):337–42. https://doi.org/10.1080/01616412.1998.11740528.
7. Polin RS, Bavbek M, Shaffrey ME, et al. Detection of soluble E-selectin, ICAM-1, VCAM-1, and L-selectin in the cerebrospinal fluid of patients after subarachnoid hemorrhage. J Neurosurg. 1998;89(4):559–67. https://doi.org/10.3171/jns.1998.89.4.0559.
8. Mijalski C, Dakay K, Miller-Patterson C, Saad A, Silver B, Khan M. Magnesium for treatment of reversible cerebral vasoconstriction syndrome: case series. Neurohospitalist. 2016;6(3):111–3. https://doi.org/10.1177/1941874415613834.
9. Sobey CG, Faraci FM. Subarachnoid haemorrhage: what happens to the cerebral arteries? Clin Exp Pharmacol Physiol. 1998;25(11):867–76. http://www.ncbi.nlm.nih.gov/pubmed/9807657. Accessed 26 Feb 2019.
10. Zimmermann M, Seifert V. Endothelin and subarachnoid hemorrhage: an overview. Neurosurgery. 1998;43(4):863–75; discussion 875–6. http://www.ncbi.nlm.nih.gov/pubmed/9766314. Accessed 26 Feb 2019.
11. Woolf CJ, Thompson SWN. The induction and maintenance of central sensitization is dependent on N-methyl-d-aspartic acid receptor activation; implications for the treatment of post-injury pain hypersensitivity states. Pain. 1991;44(3):293–9. https://doi.org/10.1016/0304-3959(91)90100-C.
12. Devlin JW, Skrobik Y, Gélinas C, et al. Clinical practice guidelines for the prevention and management of pain, agitation/sedation, delirium, immobility, and sleep disruption in adult patients in the ICU. Crit Care Med. 2018;46(9):e825–73. https://doi.org/10.1097/CCM.0000000000003299.
13. Payen JF, Bosson JL, Chanques G, Mantz J, Labarere J. Pain assessment is associated with decreased duration of mechanical ventilation in the intensive care unit: a post Hoc analysis of the DOLOREA study. Anesthesiology. 2009;111(6):1308–16. https://doi.org/10.1097/ALN.0b013e3181c0d4f0.
14. Gélinas C, Johnston C. Pain assessment in the critically ill ventilated adult: validation of the critical-care pain observation tool and physiologic indicators. Clin J Pain. 2007;23(6):497–505. https://doi.org/10.1097/AJP.0b013e31806a23fb.
15. Payen JF, Bru O, Bosson JL, et al. Assessing pain in critically ill sedated patients by using a behavioral pain scale. Crit Care Med. 2001;29(12):2258–63. https://doi.org/10.1097/00003246-200112000-00004.
16. Yu A, Teitelbaum J, Scott J, et al. Evaluating pain, sedation, and delirium in the neurologically critically Ill—feasibility and reliability of standardized tools: a multi-institutional study. Crit Care Med. 2013;41(8):2002–7. https://doi.org/10.1097/CCM.0b013e31828e96c0.
17. Echegaray-Benites C, Kapoustina O, Gélinas C. Validation of the use of the Critical-Care Pain Observation Tool (CPOT) with brain surgery patients in the neurosurgical intensive care unit. Intensive Crit Care Nurs. 2014;30(5):257–65. https://doi.org/10.1016/j.iccn.2014.04.002.
18. Dehghani H, Tavangar H, Ghandehari A. Validity and reliability of behavioral pain scale in patients with low level of consciousness due to head trauma hospitalized in intensive care unit. Arch Trauma Res. 2014;3(1):18608. https://doi.org/10.5812/atr.18608.
19. Joffe AM, McNulty B, Boitor M, Marsh R, Gélinas C. Validation of the Critical-Care Pain Observation Tool in brain-injured critically ill adults. J Crit Care. 2016;36:76–80. https://doi.org/10.1016/j.jcrc.2016.05.011.
20. Morad AH, Tamargo RJ, Gottschalk A. The longitudinal course of pain and analgesic therapy following aneurysmal subarachnoid hemorrhage: a cohort study.

Headache J Head Face Pain. 2016;56(10):1617–25. https://doi.org/10.1111/head.12908.

21. World Health Organization. Scoping document for WHO guidelines for the pharmacological treatment of persisting pain in adults with medical illnesses SCOPING DOCUMENT FOR WHO guidelines for the pharmacological treatment of persisting pain in adults with medical illnesses this scoping document is an updated and merged version of the scoping documents on chronic malignant pain and chronic non-malignant pain of 2008. https://www.who.int/medicines/areas/quality_safety/Scoping_WHO_GLs_PersistPainAdults_webversion.pdf?ua=1. Accessed 28 Apr 2019.
22. Boonstra AM, Stewart RE, Köke AJA, et al. Cut-off points for mild, moderate, and severe pain on the numeric rating scale for pain in patients with chronic musculoskeletal pain: variability and influence of sex and catastrophizing. Front Psychol. 2016;7:1466. https://doi.org/10.3389/fpsyg.2016.01466.
23. Zelman DC, Dukes E, Brandenburg N, Bostrom A, Gore M. Identification of cut-points for mild, moderate and severe pain due to diabetic peripheral neuropathy. Pain. 2005;115(1):29–36. https://doi.org/10.1016/j.pain.2005.01.028.
24. Jensen MP, Smith DG, Ehde DM, Robinsin LR. Pain site and the effects of amputation pain: further clarification of the meaning of mild, moderate, and severe pain. Pain. 2001;91(3):317–22. http://www.ncbi.nlm.nih.gov/pubmed/11275389. Accessed 1 May 2019.
25. Roberts G. A review of the efficacy and safety of opioid analgesics post-craniotomy. Nurs Crit Care. 2004;9(6):277–83. http://www.ncbi.nlm.nih.gov/pubmed/15575637. Accessed 1 May 2019.
26. Jeffrey HM, Charlton P, Mellor DJ, Moss E, Vucevic M. Analgesia after intracranial surgery: a double-blind, prospective comparison of codeine and tramadol. Br J Anaesth. 1999;83(2):245–9. https://doi.org/10.1093/BJA/83.2.245.
27. Goldsack C, Scuplak SM, Smith M. A double-blind comparison of codeine and morphine for postoperative analgesia following intracranial surgery. Anaesthesia. 1996;51(11):1029–32. http://www.ncbi.nlm.nih.gov/pubmed/8943593. Accessed 1 May 2019.
28. Stoneham MD, Cooper R, Quiney NF, Walters FJ. Pain following craniotomy: a preliminary study comparing PCA morphine with intramuscular codeine phosphate. Anaesthesia. 1996;51(12):1176–8. http://www.ncbi.nlm.nih.gov/pubmed/9038464. Accessed 1 May 2019.
29. Ng KF, Tsui SL, Yang JC, Ho ET. Increased nausea and dizziness when using tramadol for post-operative patient-controlled analgesia (PCA) compared with morphine after intraoperative loading with morphine. Eur J Anaesthesiol. 1998;15(5):565–70. http://www.ncbi.nlm.nih.gov/pubmed/9785072. Accessed 1 May 2019.
30. Houmes RJ, Voets MA, Verkaaik A, Erdmann W, Lachmann B. Efficacy and safety of tramadol versus morphine for moderate and severe postoperative pain with special regard to respiratory depression. Anesth Analg. 1992;74(4):510–4. http://www.ncbi.nlm.nih.gov/pubmed/1554117. Accessed 1 May 2019.
31. Pang W-W, Mok MS, Lin C-H, Yang T-F, Huang M-H. Comparison of patient-controlled analgesia (PCA) with tramadol or morphine. Can J Anesth. 1999;46(11):1030–5. https://doi.org/10.1007/BF03013197.
32. Kotak D, Cheserem B, Solth A. A survey of post-craniotomy analgesia in British neurosurgical centres: time for perceptions and prescribing to change? Br J Neurosurg. 2009;23(5):538–42. https://doi.org/10.1080/02688690903100595.
33. Stoneham MD, Walters FJM. Post-operative analgesia for craniotomy patients: current attitudes among neuroanaesthetists. Eur J Anaesthesiol. 1995;12(6):571–5. https://europepmc.org/article/med/8665879. Accessed 27 Jul 2020.
34. Jellish WS, Leonetti JP, Kristina S, Douglas A, Origitano TC. Morphine/ondansetron PCA for post-operative pain, nausea, and vomiting after skull base surgery. Otolaryngol Neck Surg. 2006;135(2):175–81. https://doi.org/10.1016/j.otohns.2006.02.027.
35. Nada EM, Alabdulkareem A. Morphine versus fentanyl patient-controlled analgesia for postoperative pain control in major hepatic resection surgeries including living liver donors: a retrospective study. Saudi J Anaesth. 2018;12(2):250–5. https://doi.org/10.4103/sja.SJA_625_17.
36. Zaw-Tun N, Bruera E. Active metabolites of morphine. J Palliat Care. 1992;8(2):48–50. http://www.ncbi.nlm.nih.gov/pubmed/1635007. Accessed 6 Mar 2019.
37. Christrup LL. Morphine metabolites. Acta Anaesthesiol Scand. 1997;41(1 Pt 2):116–22. http://www.ncbi.nlm.nih.gov/pubmed/9061094. Accessed 6 Mar 2019.
38. Hannam JA, Anderson BJ. Contribution of morphine and morphine-6-glucuronide to respiratory depression in a child. Anaesth Intensive Care. 2012;40(5):867–70. https://doi.org/10.1177/0310057X1204000516.
39. Egan TD. Remifentanil pharmacokinetics and pharmacodynamics: a preliminary appraisal. Clin Pharmacokinet. 1995;29(2):80–94. https://doi.org/10.2165/00003088-199529020-00003.
40. Karabinis A, Mandragos K, Stergiopoulos S, et al. Open Access Safety and efficacy of analgesia-based sedation with remifentanil versus standard hypnotic-based regimens in intensive care unit patients with brain injuries: a randomised, controlled trial [ISRCTN50308308]. Crit Care. 2004;8(4):R268–80. https://doi.org/10.1186/cc2896.
41. Yu EHY, Tran DHD, Lam SW, Irwin MG. Remifentanil tolerance and hyperalgesia: short-term gain, long-term pain? Anaesthesia. 2016;71(11):1347–62. https://doi.org/10.1111/anae.13602.
42. Rajan S, Hutcherson MT, Sessler DI, et al. The effects of dexmedetomidine and remifentanil on hemodynamic stability and analgesic requirement after craniotomy: a randomized controlled trial. J

Neurosurg Anesthesiol. 2016;28(4):282–90. https://doi.org/10.1097/ANA.0000000000000221.
43. Lexicomp | Clinical drug information. https://www.wolterskluwercdi.com/lexicomp-online/. Accessed 8 Sept 2020.
44. Maghsoudi R, Tabatabai M, Radfar MH, et al. Opioid-sparing effect of intravenous paracetamol after percutaneous nephrolithotomy: a double-blind randomized controlled trial. J Endourol. 2014;28(1):23–7. https://doi.org/10.1089/end.2013.0267.
45. Sane S, Tolumehr A, Hassani E, Mahoori A. Comparison the effects of paracetamol with sufentanil infusion on postoperative pain control after craniotomy in patients with brain tumor. Adv Biomed Res. 2015;4(1):64. https://doi.org/10.4103/2277-9175.152610.
46. Verchère E, Grenier B, Mesli A, Siao D, Sesay M, Maurette P. Postoperative pain management after supratentorial craniotomy. J Neurosurg Anesthesiol. 2002;14(2):96–101. http://www.ncbi.nlm.nih.gov/pubmed/11907388. Accessed 3 Mar 2019.
47. Muroi C, Hugelshofer M, Seule M, Keller E. The impact of nonsteroidal anti-inflammatory drugs on inflammatory response after aneurysmal subarachnoid hemorrhage. Neurocrit Care. 2014;20(2):240–6. https://doi.org/10.1007/s12028-013-9930-2.
48. Niemi T, Tanskanen P, Taxell C, Juvela S, Randell T, Rosenberg P. Effects of nonsteroidal anti-inflammatory drugs on hemostasis in patients with aneurysmal subarachnoid hemorrhage. J Neurosurg Anesthesiol. 1999;11(3):188–94. http://www.ncbi.nlm.nih.gov/pubmed/10414674. Accessed 3 Mar 2019.
49. Harirforoosh S, Asghar W, Jamali F. Adverse effects of nonsteroidal antiinflammatory drugs: an update of gastrointestinal, cardiovascular and renal complications. J Pharm Pharm Sci. 2013;16(5):821–47. https://doi.org/10.18433/j3vw2f.
50. Ong CKS, Lirk P, Tan CH, Seymour RA. An evidence-based update on nonsteroidal anti-inflammatory drugs. Clin Med Res. 2007;5(1):19–34. https://doi.org/10.3121/cmr.2007.698.
51. Grewal A. Dexmedetomidine: new avenues. J Anaesthesiol Clin Pharmacol. 2011;27(3):297–302. https://doi.org/10.4103/0970-9185.83670.
52. Zhao LH, Shi ZH, Chen GQ, et al. Use of dexmedetomidine for prophylactic analgesia and sedation in patients with delayed extubation after craniotomy: a randomized controlled trial. J Neurosurg Anesthesiol. 2017;29(2):132–9. https://doi.org/10.1097/ANA.0000000000000260.
53. Song J, Ji Q, Sun Q, Gao T, Liu K, Li L. The opioid-sparing effect of intraoperative dexmedetomidine infusion after craniotomy. J Neurosurg Anesthesiol. 2016;28(1):14–20. https://doi.org/10.1097/ANA.0000000000000190.
54. Peng K, Jin X, Liu S, Ji F. Effect of intraoperative dexmedetomidine on post-craniotomy pain. Clin Ther. 2015;37(5):1114–21.e1. https://doi.org/10.1016/j.clinthera.2015.02.011.
55. Jakob SM, Ruokonen E, Grounds RM, et al. Dexmedetomidine vs midazolamor propofol for sedation during prolonged mechanical ventilation: two randomized controlled trials. JAMA. 2012;307(11):1151–60. https://doi.org/10.1001/jama.2012.304.
56. Clinical use of pregabalin in the management of central neuropathic pain. https://www.ncbi.nlm.nih.gov/pmc/articles/PMC2656330/. Accessed 15 Jan 2020.
57. Lionel KR, Sethuraman M, Abraham M, Vimala S, Prathapadas U, Hrishi AP. Effect of pregabalin on perioperative headache in patients with aneurysmal subarachnoid hemorrhage: a randomized double-blind, placebo-controlled trial. J Neurosci Rural Pract. 2019;10(03):438–43. https://doi.org/10.1055/s-0039-1697871.
58. Cheng J-K, Chiou L-C. Mechanisms of the antinociceptive action of gabapentin. J Pharmacol Sci. 2006;100(5):471–86. http://www.ncbi.nlm.nih.gov/pubmed/16474201. Accessed 17 Apr 2019.
59. Türe H, Sayin M, Karlikaya G, Bingol CA, Aykac B, Türe U. The analgesic effect of gabapentin as a prophylactic anticonvulsant drug on postcraniotomy pain: a prospective randomized study. Anesth Analg. 2009;109(5):1625–31. https://doi.org/10.1213/ane.0b013e3181b0f18b.
60. Dhakal LP, Hodge DO, Nagal J, et al. Safety and tolerability of gabapentin for aneurysmal subarachnoid hemorrhage (SAH) headache and meningismus. Neurocrit Care. 2015;22(3):414–21. https://doi.org/10.1007/s12028-014-0086-5.
61. Von der Brelie C, Seifert M, Rot S, et al. Sedation of patients with acute aneurysmal subarachnoid hemorrhage with ketamine is safe and might influence the occurrence of cerebral infarctions associated with delayed cerebral ischemia. World Neurosurg. 2017;97:374–82. https://doi.org/10.1016/j.wneu.2016.09.121.
62. Dorhout Mees SM, Bertens D, van der Worp HB, Rinkel GJE, van den Bergh WM. Magnesium and headache after aneurysmal subarachnoid haemorrhage. J Neurol Neurosurg Psychiatry. 2010;81(5):490–3. https://doi.org/10.1136/jnnp.2009.181404.
63. van den Bergh WM, Zuur JK, Kamerling NA, et al. Role of magnesium in the reduction of ischemic depolarization and lesion volume after experimental subarachnoid hemorrhage. J Neurosurg. 2002;97(2):416–22. https://doi.org/10.3171/jns.2002.97.2.0416.
64. Feigin VL, Anderson N, Rinkel GJ, Algra A, van Gijn J, Bennett DA. Corticosteroids for aneurysmal subarachnoid haemorrhage and primary intracerebral haemorrhage. Cochrane Database Syst Rev. 2005;3 https://doi.org/10.1002/14651858.CD004583.pub2.
65. Frontera JA, Fernandez A, Claassen J, et al. Hyperglycemia after SAH: predictors, associated

complications, and impact on outcome. Stroke. 2006;37(1):199–203. https://doi.org/10.1161/01.STR.0000194960.73883.0f.

66. Nahum AM. Grant's atlas of anatomy, 7th edition. Edited by James E. Anderson, 608 pp, illus, Williams & Wilkins, Baltimore, 1978. $30.00. Head Neck Surg. 1979;1(5):465–5. https://doi.org/10.1002/hed.2890010513.
67. Ward JB. Greater occipital nerve block. Semin Neurol. 2003;23(1):59–61. https://doi.org/10.1055/s-2003-40752.
68. Osborn I, Sebeo J. "Scalp block" during craniotomy: a classic technique revisited. J Neurosurg Anesthesiol. 2010;22(3):187–94. https://doi.org/10.1097/ANA.0b013e3181d48846.
69. Sebeo J, Osborn IP. The use of "scalp block" in pediatric patients. Open J Anesthesiol. 2012;02(03):70–3. https://doi.org/10.4236/ojanes.2012.23017.
70. Manohar N, Rao KS, Chakrabarti D, Srinivas DB. Scalp block: tool for diagnosis in postoperative headache of unknown origin. J Neurosurg Anesthesiol. 2018;30(4):381–2. https://www.google.com/search?rlz=1C1GCEU_enQA881QA881&sxsrf=ALeKk03L3oY2DhkSic_k-_53lq7FCm1FCQ:1590843942725&source=univ&tbm=isch&q=17.+Manohar,+Nitin+MD,+DNB,+DM,+Rao,+Keerthi+S.+DA,+DNB,+PDF;+Chakrabarti,+Dhritiman+MD,+DM;+Srinivas,+Deepti+B.+MD.+Scalp+block:+Tool+for+diagnosis+in+Postoperative+Headache+of+Unknown+Origin.+Journal+of+Neurosurgical+Anesthesiology:+October+2018+-+Volume+30+-+Issue+4+-+p+381-382&sa=X&ved=2ahUKEwilmOXA09vpAhX27XMBHeGyCMcQsAR6BAgCEAE&cshid=1590844100991299&biw=1920&bih=937. Accessed 30 May 2020.
71. Venkatesulu KB, Nandhakumar A, Cherian M, Mehta P, Kalingarayar S, Shanmugam S. Scalp block for management of subarachnoid hemorrhage (SAH)-induced headache. J Neurosurg Anesthesiol. 2019;31(3):356–7. https://doi.org/10.1097/ANA.0000000000000523.

12 Traumatic Subarachnoid Hemorrhage

Abdulgafoor M. Tharayil, Talat Saeed Chughtai, Basil Younis, Abdulnasser Alyafei, and Vishwajit Verma

12.1 Introduction

Traumatic Brain Injury (TBI) is a major cause of mortality in those under 40 years of age. Traumatic SAH (tSAH), first described in 1859 and described as "sanguineous meningeal effusion" by Wilks [1] present unique challenges, and is associated with a worse prognosis, as shown by Head Injury Trials 1, 2, and 3. The mortality rate in patients with TBI doubles if associated with tSAH, and if the basal cisterns are involved, there is a positive predictive value of 70% for a bad outcome. Some of the reasons for the worse prognosis include complications such as: vasospasm, electrolyte disturbances, hydrocephalus, as well as endocrine dysfunctions involving the pituitary and hypothalamus. In terms of the worse outcome, according to some investigators, tSAH is a marker of severe TBI, while others stand by the theory that it is directly deleterious, leading to complications such as vasospasm and ischemia [2].

A. M. Tharayil (✉)
Surgical ICU, HMC, Doha, Qatar
e-mail: atharayil@hamad.qa

T. S. Chughtai
Trauma ICU, HMC, Doha, Qatar
e-mail: TChughtai@hamad.qa

B. Younis · A. Alyafei
Department of Neurosurgery, HMC, Doha, Qatar
e-mail: byounis@hamad.qa; athabet@hamad.qa

V. Verma
TICU, HMC, Doha, Qatar
e-mail: vverma@hamad.qa

12.2 Incidence

The incidence of SAH in TBI is reported variably between 2.9 and 53% in different studies. Mattioli et al. stated an incidence of 61% in head-injured patients admitted to intensive care units (ICUs). Computerized tomography (CT) scans obtained in 169 head-injured patients on admission to 12 Italian intensive care units during a 3-month period were examined. A review committee found this high incidence of tSAH in patients with TBI [3].

12.3 Pathophysiology

tSAH may be caused by one or more of five potential mechanisms [4].

1. Rotational acceleration causing short-lasting oscillatory movements of the brain.
2. Vertebrobasilar artery stretch due to hyperextension.
3. Sudden rise of intra-arterial pressure from a blow to the cervical carotid artery.
4. Tearing of the bridging pial veins.
5. Diffusion of blood from an intra-cerebral contusion into the subarachnoid space.

A. E. A. Ganaw et al. (eds.), *Management of Subarachnoid Hemorrhage*,
https://doi.org/10.1007/978-3-030-81333-8_12

12.4 Clinical Features and Presentations

Patients with tSAH present with same clinical features of aSAH. However, there are significant differences between traumatic and aneurysmal SAH in terms of incidence, location, vasospasm, utility of nimodipine, rate of seizure and outcome (Table 12.1). They present with severe headache, vomiting, altered conscious level, seizures, and focal neurological deficits. Sometimes patients present with clinical features of the acute complications of tSAH such as intra-cerebral clot and acute hydrocephalus. If patients developed pseudoaneurysm, they may present with neck pain, lower cranial nerve palsies, cervico-medullary compression syndrome, and Horner's syndrome. Sometimes pseudoaneurysm formed after head trauma remain silent and later rupture producing subarachnoid hemorrhage with high potential to rebleed.

Table 12.1 Comparison of traumatic and aneurysmal SAH

	Traumatic (non-aneurysmal) SAH	Aneurysmal SAH
Incidence	+++	+
Location	Cerebral convexity	Skull base
Vasospasm rate	+	+++
Vasospasm onset	12 h to 5 days	4–5 days
Vasospasm resolution	12 h to 30 days	14–21 days
Nimodipine utility	+	+++
Seizure rate	++	+
Recurrence	Rare	Common
Need for intervention (IR/OR)	+	+++
Unfavorable outcome	++	+++

IR interventional radiology, *OR* operating room

12.5 Diagnosis

12.5.1 CT Scan

A tSAH should be evident on a non-contrast CT scan of the brain. Most commonly, it is found to be involving cerebral hemispheres and basal cisterns (39.31%), followed by the cortical sulci (33.33%) and the inter-hemispheric space (11.96%) [5]. Figures 12.1 and 12.2 depict the radiological features of tSAH commonly seen in CT scan of the brain.

12.5.1.1 Advantages

(a) CT scan is easy and comparatively rapid diagnostic tool.
(b) Sensitive in first 24 h to detect SAH, highest in the first 3 days (close to 100%).
(c) Can detect Hydrocephalus and intra-ventricular hemorrhage early.

12.5.1.2 Limitations

(a) Risk of radiation.

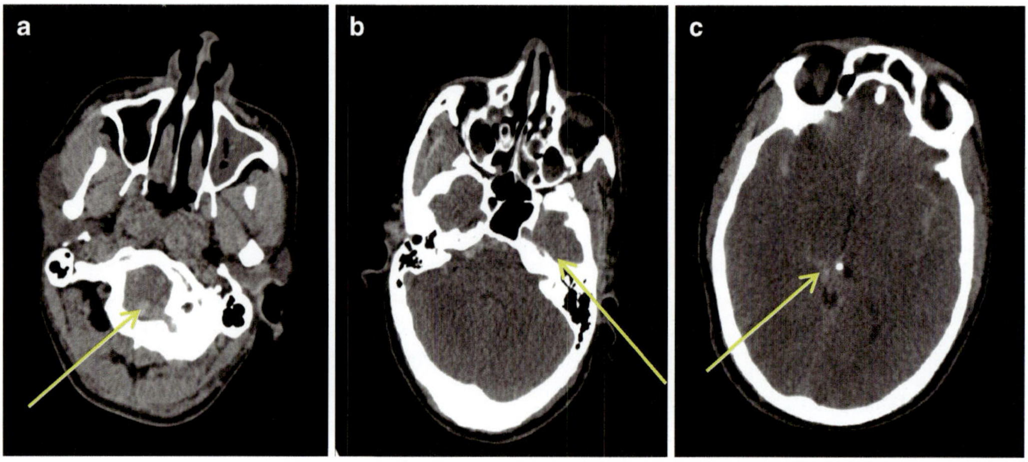

Fig. 12.1 (**a**) Cerebello-medullary {cisterna Magna}, (**b**) Prepontine, (**c**) ambient cistern

(b) Sensitivity progressively decreases over time to only 58% in the fifth day. For more details please refer to Chap. 5.

12.5.2 Magnetic Resonance Imaging and Others

Functional imaging modalities such as Positron Emission Tomography (PET), Magnetic Resonance Imaging (MRI), and Magnetic Resonance Spectroscopy are helpful in giving details of both perfusion and cerebral metabolism, and thereby have prognostic significance by defining the extent of injury and ischemia.

Fluid Attenuated Inversion Recovery (FLAIR), Gradient Reversal Echo (GRE), and Susceptibility Weighted Imaging (SWI) sequences of MRI are sensitive for the detection of acute tSAH in the first 48 h, and are complimentary to CT scan. Furthermore, SWI sequences are comparatively better in detecting IVH and tSAH in basal cisterns, which may be missed on non-contrast CT [6]. According to preliminary findings of Nikhilkumar et al., MRI FLAIR sequence delineates tSAH in the sulcal and tentorial region, which constitute 76.62% of tSAH [4]. (See Figs. 12.3 and 12.4).

12.5.2.1 Advantages

(a) No risk of radiation.
(b) MRI better sensitive than CT brain after 4 days.

12.5.2.2 Limitations

(a) Time consuming.
(b) Expensive compared to CT.
(c) May need sedation if patient is confused and uncooperative.

12.6 Grading of tSAH

There are many grading systems available to grade tSAH, for example: Fisher, modified Fisher, Morris-Marshall, and Greene.

12.6.1 Fisher Grade Classification

The Fisher scale (Table 12.2) was introduced in 1980 as an index of vasospasm risk based upon the hemorrhage pattern seen on initial head CT scan. Fisher scale was validated in a small prospective series of 41 patients with SAH, with excellent interobserver agreement. The limitation of this grading is that it is poorly correlated with outcome. For more details please refer to Chap. 6.

12.6.2 Modified Fisher's Scale [7]

This grading depicted in Table 12.3 is also based on CT scan findings. It was proposed by Classen 2001. Although this grading incorporates additional risk posed by intra-ventricular hemorrhage, this grading is also correlated with the risk of delayed cerebral ischemia and poorly correlated with clinical outcome.

12.6.3 Morris-Marshall Grading [7]

This grading system depicted in Table 12.4 is also a CT scan-based grading. This considers the distribution of SAH in the CT scan, but it was not found to be better than GCS scale on admission or contusion in the CT.

12.6.4 Greene et al. Grading [7]

This grading system (Table 12.5) proposed by Greene et al. in 1995 is also a CT based grading. This is much simpler with better interobserver agreement. The authors validated this grading against Glasgow outcome Score and found to be correlating with outcome at hospital discharge.

12.7 Complications of tSAH

Most significant complications of tSAH include post-traumatic vasospasm, hydrocephalus, and pseudoaneurysm.

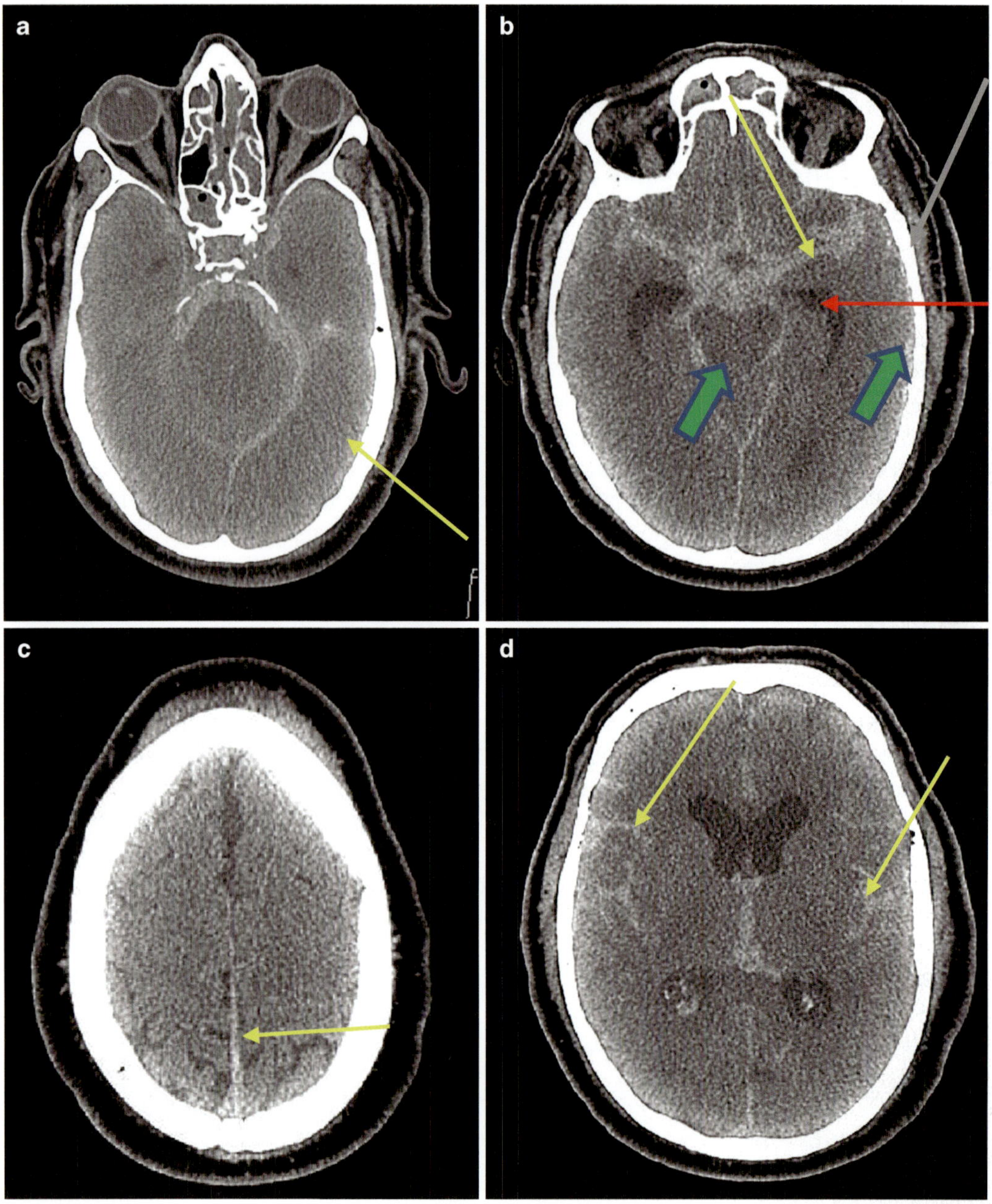

Fig. 12.2 (**a**) Tentorium cerebelli, (**b**) Enlarged temporal horn {large arrow}, suprasellar {yellow arrow}, interpeduncular {red arrow}, Sylvian {black arrow}, (**c**) Falx attenuation, (**d**) cortical sulci)

12.7.1 Post-traumatic Vasospasm (PTV)

This complication occurs up to 40% after tSAH. Unlike aneurysmal SAH [5], PTV occurs and resolves earlier; starting 12 h to 5 days after injury, and lasting for 12 h to up to 30 days. PTV is not necessarily associated with a significant amount of SAH and has been noted even without any radiographic evidence of SAH [7]. Known predictors of vasospasm include cisternal SAH and Intra-ventricular hemorrhage (IVH) [8, 9].

There are three different circulatory stages described after severe head injury [10].

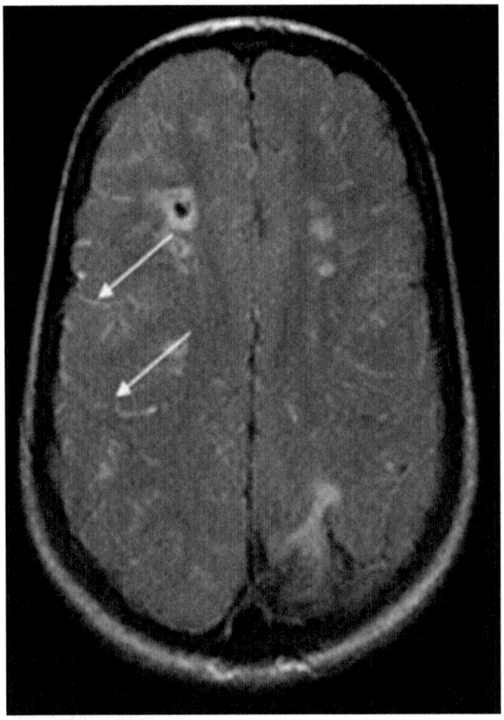

Fig. 12.3 MRI FLAIR sequence showing acute traumatic subarachnoid hemorrhage. (Adapted from: Case courtesy of Radswiki, Radiopaedia.org, rID: 11973 under creative commons License)

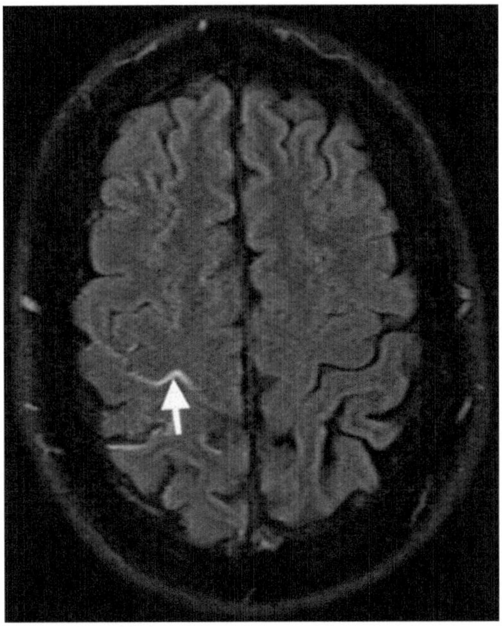

Fig. 12.4 MRI FLAIR sequence showing acute traumatic subarachnoid hemorrhage. (Adapted from: Case courtesy of Dr Amro Omar, Radiopaedia.org, rID: 32468 under creative commons License)

Table 12.2 Fisher grading

Grade	Appearance of hemorrhage
1	No subarachnoid blood detected
2	Diffuse or vertical layer <1 mm thick
3	Localized clot and/or vertical layer >1 mm thick
4	Intra-cerebral or intra-ventricular clot with diffuse (or no) SAH

Table 12.3 Modified Fisher's scale

Grade	Criteria
0	No subarachnoid hemorrhage (SAH) or ventricular hemorrhage (VH)
1	Minimal SAH, no VH in the 2 lateral ventricles
2	Minimal SAH, VH in the 2 lateral ventricles
3	Large SAH[a], no VH in the 2 lateral ventricles
4	Large SAH[a], VH in the 2 lateral ventricles

VH Ventricular hemorrhage
[a]SAH completely filling at least one cisterna or fissure

Table 12.4 Morris-Marshall grading

Grade	CT scan findings
0	No CT evidence of traumatic subarachnoid hemorrhage
1	tSAH present only in one location
2	tSAH present in only one location, but quantity of blood fills that structure, or tSAH is in any two sites, filling neither of them
3	tSAH present in two sites (including the tentorium) filled with blood
4	tSAH present in three or more sites, and being of any quantity

Table 12.5 Greene et al. grading

Grade 1	Thin SAH less than or equal to 5 mm
Grade 2	Thick SAH greater than 5 mm
Grade 3	Thin SAH with associated mass lesion
Grade 4	Thick SAH with an associated mass lesion

Phase I (hypoperfusion): This stage occurs on the day of injury (day 0) and is characterized by: low cerebral blood flow (CBF), normal middle cerebral artery (MCA) velocity, normal hemispheric index (ratio of MCA velocity to internal carotid artery velocity), and normal arteriovenous difference of oxygenation (AVDO).

Phase II (hyperemia): This stage occurs between days 1–3: CBF increases, AVDO falls, MCA velocity rises, and the hemispheric index remains less than 3.

Phase III (vasospasm): This stage occurs between days 4–15: CBF decreases, MCA velocity further increases, and there is a significant rise in the hemispheric index above 3. About 25% of vasospasm secondary to tSAH occurs by day 3 [11].

Proposed mechanisms for vasospasm include [12]:

1. Released blood products stimulating the Tyrosine Kinase pathway, causing calcium release, which results in cerebral artery smooth muscle contraction.
2. CSF oxyhemoglobin causing vasoconstriction via increased free radicals, endothelin 1, and prostaglandin, as well as reduced Nitric Oxide and Prostacyclin production.
3. Autonomic disturbance causing cerebral artery vasoconstriction.

12.7.2 Hydrocephalus

Following tSAH, there is impairment of cerebrospinal fluid (CSF) drainage and absorption resulting in hydrocephalus. Fifty percent of tSAH patients develop hydrocephalus. It is found more commonly in elderly patients, those with low GCS on admission, presence of intra-ventricular hemorrhage, and severe tSAH [13].

12.7.3 Pseudoaneurysm

Pseudoaneurysm due to traumatic brain injury comprises of only 1% of all cerebral aneurysms. The basic pathology is the loss of integrity of the arterial wall intima due to the trauma and blood seeping into the arterial wall which is confined by adventitia and surrounding tissue which is described as a "pulsating hematoma." Later the blood inside this space undergo clotting followed by fibrous tissue formation. The ongoing arterial flow results in excavation of this fibrous area and thins it out forming a pseudoaneurysm sac. Eventually this sac ruptures and results in subarachnoid hemorrhage [14].

12.7.4 Cognitive Dysfunction

Although there are many studies on cognitive dysfunction in aneurysmal SAH, there were no data on the long-term cognitive dysfunction in patients with tSAH until 2011, when Wong et al. [15] published a paper on prevalence and risk factors for cognitive dysfunction. Patients who had tSAH 3–5 years before were assessed by cognitive tests. Out of 111 patients who were recruited, 42% of them completed all assessments. Forty percent of them had at least one domain deficit and 30% had two or more domain deficits. Extended Glasgow outcome scale (GOS-E) was significantly correlated with the domain deficits and cognitive impairment. Age and Glasgow coma scale (GCS) on admission were important predictors. Extent of tSAH was found to be an independent predictor.

12.8 Management of tSAH

Patients with tSAH should be managed preferably in the neuro-intensive care unit or a Trauma Intensive Care Unit that is experienced at managing TBI. Neuro-intensive care principles such as elevation of head, avoiding compression of the neck veins, frequent turning of the patient, physiotherapy, mouth/bowel/bladder care, early enteral nutrition, analgesia, antiemetic and antiepileptic medication are essential components of care. Coagulopathy should be avoided and reversed if needed [16].

However, it has also been suggested that the presence of isolated tSAH should not by itself represent an indication to admit a patient with a clinically mild TBI to a critical care unit [17]. These cases may not necessarily require aggressive monitoring in ICU [18].

According to Bullock et al. [7], management of tSAH should be targeted at avoiding secondary injury, maintenance of cerebral perfusion pressure (CPP), optimizing cerebral oxygenation, and neuro-monitoring. Apart from routine neuro-monitoring, advanced neuro-monitoring including intracranial pressure, jugular bulb venous oxygen saturation, cerebral micro-dialysis, brain tissue oxygen tension monitoring, transcranial Doppler ultrasonography (TCD) should be used. Additional supportive management such as mechanical ventilation, hemodynamic support, hyperosmolar therapy, Lund concept, stress ulcer prophylaxis and, rarely, barbiturate coma, may be required for optimum management of tSAH patients.

12.9 Management of Specific Complications

12.9.1 Dyslectrolytemia

Maintenance of euvolemia or marginal hypervolemia, and avoidance of hypotonic solutions, are mainstays of management. A serum sodium level of 150–155 meq/L is acceptable in TBI patient with brain edema. Hyponatremia may be due to Syndrome of Inappropriate Anti-Diuretic Hormone (SIADH) or cerebral salt wasting (CSW). The former is managed by fluid restriction, while the latter is managed by replacement of volume and sodium. For more details please refer to Chap. 10.

12.9.2 Post-traumatic Vasospasm

Hypertension and hypervolemia should not be used in tSAH patients injudiciously as it may worsen cerebral edema. Use of Nimodipine, a calcium channel blocker, is controversial in tSAH. Although a 2003 Cochrane [6] review reported an improved outcome in terms of decreased mortality and severe disability, another study by Vergouwen et al. [19] did not support the routine use of nimodipine. Two studies have been done in relatively unselected head injury populations: Head Injury Trial 1, involving five British centers and Helsinki, followed by Head Injury Trial 2, including 12 centers across Europe. These studies involving a 7-day treatment with Nimodipine showed a 4% absolute improvement, and 8% relative improvement, respectively, towards favorable outcome though not statistically significant. The results were disappointing. Head Injury Trial 3, involving 123 patients with CT scan evidence of SAH, admitted to 12 centers in Germany, showed a significant difference in the rate of favorable outcome for Nimodipine-treated patients. In a meta-analysis of these studies, there was a "just-significant" improvement in mortality and disability in Nimodipine treated-patients. An ongoing trial, Head Injury Trial 4 is expected to give more insight into this issue.

12.9.3 Hydrocephalus

As with non-traumatic communication hydrocephalus, external ventricular drain (EVD) or ventriculo-peritoneal shunt (VP Shunt) is the treatment of choice [20]. For more details please refer to Chap. 10.

12.9.4 Ruptured Pseudoaneurysm

Traumatic intracranial pseudoaneurysms are rare, occurring in less than 1% of patients with cerebral aneurysms. It could be originated from the cavernous segment of ICA or middle cerebral artery (MCA). The former group present with classic triad of symptoms: massive epistaxis, unilateral blindness, and skull base fracture [14]. They are treated by endovascular occlusion. Traumatic pseudoaneurysm of MCA usually present with intracranial hemorrhage. They are best managed by surgical clipping.

12.9.4.1 Surgical Clipping

This is the most common type of intervention performed. A craniotomy is performed to locate the aneurysm, commonly utilizing a navigation system for precise localization. Often a temporary clip is placed proximally to facilitate clipping the neck of the aneurysm, to avoid bleeding [21] A permanent small clip made of titanium is placed across the "neck" of the aneurysm to block blood flow from entering, avoiding any major artery or perforators. The clip remains on the artery permanently.

For more details please review Chap. 9.

12.9.4.2 Trapping

Surgical "Complete Trapping"

Complete trapping (with concomitant flow replacement/revascularization) can be "complete classic," where the aneurysm and all the branches are occluded, or may be "complete variant," where the aneurysm is occluded, but not all the branches from the aneurysmal segment are occluded from the circulation [21].

12.9.4.3 Artery Occlusion and Bypass

If the aneurysm is large and inaccessible, or if the artery is severely damaged, the surgeon may perform a bypass surgery. A craniotomy is used for access, and then clips are placed to completely occlude the artery and aneurysm. Blood flow is then re-routed around the occluded artery by a vessel graft. The graft is commonly a small blood vessel usually taken from the leg [21].

12.9.4.4 Wrapping

If no other method is feasible, the aneurysm may be "wrapped"/coated. Several agents and wrapping techniques may be used: cotton, muscle, silastic sheet, gauze, Teflon, adhesives such as Biobond, fibrin glue, polyglactin 910 fibrin sealant, and collagen-impregnated Dacron fabric. There is no evidence that one agent is superior to the other. The common mechanism is induction of chronic inflammation and fibrosis [21].

12.9.4.5 Non-surgical Management

Endovascular Coiling

This is performed during an angiogram in the radiology department. Through the catheter, the aneurysm is packed with platinum coils or glue, which prevents blood flow into the aneurysm. This is a form of "trapping" of the aneurysm and is often used for skull base aneurysms which are difficult to clip [20].

For more details please review Chap. 8.

12.9.4.6 Follow-Up

Patients who underwent occlusive treatment for pseudoaneurysm should be followed up regularly.

In a review article by Cothren et al. [22], patients who underwent stenting for pseudoaneurysm and started on anticoagulation therapy had stenosis rate of 45% of the vessel on follow-up, whereas only 5% of the conservative treatment group had stenosis on follow-up. In another study by Berne et al. [23], stenosis was found only in one out of 7 patients who had stenting.

12.10 Prognostic Factors

In a study by Lin et al., independent predictors of poor prognosis were: age, initial Glasgow Coma Score (GCS), extensive tSAH, and IVH. They also found that statistically, patients with extensive tSAH are significantly more likely to develop vasospasm [24]. In another prospective study by Okten et al., prognosis was poorer in patients with poor admission GCS, hemorrhage in cisterna or fissures, presence of cerebral contusion or acute subdural hematoma, and patients with Fisher's grade 3 or 4 [25]. Modified fisher grade predicts vasospasm, and indirectly predicts the clinical outcome [26].

12.11 Conclusion

Traumatic subarachnoid hemorrhage is common among patients with head injury. It has a tremendous impact on the mortality of TBI patients and if survived, causes significant cognitive impairment. Neuronal loss, diffuse axonal injury (DAI), microbleed, and disruption of blood-brain barrier (BBB) contribute to the development of cognitive impairment. Early diagnosis is thus extremely important and possible with non-contrast CT in most cases; however, MRI with FLAIR, GRI, and SWI sequences are helpful in detecting missed cases. Management is conservative and supportive, with practice of standard neuro-critical care principles. Special complications encountered in these patients such as vasospasm, hydrocephalus, and electrolyte disturbances should be promptly managed. Early diagnosis and timely management are the key for successful outcome in this subset of patients with traumatic brain injury.

References

1. Ullman JS, Morgan BC, Eisenberg HM. Traumatic subarachnoid hemorrhage. Chapter 14. In: Bederson JB, editor. Textbook of subarachnoid hemorrhage: pathophysiology and management. The American Association of Neurological Surgeons; 1997. p. 225–37.
2. Armin SS, Colohan AR, Zhang JH. Traumatic subarachnoid hemorrhage: our current understanding and its evolution over the past half century. Neurol Res. 2006;28(4):445–52.
3. Mattioli C, Beretta L, Gerevini S, Veglia F, Citerio G, Cormio M, Stocchetti N. Traumatic subarachnoid hemorrhage on the computerized tomography scan obtained at admission: a multicenter assessment of the accuracy of diagnosis and the potential impact on patient outcome. J Neurosurg. 2003;98(1):37–42.
4. Modi NJ, Agrawal M, Sinha VD. Post-traumatic subarachnoid hemorrhage: a review. Neurol India. 2016;64(7):8–13.
5. Greene KA, Marciano FF, Johnson BA, Jacobowitz R, Spetzler RF, Harrington TR. Impact of traumatic subarachnoid hemorrhage on outcome in nonpenetrating head injury. Part I: a proposed computerized tomography grading scale. J Neurosurg. 1995;83:445–52.
6. Langham J, Goldfrad C, Teasdale G, Shaw D, Rowan K. Calcium channel blockers for acute traumatic brain injury. Cochrane Database Syst Rev. 2003;(4):CD000565.
7. Bullock MR, Hovda DA. Introduction to traumatic brain injury. Chapter 322. In: Richard Winn H, editor. Textbook: Youmans neurological surgery. 6th ed. Saunders. p. 3267.
8. Claassen J, Bernardini GL, Kreiter K, Bates J, Du YE, Copeland D, et al. Effect of cisternal and ventricular blood on risk of delayed cerebral ischemia after subarachnoid hemorrhage: the Fisher scale revisited. Stroke. 2001;32:2012–20.
9. Kawamoto S, Tsutsumi K, Yoshikawa G, Shinozaki MH, Yako K, Nagata K, et al. Effectiveness of the head-shaking method combined with cisternal irrigation with urokinase in preventing cerebral vasospasm after subarachnoid hemorrhage. J Neurosurg. 2004;100:236–43.
10. Martin NA, Patwardhan RV, Alexander MJ, Africk CZ, Lee JH, Shalmon E, et al. Characterization of cerebral hemodynamic phases following severe head trauma: hypoperfusion, hyperemia, and vasospasm. J Neurosurg. 1997;87:9–19.
11. Rozsa L, Gombi R, Szabo S, Sztermen M. Vasospasm after head injury studied by transcranial Doppler sonography. Radiol Diagn. 1989;30(2):151–7.
12. Kolias AG, Sen J, Belli A. Pathogenesis of cerebral vasospasm following aneurysmal subarachnoid hemorrhage: putative mechanisms and novel approaches. J Neurosci Res. 2009;87(1):1–11. https://doi.org/10.1002/jnr.21823.
13. Tian HL, Xu T, Hu J, Cui YH, Chen H, Zhou LF. Risk factors related to hydrocephalus after traumatic subarachnoid hemorrhage. Surg Neurol. 2008;69:241–6.
14. Moon TH, Kim SH, Lee JW, Huh SK. Clinical analysis of traumatic cerebral pseudoaneurysms. Korean J Neurotrauma. 2015;11(2):124–30. https://doi.org/10.13004/kjnt.2015.11.2.124. Published online 2015 Oct 31. PMCID: PMC4847513.
15. Wong GKC, Ngai K, Wong A, et al. Long-term cognitive dysfunction in patients with traumatic subarachnoid hemorrhage: prevalence and risk factors. Acta Neurochir. 2012;154:105–11. https://doi.org/10.1007/s00701-011-1198-8.
16. Von der Brelie C, Schneegans I, van den Boom L, Meier U, Hedderich J, Lemcke J. Impaired coagulation is a risk factor for clinical and radiologic deterioration in patients with traumatic brain injury and isolated traumatic subarachnoid hemorrhage. J Trauma Acute Care Surg. 2015;79(2):295–300. https://doi.org/10.1097/TA.0000000000000722.
17. Witiw CD, Byrne JP, Nassiri F, Badhiwala JH, Nathens AB, da Costa LB. Isolated traumatic subarachnoid hemorrhage: an evaluation of critical care unit admission practices and out-comes from a North American perspective. Crit Care Med. 2018;46(3):430–6. https://doi.org/10.1097/CCM.0000000000002931.
18. Albertine P, Borofsky S, Brown D, Patel S, Lee W, Caputy A, Taheri MR. The clinical significance of small subarachnoid hemorrhages. Emerg Radiol. 2016;23(3):207–11. https://doi.org/10.1007/s10140-016-1377-2. Epub 2016 Feb 12.
19. Vergouwen MD, Vermeulen M, Roos YB. Effect of nimodipine on outcome in patients with traumatic subarachnoid haemorrhage: a systematic review. Lancet Neurol. 2006;5:1029–32.
20. Ringer A, Kilburg C. Mayfield Clinic, Cincinnati, Ohio, Mayfield Certified Health Info materials are written and developed by the Mayfield Clinic. updated > 1.2020.
21. Greenberg MS. Handbook of neurosurgery. 8th ed; 2016. ISBN 978-1-62623-241-9123456.

22. Cothren CC, Moore EE, Ray CE Jr, et al. Carotid artery stents for blunt cerebrovascular injury: risks exceed benefits. Arch Surg. 2005;140(5):480–6.
23. Berne JD, Reuland KR, Villarreal DH, McGovern TM, Rowe SA, Norwood SH. Internal carotid artery stenting for blunt carotid artery injuries with an associated pseudoaneurysm. J Trauma. 2008;64(2):398–405.
24. Lin TK, Tsai HC, Hsieh TC. The impact of traumatic subarachnoid hemorrhage on outcome: a study with grouping of traumatic subarachnoid hemorrhage and transcranial Doppler sonography. J Trauma Acute Care Surg. 2012;73(1):131–6.
25. Okten AI, Gezercan Y, Ergün R. Traumatic subarachnoid hemorrhage: a prospective study of 58 cases. Ulus Travma Acil Cerrahi Derg. 2006;12(2):107–14.
26. Hussain F, Rafay M, Gulzar F, Sharif S. Traumatic subarachnoid hemorrhage comprising outcome with modified fisher grade. Surgery Curr Res. 2019;9:330. https://doi.org/10.35248/2161-1076.19.9.330.

13 Prognosis of Aneurysmal Subarachnoid Haemorrhage: Facts and Figures

Nissar Shaikh, Shoaib Nawaz, Arshad Chanda, Alisha Alkubaisi, Ali O. M. Bel Khair, Sami M. Belhaj, Mohamed Elgamudi, Adel E. Ahmed Ganaw, Marcus Lance, and Ali Ayyad

13.1 Introduction

Aneurysmal subarachnoid haemorrhage (aSAH) has remained a global health and financial burden with a higher fatality rate and permanent disabilities [1]. Most of these patients are in the productive stage of their life, and less than 16% of patients will return to their premorbid status. In forecasting the prognosis indicators of aSAH like the age, comorbidities, clinical-grade of aSAH on presentation, location, size of the aneurysm, early and late complication related to aSAH has to be given due consideration.

The outcome also depends on the treating facility. In facilities managing a significant volume of aSAH patients, receiving both microsurgical and endovascular intervention and dedicated Neurointensive Care Unit have a better outcome.

The prognosis of aSAH is influenced by several non-modifiable factors as well as factors that can be manipulated by prompt interventions and proper management. Early prognostication of subarachnoid haemorrhage patients is important as the bulk of evidence indicates that brain injury begins at the aneurysm rupture, evolves with time, and plays an essential role in patients' outcome [2]. It may help the treating physicians to decide the level of care, wisely utilize the resources, and give families clear picture of disease process and expected outcome.

13.2 Mortality in aSAH

Although the mortality of spontaneous aneurysmal subarachnoid haemorrhage (aSAH) is showing a decreasing trend in the last three decades, aSAH still has a high fatality rate [1]. Approximately up to 15% of aSAH patients die before reaching the

Note: Figures and tables are original and have been not be published anywhere else.

N. Shaikh (✉) · A. E. A. Ganaw
Anesthesia, ICU, Perioperative Medicine, Hamad Medical Corporation, Doha, Qatar
e-mail: Smaheboob@hamad.qa; aganaw@hamad.qa

S. Nawaz · A. Chanda · A. O. M. Bel Khair
M. Lance
Surgical Intensive Care Unit, Hamad Medical Corporation, Doha, Qatar
e-mail: snawaz1@hamad.qa; achanda@hamad.qa; akhair2@hamad.qa; mlance@hamad.qa

A. Alkubaisi · A. Ayyad
Department of Neurosciences, Neurosurgery Section, Hamad Medical Corporation, Doha, Qatar
e-mail: aalkubaisi8@hamad.qa; aayyad@hamad.qa

S. M. Belhaj
Department of Anaesthesia, Yarmouth Regional Hospital, Yarmouth, NS, Canada

M. Elgamudi
Department of Psychiatry, Hamad Medical Corporation, Doha, Qatar
e-mail: Melgamudi@hamad.qa

A. E. A. Ganaw et al. (eds.), *Management of Subarachnoid Hemorrhage*,
https://doi.org/10.1007/978-3-030-81333-8_13

health care facility, and 25% die within 24 h of haemorrhage with or without medical therapy. The early mortality is a result of complications of aneurysmal SAH. Mortality can be secondary to early neurological injury, re-bleeding, hydrocephalus, increased intracranial pressure, seizures, and non-neurological conditions like cardiac complications. In all hospitalized aSAH patients, 40% die within 1 month, and around 60% die within 6 months [1]. The decrease in aSAH case fatality over the last decades is mainly due to improved technologies to diagnose, endovascular or surgical treatment with recent parallel development in critical care management [1]. The long term survivors' of the aSAH have a higher mortality rate than the general population, mostly due to cerebrovascular events.

13.3 Morbidity in aSAH

The morbidity among survivors of aSAH is related mainly to two groups of dysfunctions. The neurophysical dysfunctions like motor and sensory deficits, epilepsy and the neuropsychological i.e., the cognitive dysfunctions such as loss of memory, sleep disturbances, language, and executive function.

13.3.1 Neurophysical Dysfunction

The neurophysical dysfunctions is due to the primary insult from the subarachnoid haemorrhage or secondary insults such as brain oedema, re-bleeding, cerebral vasospasm, brain ischaemia, hydrocephalus, and seizures. These are major determinants of the functional outcome. They may be seen at the time of presentation or newly developed in the postoperative period. The new postoperative deficits have poor outcome and are associated with multiple factors related to the aneurysm and intraoperative events. While, the neurophysical deficits that detected at the initial presentation improve with time.

Early diagnosis and interventions may prevent secondary neurological complications like rebleed, vasospasm, hydrocephalus, and seizures in patients with aSAH.

Treating physicians should concentrate on preventing ischaemic complications by using various therapies to maintain adequate cerebral perfusion such as induced hypertension [3]. Nimodipine is the only drug approved by the US Food and Drug Administration for use in the treatment of vasospasm. It is safe, cost-effective, and reduces the poor outcome as well as secondary ischaemia after aSAH [4]. The seizure prophylaxis is controversial in patients with SAH, but the use of phenytoin is documented to be associated with worse outcomes, especially when it is used for a longer duration [5]. The most common comorbidities in these patients are hypertension and diabetes mellitus. They require proactive management to improve outcome [6].

13.3.2 Neuropsychological Dysfunction

The neuropsychological, i.e., the cognitive dysfunctions, are well known but underreported. Al-Khindi and colleagues reported that more than 33% of aSAH patients had a significant neurocognitive disturbance upon discharge from the hospital. These patients commonly present with memory, language, and executive day-to-day functional disorders [7]. Memory loss is mainly verbal memory; executive functions like attention, inhibition, strategizing, planning, problem-solving, and decision making are impaired. The neurocognitive disturbances, in combination with depression, anxiety, and sleep disturbances, will significantly hamper the day-to-day essential functional abilities [2]. The recovery time of cognitive dysfunction is variable, but it improves with time. During the evaluation of cognitive performance, symptoms such as headache, sleep disorders, fatigue, depression, etc., affect the outcome score.

13.3.3 Neuropsychiatric Manifestation in Post aSAH

Neuropsychiatric manifestations are common after aSAH. The most common being depression. The manifestations of depression are similar to those of the frontal lobe syndrome. Sometimes depression and frontal lobe syndrome may overlap. It takes considerable time for improvement when compared to neurocognitive impairment. The other neuropsychiatric manifestations are anxiety, apathy, and denial, catastrophic reaction, and sleep impairment.

13.4 Prediction and Monitoring the Prognosis in aSAH

Prediction and monitoring the prognosis in aSAH is usually done by neurological examination on presentation to hospital, daily till discharge and then periodically. This helps in clinical grading and assessment of progress or deterioration of the clinical condition and the neurophysical prognosis. The second most important tool is neuroimagining, especially the Computed tomography scan grade. Other tools are the neuropsychological tests, modified Rankin score, Glasgow outcome score. The functional outcome assessment comprises daily living, instrumental activities of daily living, and the ability to return to work.

The unexplored domains are the Biomarkers assays. Biomarkers assays in combination with neurological examinations and imaging may predict high-risk patients; thus, the treating physicians use all the available resources and mandatory interventions to prevent expected complications and improve the outcome [8].

In aSAH patients, certain biomarkers like CRP, selectin, thrombin antithrombin complex (TAT), creatine kinase-BB (CK-BB), malondialdehyde (MDA), S100β protein, ubiquitin C terminal hydrolase 1 (UCHL1), and D-dimer are considered as best specific and sensitive biomarkers to predict the outcome as well as possibilities of recovery. However, the sensitivities and specificities of all these biomarkers are less than 90%.

Because of a lack of evidence, lower sensitivities, and specificities of any given single biomarker, their utilization in the standard of care in the acute phase of SAH has not been adopted. Further research must be conducted to identify specific biokinetics of these biomarkers, including appropriate ranges, specific peaks, and half-lives, to improve their sensitivities and specificities [8].

13.4.1 Severity of aSAH

Traditionally the severity of aSAH is assessed by two scoring systems, namely Hunt and Hess (H&H) and World Federation of Neurological Surgeons (WFNS) scores. These scores are inversely related to the aSAH patient's prognosis, morbidity, and mortality. The lower are the scores better is the prognosis. It is well documented in the literature that these scores predict the aSAH patient's outcome [9]. Relation between the Hunt and Hess (H&H) score and mortality are shown in Table 13.1.

13.4.2 Re-bleeding

Re-bleeding in patients with aSAH is an ominous sign. It frequently occurs within 24–48 h of the aSAH, but it can occur up to 2 weeks in 30% of unsecured aneurysms. The re-bleeding in aSAH patient is a major complication and usually fatal with a mortality rate of 51–80% [9]. Table 13.2 describes the risk factors for re-bleeding [9].

Table 13.1 Hunt and Hess score and patient outcome (Courtesy of Dr. Nissar Shaikh)

Hunt and Hess score	Mortality (%)
Grade I	30
Grade II	40
Grade III	50
Grade IV	60–70
Grade V	80–90

Table 13.2 Risk factors for re-bleeding in aSAH patients (Courtesy of Dr. Nissar Shaikh)

Delay in securing the aneurysm
Loss of consciousness
High grades of aSAH
Large size aneurysms
Sentinel headache
Anxiety/agitation
Hypertension
Seizures
EVD insertion before securing the cerebral aneurysm

Table 13.3 Showing risk factors for cerebral vasospasm and brain ischaemia

Smoking
Young patients
Female gender
Hyperglycaemia
High-grade Fisher scale

13.4.3 Degree of Cerebral Vasospasm and Cerebral Ischaemia

The delayed cerebral ischaemia due to recurrent or persisting cerebral vasospasm is a frequent cause of morbidity and mortality in patients with aSAH. Up to 20% of aSAH patients have a poor outcome and a mortality of up to 32% due to cerebral ischaemia [10]. Table 13.3 shows the risk factors for cerebral vasospasm and brain ischaemia [10].

13.4.4 Role of Nimodipine

It is L-type calcium channel blocker—it is the only drug that has been approved for SAH in European countries and the USA. It improves long-term neurological outcomes if it is started on admission and administered for 21 days. The recommended oral dosage is 60 mg 4 hourly orally (maximum daily dose of 360 mg). The role of nimodipine is based on general brain protective mechanism as there is no proof to suggest that it treats angiographically diagnosed vasospasm, and it also increases fibrinolytic activity and inhibits cortical spreading ischaemia. For more details, please refer to Chap. 10.

13.4.5 Recreational Drug Abuse

Aneurysmal SAH patients with acute cocaine abuse have a three-fold increase in in-hospital mortality. In a retrospective aSAH study, acute cocaine abuse was associated with significant mortality compared to the control group. The cocaine with aSAH have a higher chance of cerebral vasospasm thus at a higher risk of morbidity and mortality [11].

Table 13.4 The location of cerebral aneurysms and chances of intraventricular haemorrhage (Courtesy of Dr. Nissar Shaikh)

Anterior cerebral artery	40%
Internal carotid artery	25%
Middle cerebral artery	21%
Vertebrobasilar arterial system	14%

13.4.6 Intraventricular Haemorrhage (IVH)

Intraventricular haemorrhage (IVH) occurs in 28% of aSAH patients and is detected in up to 54% in the post-mortem examination in these patients. Intraventricular haemorrhage may interfere with CSF circulation leading to obstructive hydrocephalus. The mortality rate may reach 60% in patients with IVH [12]. Table 13.4 shows the percentage risk of intraventricular haemorrhage according to the aneurysms location. IVH is one of the causes of anosmia in post aSAH patients.

13.4.7 Seizures

The seizure occurs in up to 18% of the aSAH patients. The risk of seizure increases with middle cerebral artery aneurysm, intracerebral haemorrhage, re-bleed, and delayed cerebral ischaemia. Non-convulsive status epilepticus and subclinical seizures should be considered if there is a prolonged deterioration of conscious level, which associated with the worst outcome in aSAH patients [13].

13.4.8 Hydrocephalus

Hydrocephalus occurs in up to 30% of aSAH patients. It may develop acutely within minutes to hours of insult, which is non-communicating and obstructive. While communicating, normal pressure hydrocephalus develops after or around 2 weeks of the insult; it is due to blockage of subarachnoid villi by blood and blood products [14]. Table 13.5 shows the risk factors for developing hydrocephalus in patients with aSAH. The hydrocephalus increases morbidity, hospital, and intensive care unit stay [15].

Table 13.5 Risk factors associated with hydrocephalus development [15]

Low Glasgow Coma Scale at presentation
Elderly
Subdural hematoma
Large amount of intraventricular blood
Vasospasm
Administration of antifibrinolytic medications
Seizures
Posterior circulation aneurysms

13.4.9 Cerebral Aneurysmal Diameter

Both extreme size of the cerebral aneurysm, i.e., small <4 mm and giant >9 mm is associated with the worst prognosis, as these extreme sizes related to difficulty in securing of cerebral aneurysm and increase the risk of re-bleeding [16].

13.4.10 Patient Age

As the patient's age increases, the prognosis of aSAH is guarded. Younger patients (age <40 years) have complication rate of 28% when compared to elderly patients (age >70 years) who have a complication rate of 46%. The elderly patients with aSAH present with high WFNS and Fisher grades. Furthermore, their brain has less capability to tolerate the secondary insults after acute aSAH; the risk of hydrocephalus and re-bleeding is exceptionally high. Apart from the above mentioned high risks, this group of patients has low cardiopulmonary reserves and metabolic dysfunctions, which increases the risk of poor prognosis [16].

13.4.11 Medical Complications or Organ Dysfunction and Association with Morbidity and Mortality

The following medical complications and organ dysfunction of aSAH patients (Fig. 13.1).

13.4.11.1 Electrolyte Disturbance

Dysnatraemia, which comprises both hyponatraemia and hypernatraemia is frequently observed in patients with aSAH, Hyponatraemia occurs in up to 30% of aSAH patients and is believed to be caused by a hypothalamic injury. Hyponatraemia in these patients could be due to the syndrome of inappropriate secretion of antidiuretic hormone (SIADH) or salt-wasting syndrome. While, Hypernatremia is reported in 22% of the aSAH cases. Although hyponatraemia is frequent in aSAH, the hypernatremia is found to be associated with the poor outcome in these patients [17].

Hypomagnesemia; Van den Bergh et al. proposed that hypomagnesemia following rupture of cerebral aneurysm was a risk factor for vasospasm as well as DCI, administration of magnesium might be worthy to prevent cerebral vasospasm [18].

13.4.11.2 Fever

Fever is the most frequent medical complication in patients with aSAH. It develops in up to 54% of aSAH patients. In general, fever is found to increase the sensitivity of the brain to develop cerebral vasospasm, ischaemic injuries, and cerebral oedema. Thus, it is associated with increased morbidity and mortality in aSAH patients [19].

13.4.11.3 Anaemia

Anaemia occurs in 36% of aSAH patients. Most of the literature describes that anaemia is associated with poor outcome in patients with aSAH. However, it is also reported in the literature that treating anaemia by red blood cell transfusions in patients with aSAH increases morbidity and mortality, may be associated with changes in blood rheology [20]. In that sense, it seems justified to be critical with the indication to correct anaemia by blood transfusion. Oliver et al. consider anaemia with haemoglobin levels less than 10 g/dL, and blood transfusion was associated with better neurological outcome [21].

13.4.11.4 Hyperglycaemia

Hyperglycaemia occurs in 90% of aSAH patients. It is found to be associated with poor outcomes in these patients. The aggressive management of hyperglycaemia should be avoided; it may lead

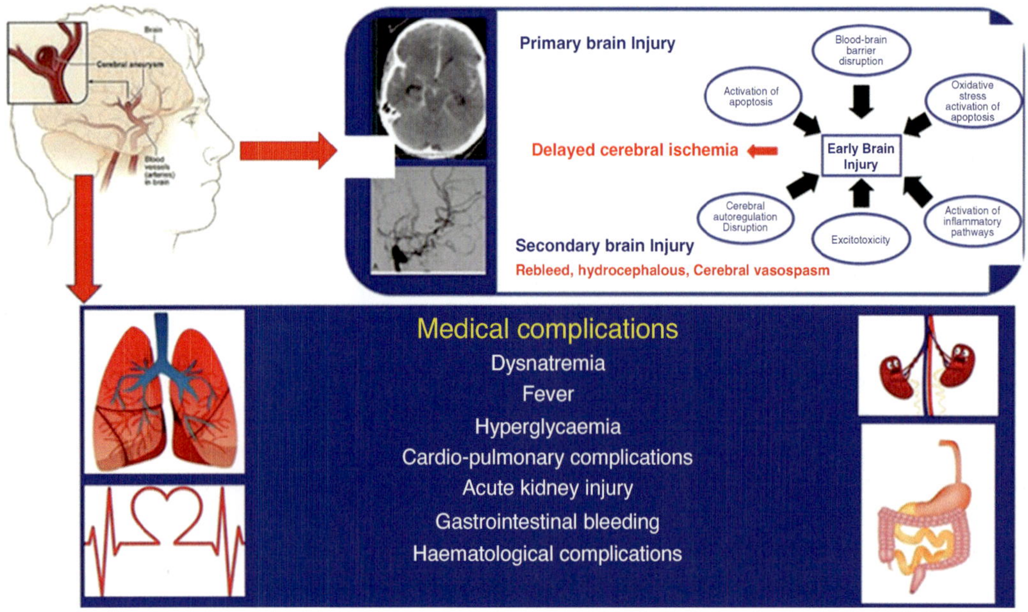

Fig. 13.1 Medical Complications and Multi-organ dysfunction associated with aSAH. (Courtesy of Dr. Nissar Shaikh and Dr. Arshad Chanda)

to frequent hypoglycaemia, which has a detrimental effect on the brain tissue [19]. Moderate hypoglycaemia is associated with vasospasm, cerebral infarction, and a 3-month disability after SAH. Determination of optimal glucose level is extremely difficult, and the literature does not recommend a single optimal glucose target [22].

13.4.11.5 Pulmonary Complications

Pulmonary complications are reported in 20% of aSAH patients. Pulmonary dysfunctions contribute to an increased incidence of cerebral vasospasm and 50% of all fatal medical complications in patients with aSAH. Pneumonia accounts for up to 20% of the pulmonary complications, pulmonary oedema is seen in 14–23%, and pulmonary embolism in 0.3%. Pneumonia was found to be associated with a three-fold increase in mortality in ischaemic stroke patients [19]. However, it is not clear whether this is a consequence of the severity of neurological dysfunction or an active contribution by the inflammation itself.

13.4.11.6 Cardiac Complications

The neurocardiogenic injuries in patients with aSAH vary from stunned myocardium to fatal cardiac arrhythmias. The cardiac dysfunction

Table 13.6 Cardiac dysfunction in aSAH patients (Courtesy of Dr. Nissar Shaikh)

ECG changes	ST-segment depression
	T wave-inversion
	Prolonged QT interval
	U waves
	Tachycardia/bradycardia
Changes in echocardiogram	Decrease in ejection fraction
	Wall motion abnormalities
Cardiac biomarkers	Increased levels of serum troponin & NT-pro BNP levels

as well as wall motion abnormalities after the aSAH is associated with an increased incidence of delayed cerebral ischaemia and poor outcome. The details of cardiac changes are mentioned in Table 13.6.

13.4.11.7 Renal Dysfunctions

Renal dysfunction in aSAH can be multifactorial, the most common important etiologies are the repeated use of intravenous contrast, use of nephrotoxic antibiotics in infected SAH patients as well as hypervolemia and induced hypertension. Chen et al. have reported the incidence of 0.8–7% of renal dysfunction. A deteriorated renal function had an adverse outcome at 3 months.

Furthermore, the 1-year mortality is significantly higher in stroke patients with acute kidney injury compared to the normal renal function stroke patients [23].

13.4.11.8 Coagulation Disorders

Activation of the coagulation cascade and impairment of the fibrinolytic cascade are the two coagulation disorders that are observed in aSAH. There is an elevation in the von Willebrand factor, thrombin, antithrombin, CSF tissue factor, and Platelet-activating factors. Fibrin degradation products and D-dimer are elevated in CSF [23]. The development of the microthrombi is seen in cerebral vessels. Though the prothrombin time (PT), activated partial thrombin time (aPTT), and fibrinogen levels were observed to be normal in aSAH Patients. These derangements in the coagulation system in patients with aSAH are associated with poor outcomes [24].

13.4.11.9 Gastrointestinal Bleeding

The raised intracranial pressure and hydrocephalus in patients with aSAH potentially induce a surge in stress hormones, thus putting these patients at the risk of stress ulcer and gastrointestinal (GI) bleeding. The in-hospital mortality of aSAH patients with GI bleeding is significantly higher than those without GI bleed. O'Donnell et al. reported that the GI bleeding was strongly associated with in-hospital death and 6-month mortality in stroke patients [25].

13.4.11.10 Aneurysm Recurrence and Late Re-bleeding

Recurrence of SAH can occur in survivors of aneurysmal aSAH. This could result from the rebleed of a previously coiled or clipped aneurysm. Rupture of non-coiled or non-clipped aneurysm, from multiple aneurysms or formation of a new aneurysm. This risk is very low but may happen.

13.5 Conclusion

Aneurysmal SAH is a devastating disease associated with high morbidity and mortality. More than 60% of aSAH patients die within 6 months of acute insult. Various complications occur in patients with aSAH increasing the morbidity and mortality in these patients. A combination of primary neurological insult due to the aneurysm rupture and secondary neurological and nonneurological complications worsens the overall clinical outcome of aSAH patients. Prediction of the outcome is extremely important, the use of biomarkers for prognostication of aSAH needs further studies. Extreme size cerebral aneurysms and elderly patients have a guarded prognosis. Early diagnosis, proper intervention, and early administration of nimodipine may prevent secondary brain injury and improve the patient's outcome.

References

1. D'Souza S. Aneurysmal subarachnoid haemorrhage. J Neurosurg Anesthesiol. 2015;27:222–40.
2. Rosengart AJ, Schultheiss KE, Tolentino J, Macdonald RL. Prognostic factors for outcome in patients with aneurysmal subarachnoid haemorrhage. Stroke. 2007;38:2315–21.
3. Marcolini E, Hine J. Approach to the diagnosis and management of subarachnoid haemorrhage. West J Emerg Med. 2019;20(2):203–11.
4. Keyrouz SG, Diringer MN. Clinical review: prevention and therapy of vasospasm in subarachnoid hemorrhage. Crit Care. 2007;11(4):220.
5. Lanzino G, D'Urso PI, Suarez J. Seizures and anticonvulsants after aneurysmal subarachnoid hemorrhage. Neurocrit Care. 2011;15:247.
6. Avdagic SS, Brkic H, Avdagic H, Smajic J, Hodzic S. Impact of comorbidity on early outcome of patients with subarachnoid hemorrhage caused by cerebral aneurysm rupture. Med Arch. 2015;69(5):280–3.
7. Al-Khindi T, Macdonald RL, Schweitzer TA. Cognitive and functional outcome after aneurysmal subarachnoid haemorrhage. Stroke. 2010;41(8):e519–36.
8. Hong CM, Tosun C, Kurland DB, Gerzanich V, Schreibman D, Simard JM. Biomarkers as outcome predictors in subarachnoid hemorrhage—a systematic review. Biomarkers. 2014;19(2):95–108.
9. Naidech AM, Janjua N, Kreiter KT, et al. Predictor and impact of aneurysm re-bleeding after subarachnoid haemorrhage. Arch Neurol. 2005;62:410.
10. Gross BA, Rosalind Lai PM, Frerichs KU, Du R. Treatment modalities and vasospasm after aneurysmal subarachnoid haemorrhage. World Neurosurg. 2014;82:e725.
11. Lucerna A, Espinosa J. Subarachnoid hemorrhage in association with heroin overdose. M J E-Med. 2016;1(2):011.
12. Rosengart AJ, Schultheiss KE, Jocelyn Tolentino J, Macdonald RL. Prognostic factors for outcome in

patients with aneurysmal subarachnoid hemorrhage. Stroke. 2007;38:2315–21.
13. O'Connor KL, Westover MB, Phillips MT, et al. High risk for seizures following subarachnoid hemorrhage regardless of referral bias. Neurocrit Care. 2014;21(3):476–82.
14. Chen S, Luo J, Reis C, Manaenko A, Zhang J. Table 5 shows the risk factors for the development of hydrocephalus in patients with aSAH. Hydrocephalus after subarachnoid hemorrhage: pathophysiology, diagnosis, and treatment. Bio Med Res Int. 2017;2017:8.
15. Hao X, Wei D. The risk factors of shunt-dependent hydrocephalus after subarachnoid space hemorrhage of intracranial aneurysms. Medicine (Baltimore). 2019;98(27):e15970.
16. Shukla DP. Outcome and rehabilitation of patients following aneurysmal subarachnoid haemorrhage. J Neuroanesthesiol Crit care. 2017;4:S65–75.
17. Tam CW, Shum HP, Yan WW. Impact of dynatremia and dyskalemia on prognosis in patients with aneurysmal subarachnoid haemorrhage. Ind J Crit Care Med. 2019;23(12):562–7.
18. van den Bergh WM. Magnesium sulfate in aneurysmal subarachnoid hemorrhage: a randomized controlled trial. Stroke. 2005;36(5):1011–5.
19. Wartenberg KE, Schmidt JM, Claasen J, Tomes RE, Frontera JA, Ostapkovich N, et al. Impact of medical complications after subarachnoid haemorrhage. Crit Care. 2006;34:617–23.
20. Broesser G, Lackner P, Hoefer C, et al. Influence of red blood cell transfusion on mortality and long-term functional outcome in 292 patients with spontaneous subarachnoid haemorrhage. Crit Care Med. 2009;37:1886.
21. Ayling OGS, Ibrahim GM, Alotaibi NM, Gooderham PA. Anemia after aneurysmal subarachnoid hemorrhage is associated with poor outcome. Stroke. 2018;49:1859–65.
22. Schmutzhard E, Rabinstein AA. The participants in the international multi-disciplinary consensus conference on the critical care management of subarachnoid hemorrhage. Neurocrit Care. 2011;15:281–6.
23. Chen S, Li Q, Wu H, Krafft DR, Wang Z, Zhang JH. Harmful effects of subarachnoid haemorrhage on extracerebral organs. Bio Med Res Int. 2014;2014:12.
24. Rowland MJ, Hadjipavlou G, Kelly M, Westbrook J, Pattinson KT. Delayed cerebral ischaemia after subarachnoid haemorrhage: looking beyond vasospasm. Br J Anaesth. 2012;109(3):315–29.
25. O'Donnell MJ, et al. Gastrointestinal bleeding after acute ischemic stroke. Neurology. 2008;71:650–5.

Brain Death

14

Vishwajit Verma and Yash Verma

14.1 Introduction

Brain death or diagnosing death by irreversible cessation of brain stem function is a relatively new concept in medical sciences. Death is defined as the irreversible loss of functions that are essential for the existence of a living organism. A patient without life-sustaining respiratory functions would die within minutes of a cardiac arrest unless these functions are supported by artificial means. Progress made in cardiorespiratory resuscitation, and mechanical ventilation has made it possible to sustain organ support despite the loss of spontaneous life-sustaining cardio-respiratory controls from the injured brain. It is not surprising, therefore that the concept and the need for defining death by neurological criteria emerged after the advent of sophisticated organ support measures in intensive care.

Diagnosing death by neurological criteria is important, to stop the unnecessary and futile organ support in patients who have an irreversible loss of brain stem reflexes that are essential for the existence. The diagnosis is also necesary for determining the mode of end of life care and organ donation. In countries where organ donation programmes involve donation after cardiac or brain death, the distinction is vital to decide the mode of organ donation. The determination of brain death may also provide family members with a robust prognosis of the condition removing any uncertainty.

V. Verma (✉)
Neurocritical Care, Department of Trauma Surgery, Hamad General Hospital, Doha, Qatar
e-mail: vverma@hamad.qa

Y. Verma
Humanitas University, Milan, Italy
e-mail: yash.verma@st.hunimed.eu

14.2 Historical Perspective

The earliest record of clinical states resembling what we now know as brain death goes back to the late nineteenth century. As reported by many authors, an increase in the intracranial pressure (ICP) both in experimental animals and patients was associated with cessation of breathing before heart stopped. In 1902 Cushing reported that when death resulted from a fatal increase in intracranial tension, the arrest of respiration precedes that of the heart. Prompt surgical relief, with a wide opening of the calvarium, may save a life even in desperate cases with pronounced medullary involvement [1].

In 1954 two French neurologists Mollaret and Goulon described a pathological state in a cohort of 23 patients which they called "coma dépassé" meaning "beyond coma" [2]. These patients were characterised not only by a lack of awareness but also by the loss of vegetative functions like breathing.

A. E. A. Ganaw et al. (eds.), *Management of Subarachnoid Hemorrhage*,
https://doi.org/10.1007/978-3-030-81333-8_14

Table 14.1 Harvard criteria for brain death [3]

1	Unresponsive coma
2	Apnoea
3	Absence of brain stem reflexes
4	Absence of spinal reflex
5	Isoelectric electroencephalogram (EEG)
6	Persistence of conditions for at least 24 h
7	Absence of drug intoxication or hypothermia

In 1968, Ad Hoc committee of the Harvard medical school published its report "A definition of irreversible coma" to propose a new concept of defining death by a state of irreversible coma, which required the absence of spontaneous movements or breathing, lack of brainstem reflexes, and an isoelectric EEG (Table 14.1) [3].

In the UK, the Conference of the Medical Royal Colleges and their faculties produced guidance for diagnosing brain (stem) death in 1976, and a subsequent memorandum three years later, equated brain death with the death of a person for the first time.

The 1981 Uniform Determination of Death Act (UDDA) in the USA stipulated that death can be determined by either neurological or cardiovascular criteria but stopped short of mandating a standard by which brain death should be determined.

Currently, in the USA, UDDA enshrines the principle of equivalence of cardiac and neurological criteria for declaration of death and is adopted by many states as the legal definition of death.

The early and prompt diagnosis of brain death in critical care is significant, mainly due to two reasons. Firstly, with the advances in organ support, it is possible to keep a body functioning for an extended period, leading to expensive and futile procedures accompanied by considerable emotional stress on the family and staff looking after the patient. Secondly, with the shortage of organs available for transplant worldwide, an early diagnosis helps the retrieval of organs before the collapse of the systemic circulation. Prolonged treatment of a patient who is brain dead poses a considerable drain on otherwise limited and expensive resources of critical care beds.

Brain death can be conceptualised as whole brain or only brain stem death. Whole brain death concept requires irreversible cessation of whole entire brain including the functions of the brain stem. Brain stem death on the other hand requires proof of irreversible cessation of brain stem functions only. At practical level the clinical tests required for both formulations are the same except that former requires additional confirmatory tests such as electroencephalogram (EEG) or lack of cerebral blood flow to confirm brain death. A patient who has preserved cortical electrical activity or intracranial blood flow but no brain stem reflexes will be considered to be dead in legal systems that utilise a brainstem approach but not in those where a whole brain concept is applied [4]. From a legal perspective, each country, and in the USA, each State, has its legal regulations for death by brain criteria.

14.3 Preconditions for Diagnosis

The cornerstone of brain death is a meticulous neurological examination of the patient with careful review of medical history, neuroradiologic examination, and lab results. The diagnosis of brain death relies on two primary and indispensable preconditions. Firstly, the cause of unresponsive coma must be an irreversible structural or metabolic injury. Secondly, the anatomical apparatus of the brain needed to sustain vegetative functions and consciousness must be damaged beyond recovery. An overview of diagnostic algorithm for diagnosing brain death is shown in Fig. 14.1.

14.3.1 Aetiology

The clinical testing for brain death begins with the indispensable precept of demonstrating that the cause of brain damage is a known irreversible structural or metabolic disease. The precept is critical, and clinical testing for brain death cannot be considered until it is satisfied. The emphasis on this point lies in the fact that coma of unknown cause is often due to toxicity of a depressant drug. A collaborative study sponsored by the National Institutes of Health reported that deep coma in many patients was caused by drug toxicity. The drug toxicity was revealed only on toxicological analysis and was not suspected clinically by the treating physicians [5]. Therefore, doctors involved

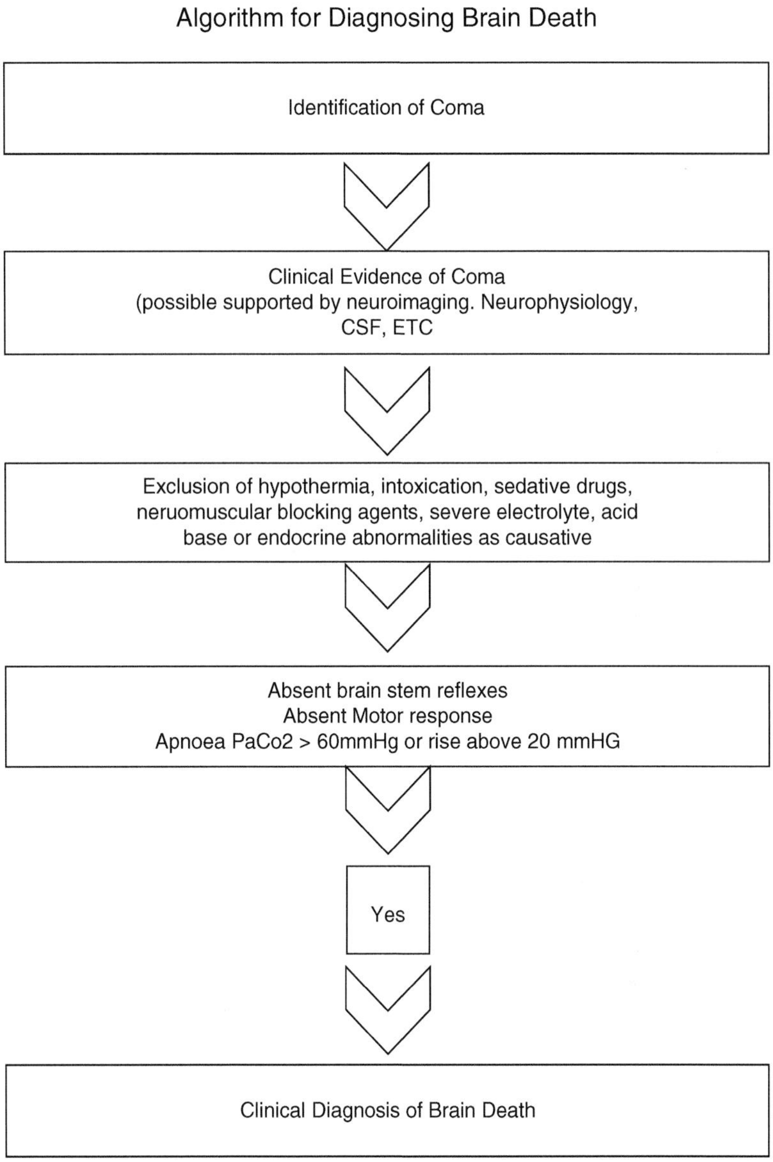

Fig. 14.1 Diagnostic algorithm for brain death

in diagnosing brain death document the cause of brain injury with the relevant reference to anatomical correlate of brain injury or herniation on CT or MRI scan of the brain.

14.3.2 Exclusion of Reversible Causes of Coma

14.3.2.1 Drugs

A good thorough history of drug usage and administration is essential before proceeding with the clinical testing of the patient. Sedative and anaesthetic drugs may cause a prolonged period of unresponsive coma, especially in hypothermic subjects or patients with renal and hepatic dysfunction. Some anaesthetic drugs like midazolam and fentanyl show an increase in context-sensitive half-life due to accumulation of the drug in fat or muscle compartments.

Special care must be taken when approaching patients for brain death criteria who were managed with the thiopentone infusion.

Infusion and multiple doses of thiopentone metabolism follow zero-order kinetics due to saturation of hepatic enzymes, thus prolonging its elimination from the body. Also, continuous infusion of thiopentone without continuous EEG monitoring can notoriously cause an isoelectric EEG with or without suppression of the brain stem reflexes.

The length of time between discontinuation of a depressant drug and brain stem testing depends upon multiple factors such as the total dose, duration of treatment, and the hepatic or renal functions of the patient. If plasma drug assays are available, plasma concentrations of the depressant medications should be measured to exclude the effect of depressant drugs. It is not considered safe to undertake brain stem testing if serum level is above 5 mg/L for thiopentone and 10 μg/L for midazolam [6]. If the treating physicians suspect or confirm alcohol intoxication, the alcohol blood level should be ≤80 mg/dL [7].

In circumstances where the facility for drug assays is not available, the residual sedative can be predicted according to pharmacokinetic profile of the drug. In some organisations, it is mandatory to wait for five elimination half-lives before proceeding with the clinical testing. However, such a strategy lacks both accuracy and precision due to multiple pharmacokinetic factors such as redistribution into multiple compartments.

In exceptional circumstances, ancillary brain death tests can be used, if doubt remains regarding the residual effects of sedatives [7].

14.3.2.2 Primary Hypothermia

Core temperatures between 32 and 34 °C are occasionally associated with an impaired level of consciousness but with intact brain stem reflexes. Brain stem reflexes are reversibly lost below 28 °C. In clinical practice, patient remains awake and conscious above the temperature of 34 °C.

The current recommendation is, therefore, to ensure that the core temp is above 36 °C before attempting clinical tests for brain death [7].

14.3.2.3 Metabolic and Endocrine Disturbance

Encephalopathies caused by acute and metabolic conditions may mimic brain death by abolishing some or all brain stem reflexes. Therefore, meticulous attention must be paid to medical history, and lab results rule out these conditions.

Endocrine Disorders

Hyperglycaemia caused by diabetic ketoacidosis or hyperosmolar non-ketotic coma may cause a state with absent brain stem functions that may mimic brain death. Likelihood of this happening increases with blood glucose levels above 20 mmol/L. Severe hypoglycaemia may also result in coma or stupor. In this situation, brain death testing should be deferred below a blood glucose level of 3.0 mmol/L [6]. Both myxoedema and thyrotoxicosis can produce a comatose state. Addisonian crisis may also be associated with severe myopathy and ascending paralysis leading to coma. If these conditions are suspected, then additional lab tests are required to rule out these conditions [6].

Electrolyte Disorders

Hypernatremia is frequently seen in patients with brain death. In most patients hypernatremia is caused by diabetes insipidus induced by the changes in intracranial pressure. Serum sodium concentration greater than 160 mmol/L may cause deep coma and unresponsiveness and should be corrected before brain death testing.

Hyponatremia can also cause coma, but it is the rate of sodium decline rather than the absolute level that determines the development of an unresponsive state. It is rare for a patient to be unresponsive above the sodium of 115 mmol/L. Caution should be exercised during correction of sodium in patients with severe hyponatremia as the rapid changes in sodium concentration may result in a state of decreased consciousness and quadriparesis caused by osmotic demyelination in pons.

Low serum potassium may cause myopathy, and levels below 1 mmol/L are reported to cause flaccid quadriplegia. It is not advisable to proceed with testing below the potassium level of 2.0 mmol/L [6].

Extremely low or high serum levels of Phosphate and Magnesium may also cause severe neuromuscular weakness and generalised flaccid paralysis. There is currently no agreement on precise values at which brain stem testing can be undertaken. A clinically significant weakness is unlikely unless serum levels of magnesium or phosphate are below 0.5 or above 3.0 mmol/L [6].

Exclusion of Reversible Causes of Apnoea

It is crucial to rule out reversible causes of apnoea before proceeding to the clinical tests. Most patients receive neuromuscular blocking during their course of stay in ICU. The residual effect of these drugs must be ruled out by meticulous attention to the history and timing of medications received by the patient. A train of four examination by the nerve stimulator can be used to rule out the presence of neuromuscular blockade. Some neurological disorders, for e.g., Guillain Barre, Botulism can cause symmetrical cranial nerve dysfunction with respiratory muscle paralysis. It is therefore vital to establish a definite diagnosis of irreversible brain damage of known aetiology.

In a head-injured unresponsive patient, the presence of a high spinal cord injury should be ruled out and documented. If the diagnosis of high spinal cord injury is established or suspected, then the apnoea test becomes invalid. In this situation diagnosis of brain, death can only be established by the use of ancillary investigations [7].

14.4 Clinical Tests

The clinical diagnosis of brain death is based on confirming beyond doubt three cardinal features: unresponsive coma, absence of brain stem reflexes, and apnoea. In most legal systems, tests are performed by two senior doctors who are not part of the transplant team. The tests are repeated after the initial testing to confirm the findings of the first sets of tests. The time between the first and second tests varies in different countries and legislation. In the UK second set of tests can be repeated immediately after the first test, once the $PaCO^2$ is normalised from the first apnoea test [6].

A recent consensus statement made by The World Brain Death Project concluded that an intervening period between the two tests is unnecessary if the pre-requisite for irreversibility has been met undeniably. Readers are encouraged to review their local guidelines for specific instances [7].

14.4.1 Unresponsive Coma

The presence of unresponsive coma is confirmed by the absence of a motor response in the cranial nerve distribution to a noxious stimulus applied in the supraorbital area. A common pitfall of this test is the presence of spinal reflexes, spontaneous and myokymic movements seen in the area of cranial nerve distribution.

Spinal reflexes can pose challenge for the clinicians performing the test and make it difficult for the grieving family to accept brain death. Diverse varieties of poly, oligo or mono-segmental reflexes are seen in patients after brain death. These spinal reflexes represent phylogenetically old motor patterns that are set free from descending cortical influences after brain death. Spinal reflexes usually manifest 48 h after brain death. Spinal reflexes can be differentiated from volitional and brain stem activity by being triggered by stimuli of limited variations, a consistent latency, duration and fade after the repeated triggers [8]. These movements are stereotypical and non-purposeful but can confuse inexperienced clinicians and family members by giving an impression of vitality. A summary of different types of spinal reflexes is shown in Table 14.2 [8].

Myokymia are fine tremulous or quivering movements that are sometimes seen in the area of facial nerve distribution. There are other automatic movements that have been described such as flickering of eyelids, transient eyelid opening and rhythmic dilation, constriction of pupils.

A group of British investigators reported a case of women who showed periodic constriction and dilation of the iris with absent brain stem reflexes [9]. In another case, investigators reported a patient with the slow opening of the

Table 14.2 Types of spinal reflexes in brain-dead patients [8]

1	Mono-segmental muscle stretch reflexes
2	Oligo-segmental cutaneo-muscular reflexes: Cremasteric, plantar extensor response, tonic penile erections/vaginal contractions, tonic plantar flexion
3	Poly-segmental spinal reflexes: Embrace (Moro) response Neck-flexion abdominal-contraction, neck-flexion hip-flexion, neck-flexion arm-flexion reflex Endotracheal suction arm-flexion reflex, leg strike leg-flexion reflex Undulating toe flexion sign Head tilt upon noxious stimuli on upper limb
4	Poly-segmental spinal automatism patterns (PSAP) Embrace automatism/Moro automatism

eyelid in response to pinching the ipsilateral nipple. The exact mechanism of these movements is not known. However, a plausible explanation is that they are caused by deafferentation of the supranuclear fibres of the facial nerve or hypersensitivity to neurotransmitters in the ciliary muscles in the setting of denervation.

14.4.2 Brain Stem Reflexes

14.4.2.1 Pupils

The pupils should be fixed and unresponsive to bright light. Ideally, mid-sized pupils are more reliable for the diagnosis of brain death.

Pupillary reflex is maintained by the opposing effects of sympathetic and parasympathetic activity. The parasympathetic pupillo-constrictor fibres originate from the Edinger–Westphal nucleus or accessory third nerve nucleus in the midbrain. Pupillo-dilator muscles in the iris are innervated by sympathetic fibres arising from the superior cervical ganglion. The preganglionic sympathetic fibres which regulate the pupillary response derives its input from ipsilateral hypothalamus (Fig. 14.2). Descending hypothalamic fibres descend in the lateral pons and medulla, where they can be interrupted by an injury to the brain stem. After the brain death, due to destruction of the brain stem, both sympathetic and parasympathetic fibres are destroyed, resulting in the cadaveric or mid-sized pupils between 4 and 6 mm. In early stages after the brain death, the agonal release of the noradrenaline causes dilation of the pupils [10]. However, as catecholamine are metabolised, the pupils should return to mid or cadaveric size.

Current guidelines recommend that there should be an absence of ipsilateral and contralateral pupillary response to bright light with pupils fixed in midsize or dilated position (4–6 mm) in in both eyes [7].

14.4.2.2 Pitfalls

Many drugs and medical conditions can influence the pupils. Anticholinergic drugs, adrenaline, and local injury to oculomotor (CNIII) nerve can also cause fixed and dilated pupils. In these situations, pupils are usually larger than 5–6 mm (midbrain pupils) in size.

14.4.2.3 Ocular Movements

Ocular movements are assessed by the demonstration of oculocephalic or vestibulo-ocular (caloric) responses (VOR). The oculocephalic response is assessed by moving the head side to side in the horizontal plane, followed by up and down movement in a vertical plane. The normal reflex is a tonic, brisk eye movement in the contralateral direction to that of the head movement. Oculocephalic reflex is a complex reflex which requires afferent input from ear canals and proprioceptors of neck muscles. In comatose and anaesthetised patients, it is often difficult to elicit this response. The spinal injury must be excluded before attempting a demonstration of oculocephalic response.

The vestibulo-ocular response, also known as the caloric response, is performed by irrigating ice-cold saline in the ear canal. In awake subjects, the injection of cold water causes a reduction of tonic neural output from the semicircular canals present in the inner ear of the same side. The unilateral decrease in neural output causes an asymmetry which is similar to turning the head opposite to the side of the injectate. Consequently, the ipsilateral, lateral rectus and contralateral, medial rectus muscles contract, leading to a slow movement of eyes towards the side of cold water injection. A fast corrective saccade follows this

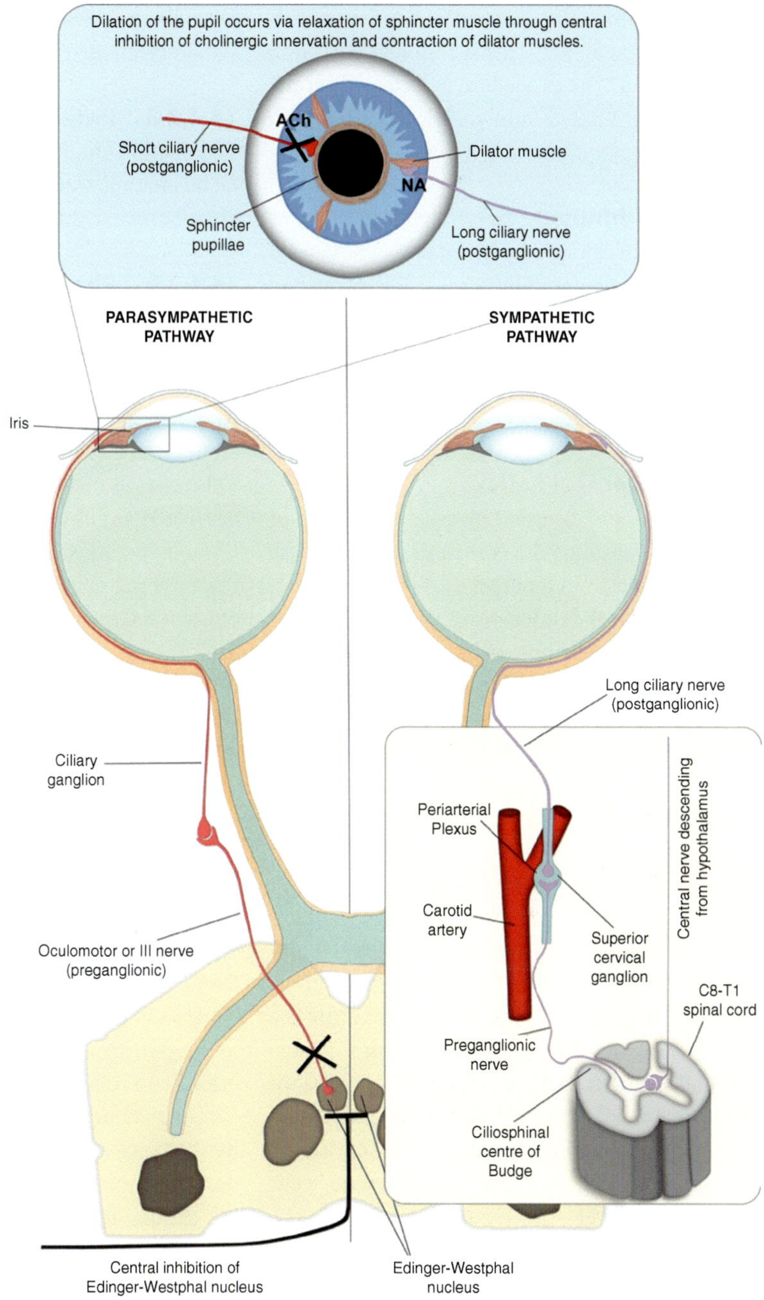

Fig. 14.2 Parasympathetic and sympathetic nervous system pathways involved in pupillary light reflex. (Figure reproduced under creative common licence, [74])

slow drift in the opposite direction initiated from the frontal eye fields. The fast component by convention defines the direction of the nystagmus leading to the well-known mnemonic COWS (cold opposite warm same). However, in anaesthetised or comatose patients with an intact brainstem, the corrective fast saccadic movement is absent, and only the slow tonic drift towards the side of injection is seen. In brain-dead subjects, VOR is absent [10].

Before performing test for vestibulo-ocular reflex, auditory canals on both side should be examined for patency and intact tympanic membrane. Caloric test is performed injecting 50 mL of ice-cold saline in the ear canal for 5 min with patient reclined at 30°. This is followed by 1 min of observation. The procedure is repeated on the opposite side after 5 min to allow endolymph temperature to equilibrate.

14.4.2.4 Pitfalls

The absence of caloric response can also be caused by bilateral vestibular failure due to Phenytoin and Tricyclic antidepressant toxicity. In such patients instead, an oculocephalic response may be elicited as the stimulatory afferents derived from the neck muscles are usually present.

14.4.2.5 Corneal Reflex

The corneal reflex is tested by brushing a wisp of cotton lightly against the cornea or dropping few drops of saline from a height of 4–5 in. The normal reflex results in closure of both eyelids followed by upward rolling of both eyeballs (Bell's phenomenon). An intact response affirms the integrity of the reflex pathway comprising of efferent supply from sensory division of trigeminal nerve via lateral tegmental connections to third nerve nuclei in midbrain and seventh nerve nuclei in pons.

14.4.2.6 Pitfalls

In comatose patients eliciting the reflex usually requires more vigorous stimulation as compared to awake subjects. But care must be taken to avoid causing trauma to the cornea during the testing. A lesion in the course of facial nerve may abolish the blink but Bell's phenomenon should still occur. Corneal reflex may be abolished in some subjects who wear contact lenses [11].

14.4.2.7 Motor and Sensory Response

All motor responses mediated by the brain stem must be absent in a patient who is brain dead. These include corneal response, jaw jerks, and cutaneous response such as snout and rooting reflex. Motor response within the cranial nerve distribution should be checked by application of a noxious stimulus to the supraorbital ridge and nail. No motor response in the cranial nerve distribution should be elicited in brain-dead patients [7].

14.4.2.8 Pitfalls

The caution should be exercised in patients with facial trauma. An injury to the facial nerve can blunt corneal response in some patients.

14.4.2.9 Pharyngeal and Tracheal Reflex

Gag response is elicited by gently touching the post-pharynx by the tongue depressor. Normal response results in the elevation of the palate and bilateral contraction of the pharyngeal muscles. This reflex is mediated by Glossopharyngeal (IX) nerve and Vagus (X) nerve.

Cough reflex is tested by observing the response to tracheal suctioning. Both afferent and efferent are mediated by Vagus nerve [7].

14.4.2.10 Pitfalls

Gag reflex may be difficult to elicit or observe in intubated patient.

14.4.3 Apnoea Test

Absence of spontaneous respiratory effort is a cardinal finding in brain-dead subjects. Demonstration of apnoea requires some prerequisites and preparation. Apnoea test is the last test to be performed and is only performed if the brain stem reflexes are absent.

The patient should have cardiovascular stability. Patients with multiorgan failure, on high doses of inotropes, may become unstable during the apnoea test. Patients who have severe lung injury, pulmonary oedema with low P/F ratio, run the risk of becoming hypoxic during the test.

Most countries or regions have specific procedural guidelines for the conduct of the apnoea test. The patient should be exposed from the chest up to the pubic symphysis to evaluate the slightest of respiratory movements. The ventilator is then adjusted to ensure normocarbia. The patient is preoxygenated with 100% oxygen for 10–15 min. Arterial blood gases should be done to ensure the

$PaCO_2$ between 35 and 45 mmHg and PaO_2 >200 mmHg. The patient is then connected to a 6 L/min oxygen via a suction catheter inserted via an endotracheal tube (ETT) up to the level of the carina, alternatively, a T-piece with continuous positive airway pressure at 10 cmH_2O. Once the ventilator is disconnected, the patient is observed for 8–10 min for signs of spontaneous respiration. Arterial blood gasses are repeated at the end of the observation period, and the patient is reconnected to the ventilator. Apnoea test is deemed positive (supports the diagnosis of brain death) if no spontaneous breathing is detected and $PaCO_2$ is above 60 mmHg or risen by 20 mmHg the baseline [6, 7].

14.4.3.1 Pitfalls

Cardiac pulsations, shoulder elevation and adduction, back arching and intercoastal expansion without significant tidal volume can give the impression of spontaneous breathing.

Clinical tests and pitfalls are summarised in Table 14.3.

Table 14.3 Clinical test, pitfalls, and possible solutions (Courtesy of Dr. V. Verma)

Clinical tests	Pitfalls	Solutions
Identify a clear cause of coma	Cause unknown	Further radiology or lab testing
Preconditions Depressant drugs Neuromuscular blocking drugs Hypothermia Metabolic & Endocrine	Drug intoxication Unknown drugs Severe metabolic disturbances	Wait for drug clearance Check plasma levels Correction of underlying condition. Lab tests and ancillary tests
Brain stem tests Pupillary response Corneal reflex Caloric response Motor response in cranial nerve distribution	Anticholinergic drugs Facial nerve injury Ototoxic drugs Base of skull fracture Facial fractures Locked in syndrome	Ancillary tests Evidence of pontine injury on MR
Apnoea test	Presence of neuromuscular blocking drugs High spinal cord injury Pre-existing respiratory illness, e.g. COPD Unstable patient Spinal reflexes triggering the ventilator	Nerve stimulation Ancillary testing Starting apnoea test with a high baseline CO_2 which is normal for patient

14.5 Ancillary Tests

Brain death is a clinical diagnosis. Some ancillary tests are mandated to support clinical examination in some countries. While in others they are only necessary if a certain part of the neurological examination or apnoea test cannot be performed or validated reliably.

Ancillary tests used are aimed at confirming two physiological sequelae that accompany the process of brain death. These sequelae are an absence of bioelectrical activity in the brain and blood flow in the cerebral circulation. This cessation of cerebral blood flow results from a sudden and large surge in the intracranial pressure above the mean arterial pressure, reducing the cerebral perfusion pressure to near zero and causing circulatory arrest. However, in the majority of the patients, the cessation of the cerebral circulation results from a progressive increase in the tissue oedema that elevates the tissue pressure above the capillary perfusion, starting a vicious cycle of increasing vascular stasis and oedema. If the organ support is continued after the brain death that prevents or delays somatic death, the lack of cerebral blood flow results in autolysis of the brain at the body temperature turning it into a soft necrotic tissue mass.

Commonly used tests are digital subtraction angiography, CT or MRI angiography which rely on the absence of contrast filling in intracranial blood vessels or the transcranial Doppler that shows characteristic flow pattern of systolic spikes or reverse flow.

Radionuclide tests such as Technitium -99m Hexamethyl-Propylene Amine oxime (99mTc-

HMPAO) with single-photon emission computed tomography (SPECT) scan show an absence of brain uptake of tracer in brain-dead patients. Somatosensory evoked potential (SSEP) are EEG based bedside tests that evaluate the cortical electrical response to stimulation of median nerves. In brain-dead patient cortical response is characteristically absent bilaterally 22 ms after the stimulation.

14.6 Techniques to Confirm Cerebral Circulatory Arrest

14.6.1 Cerebral Digital Subtraction Angiography (DSA)

This technique involves the injection of a radio-opaque dye into the anterior and posterior cerebral vessels under high pressure. The procedure involves injecting each of the main intracranial arteries separately with a radio-opaque dye approximately 20 min apart. In patients who are brain dead, no contrast is seen in the intracranial courses of internal carotid and vertebral arteries on both sides [12] (Fig. 14.3).

While DSA is regarded as a gold standard, it suffers from major disadvantages. Angiography is a time consuming, and resource-intensive procedure which can only be performed in large neuroscience centres. Complications include anaphylactic reaction, nephrotoxicity or vascular injury related to the procedure [12].

14.6.2 Cerebral Computerized Tomographic Angiography (CTA)

CTA involves a rapid intravenous injection of a contrast media followed by volume scanning of the whole brain. CTA in brain-dead subjects will reveal an absence of opacification in the intracranial course of the arteries (Fig. 14.4). This technique has the advantage of being widely available and shorter in duration. High-quality large studies to validate CTA are not available. The sensitivity of CTA is reported to be poor (52.4%) in one series. The reason for low sensitivity is due to persistent enhancement of cerebral vessels. More recently attempts have been made to use a 7- or 4-point scoring system to improve the sensitivity of CTA to confirm brain death [13]. These scoring systems are based on lack of opacification of peri-callosal and cortical segments of the middle cerebral arteries, internal cerebral veins, and the great cerebral vein [13]. Various studies have reported that the use of the scoring system increases the sensitivity to 85.7%. There have been no case reports of false-positive detection of brain death by the CTA.

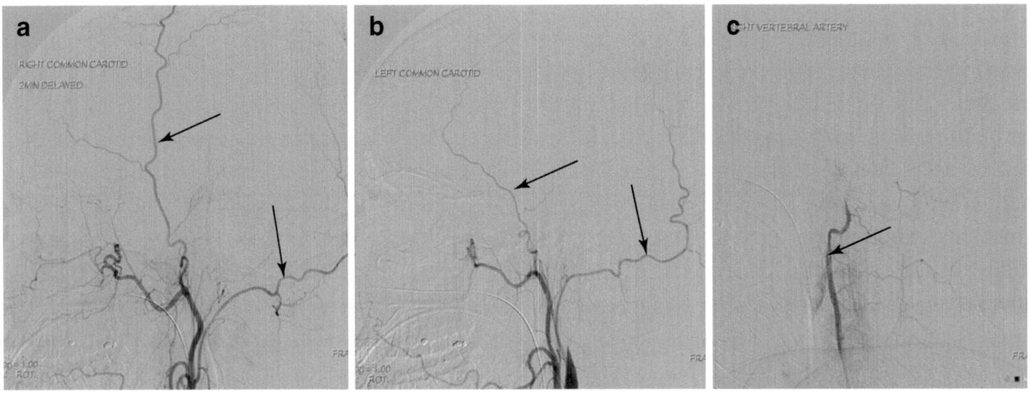

Fig. 14.3 4-vessel digital subtraction angiography in a brain-dead patient. (**a** and **b**) Shows contrast media in right and left common carotid artery (arrows). Contrast is also seen in the branches of external carotid artery but none in internal carotid artery. (**c**) Shows contrast only in extra-cranial portion of the right vertebral artery (arrow). No contrast is seen in the intracranial portion. (Image Source: Reproduced under creative common licence courtesy of Dr. Chris O'Donnell, Radiopaedia.org, rID: 16808)

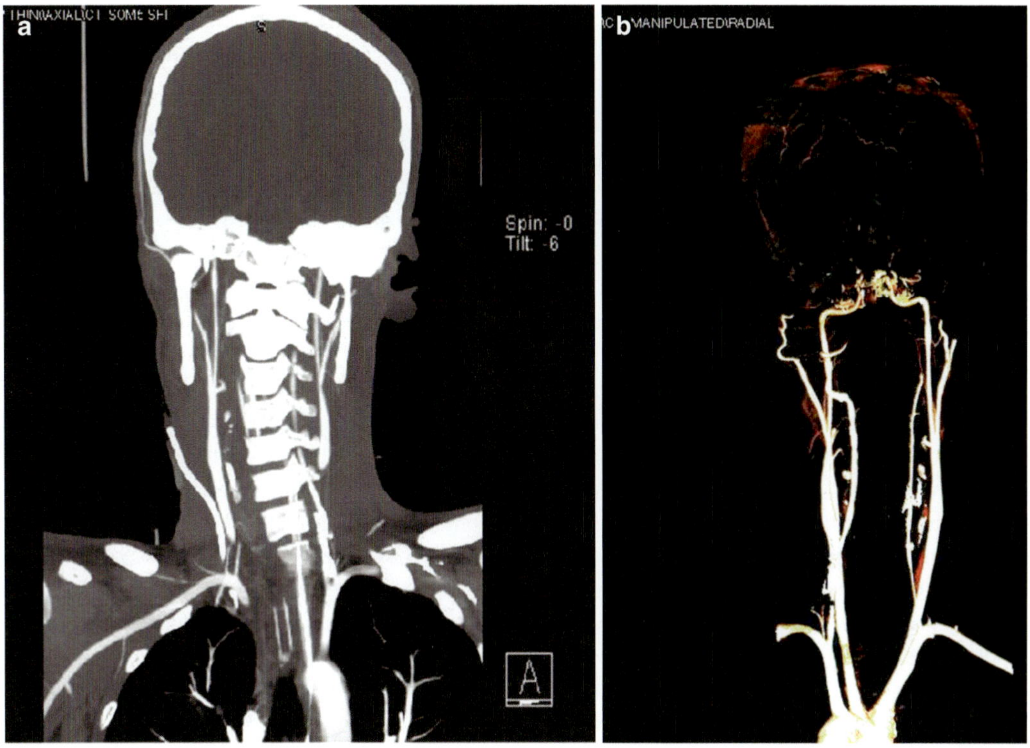

Fig. 14.4 CTA showing absence of opacification of intracerebral arteries. Extracranial internal carotid arteries and vertebral arteries show contrast uptake. (**a**) Coronal MIP; (**b**) 3D-Volume rendering reconstruction in the same patient. (Image source: Authors own image)

14.6.3 MRI and MR Angiography (MRA)

MRI and MRA can also be used for confirming the diagnosis of brain death. In normal circumstances, low or dark signal (void) is seeing in the blood vessels due to vigorous blood flow. Loos of the signal void above the supra-clinoid internal carotid artery is suggestive of brain death. MRI can be useful to detect anatomical correlates of herniation syndromes like central, tonsillar, and Uncal herniations. At this moment, due to lack of robust evidence, MRI is not considered a valid ancillary test [7].

14.6.4 Transcranial Doppler Ultra sonography (TCD)

TCD is a non-invasive ultrasound technique that uses sound waves in the range of 2 MHz to detect and measure blood flow velocity in the intracerebral vessels.

As the intracranial pressure rises, there is a progressive reduction in the diastolic flow velocity. This is followed by loss of anterograde diastolic blood flow and appearance of a biphasic flow with the retrograde diastolic flow. Eventually, diastolic flow is completely abolished, and all that remains are systolic spikes (Fig. 14.5). Middle cerebral arteries are insonated on both sides using temporal windows just above the zygomatic arch. Similarly, supra-clinoid internal carotid arteries can be studied using orbital windows. The basilar artery is studied using occipital windows just below the occipital protuberance.

TCD has many advantages. It is a non-invasive, portable test and is usually done on the bedside. One major drawback is the lack of insonation windows in the skull, which is found in 5–10% of the population. In this case, a non-diagnostic study due to lack of insonation win-

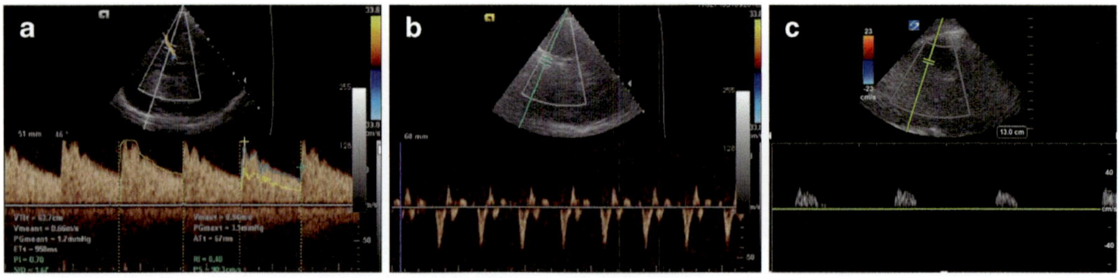

Fig. 14.5 Changes in TCD signal as intracranial pressure increases. (**a**) Normal TCD signal; (**b**) Reverberating or biphasic flow; (**c**) Systolic spikes. Last (**b** and **c**), flow patterns are indicative of cerebral circulatory arrest. (Image source: Authors own image)

dows may be misinterpreted as an absence of blood flow in the artery.

The sensitivity of TCD for diagnosing brain death is in the range of 70–100% and specificity of 97–100%. False-positive tests are rare, but false-negative tests are frequently reported. It is reported that in 17.4% of patients who fit the clinical criteria for brain death, persistent blood is observed in the intracranial arteries [14, 15]. Sometimes signal may also be normal in the infratentorial compartment while it is absent in the supratentorial compartment.

14.6.5 Cerebral Scintigraphy

This technique measures the failure of uptake of the radioisotope nuclide technetium (Tc) 99m hexamethyl-propyleneamine oxime (HMPAO) in brain parenchyma.

The test is done at the bedside using a portable gamma camera after injection of the isotope. A static image of 500,000 counts is obtained at several time points. A slight modification of the technique uses static single-photon emission tomography to detect intracranial radionuclide activity of TC-99m-HMPAO. This technique creates a characteristic image which is called a "hollow skull sign" (Fig. 14.6a) in patients who are brain dead. In addition to an anterior static image, flow image reveals a lack of cerebral perfusion and uptake.

In brain-dead patients, the nuclear blood flow shows the diversion of blood from the internal carotid artery to the external carotid artery supplying the face. This phenomenon results in another characteristic "hot nose" sign [16] (Fig. 14.6b), implying a high concentration of the tracer in the nose. A study that compared SPECT and cerebral angiography showed that both techniques confirmed the brain in 95% of patients on initial examination and 100% after 48 h [17].

14.7 Neurophysiological Methods: EEG and Evoked Potentials

EEG is required to show the absence of electrical activity at a sensitivity of 2 μV for 30 min in order to diagnose brain death. EEG can be a reliable adjunct to the clinical tests if isoelectric activity is detected and confirmed, but there are distinct disadvantages which makes it usefulness limited. Firstly, EEG only records the cortical electrical activity and not brain stem activity. So, it is possible to have an isoelectric EEG but with residual brain stem activity.

A group of researchers reported a case report of a patient with isoelectric EEG due to cardiac arrest who showed residual brain stem functions, including breathing and a SPECT evidence of cerebral blood flow 7 weeks prior to death [18]. Secondly, EEG is likely to produce false positives due to the effect of sedative drugs, hypothermia or metabolic factors. EEG is also prone to interference by electromagnetic fields especially com-

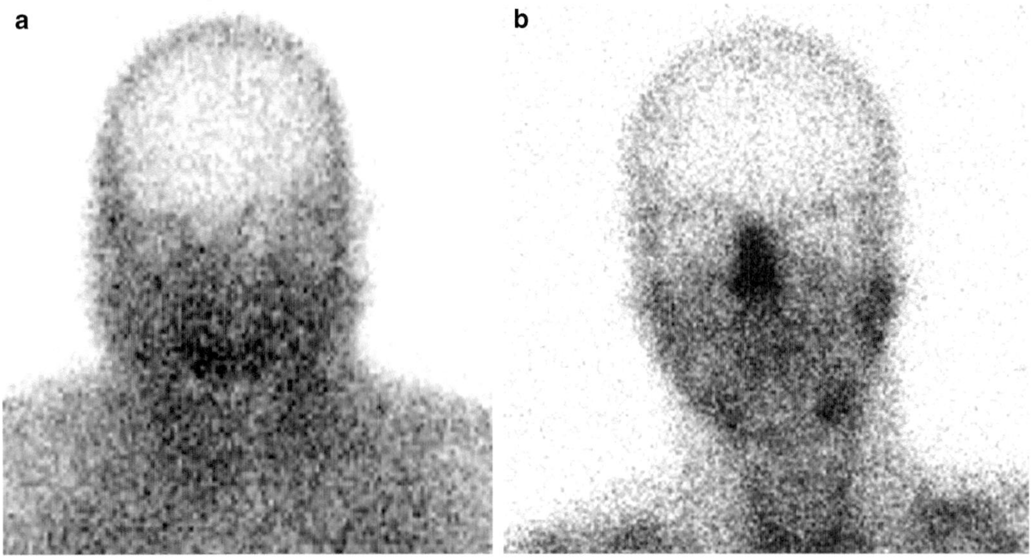

Fig. 14.6 HMPAO spect scan in a brain-dead patient. (**a**) Shows empty skull sign; (**b**) 'Hot Nose" sign. (Image source: (**a**) Reproduced under Creative Common License Case courtesy of Dr. Yair Glick, Radiopaedia.org (**b**) Reproduced under Creative Common License Case courtesy of Dr. Andrew Dixon, Radiopaedia.org)

mon in intensive care units and electromyographic activity which is enhanced in the absence of brain electrical activity. Inter and intra-rater variability can give rise to diagnostic uncertainty in 20% of the patients [19]. Overall the usefulness of EEG in diagnosing brain death at best remains limited due to myriad confounding factors.

Somatosensory Evoked potential (SSEP) assess the functional integrity of posterior columns, medial lemniscus, thalamus, and the sensorimotor cortex. SSEPs are indicative of brain death if bilateral cortical responses, 20 s (N20-P22) after median nerve stimulus are absent [20] (Fig. 14.7). However, in the early stages of brain death, SSEP can be normal. This is thought to be due to residual activity of the damaged neurons still capable of generating a response. This activity usually fades over a period of 24–48 h [21]. Patients who have upper cervical spinal cord injury or lesion can produce the same absent cortical response as in brain death. Placement of additional nasopharyngeal electrodes has been proposed to detect activity in the lower brain stem and upper cervical spinal cord. This technique still requires further validation.

The distinct advantages of evoked potentials are that they are widely available, non-invasive, cheap, and feasible in hypothermic and sedated patients. Disadvantages include the need for expertise in interpretation and performance, false-negative results thus delaying the diagnosis of brain death, possibly of false positive due to lesion or injury in the cervico-medullary junction.

Table 14.4 summarises ancillary tests, their reliability and limitations.

14.8 Diagnosis of Brain Death in Infants and Children

The criteria for diagnosing brain death and preconditions are same as in adult patients, but certain caveats exist pertaining to age group the patient belongs to. The need for this distinction is due to varying level of brain maturation and resil-

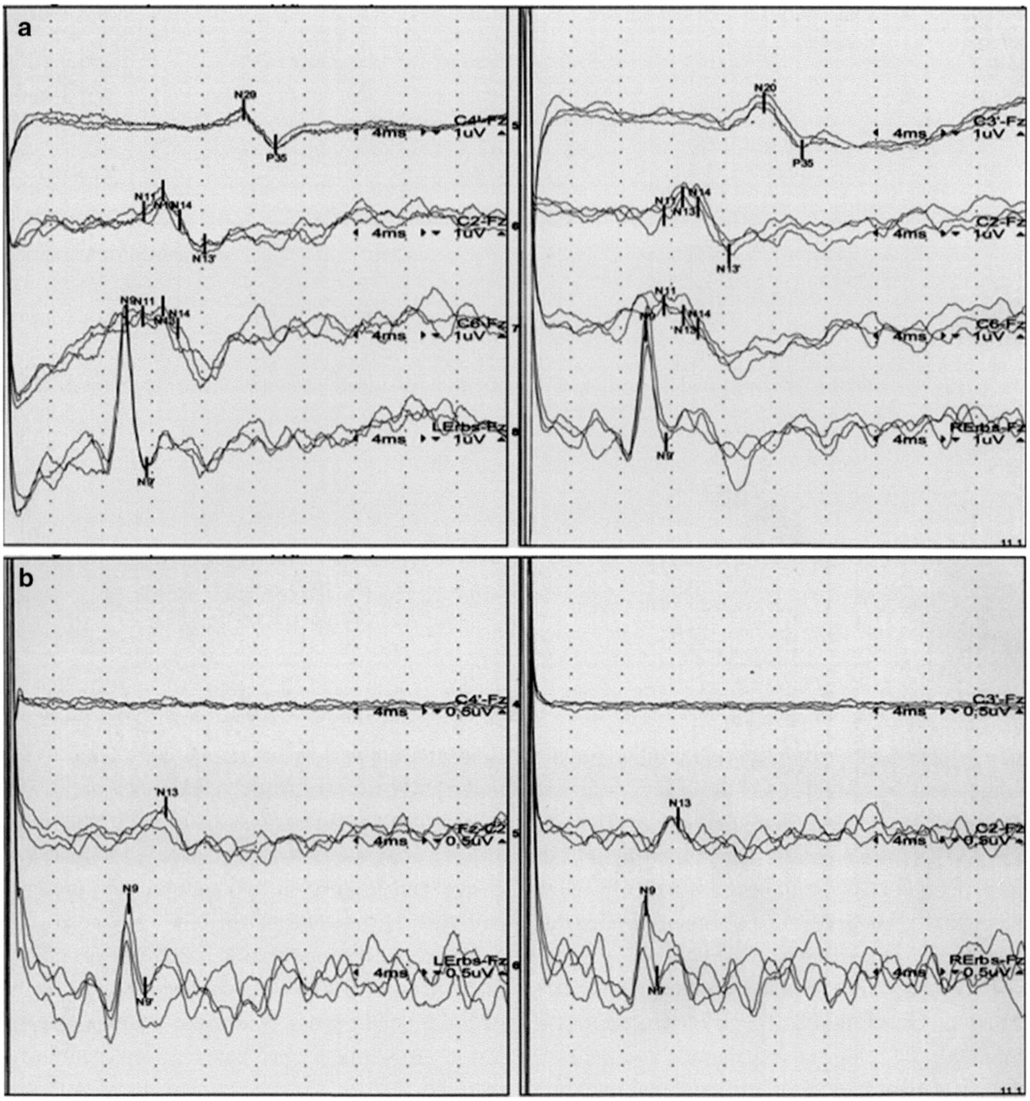

Fig. 14.7 (**a**) Showing normal bilateral somatosensory evoked response N20. (**b**) Showing absent bilateral somatosensory evoked potential N20 response in a brain-dead patient. (Image source: Authors own image) [74]

ience to a certain type of brain injury. This results in age-dependent observation period and criteria.

14.8.1 Children Older Than 2 Months

There is a general agreement that criteria for assessing brain death criteria in adults are applicable. All preconditions should be met with and the cause of irreversible coma should be unequivocally confirmed. It is recommended plasma drug levels of barbiturates, and other sedatives should be measured to rule out their effect on coma. Reversal form neuromuscular blockade must be demonstrated by peripheral reflexes or nerve stimulation [6].

Table 14.4 Reliability and pitfalls of ancillary tests (Courtesy of Dr. V. Verma)

Test	Reliability	Limitations
4 Vessel angiography	Good	Requires transport, invasive, contrast nephropathy, and anaphylaxis. Requires injection of all four vessels
HMPAO SPECT	Good	Post fossa difficult to visualise, uptake affected by barbiturates and hypothermia
TCD	Mixed	Operator dependent, lack of insonation window in 5–10% of subject
CT angiography/ MR angiography	Not known	Not validated, may show residual flow in proximal vessels despite lack of brain stem reflexes, resource-intensive specially MRA
EEG	Mixed	Measures surface activity, subject to artefacts
SSEP	Good	False negatives in early stages and high cervical cord injury may mimic brain death

14.8.2 37 Weeks Gestation to 2 Months of Age

The most common cause of coma in this age group is a hypoxic-ischemic encephalopathy, especially that occurs in utero or at the time of birth. Such infants are very difficult to assess. It may not be possible satisfactorily to demonstrate structural brain damage, and the infant may have a multisystem failure.

In the USA, the task force considers that in certain infants, it may be possible to satisfy all the preconditions before the brain death exam. It is recommended that two formal brain death exam performed 48 h apart with an isoelectric EEG should be enough to diagnose brain death [22].

14.8.3 Infants Below 37 Weeks Gestation

It is challenging to demonstrate irreversible brain injury in this age group as coma and apnoea problems are common in this age group. The other issue that the development of brainstem reflexes in the pre-term infant has not been systematically studied. Brain myelination starts caudally and posteriorly during the gestational period. It is possible that brain stem damage will have different effects than those seen in older children or adult. Use of brain death concept in this age group may not be appropriate and the decision to continue support in intensive care should be based on likely outcome after closed and unhurried discussion with the family [6].

14.9 Diagnosis of Brain Death in Patients with Extra-Corporeal Membrane Oxygenation (ECMO)

Patients with respiratory and cardiac failure who are managed on ECMO are at an increased risk of developing cerebral complications leading to brain death. Presence of ECMO possess a particular challenge for performing and interpretation of apnoea test. There is also a lack of consistent guidelines on the practical aspect of the apnoea test in this group of patients.

In August 2020, the steering committee of The World Brain Death Project published their recommendations in order to consolidate practice and set standards for declaration of death by neurological criteria. The committee stipulated that the preconditions and clinical tests remain same as for non-ECMO patient. In addition, following recommendations be adhered to while performing the apnoea test [7].

1. Apnoea test must be performed in order to pronounce brain death, in patients receiving veno-venous (VV) or veno-arterial (VA) ECMO. If apnoea test cannot be completed or conducted due to cardio-respiratory instability, then an ancillary test be considered.
2. In patients receiving VA ECMO, the extracorporeal flow be maintained during the clinical evaluation and apnoea test to maintain a minimum mean arterial pressure (MAP) at 60 mmHg in adults or at an age appropriate

target for a paediatric patient. The VA flow may be increased to support the MAP before or during the test is needed.
3. Pre-oxygenation must be provided prior to testing for all patients receiving ECMO. This can be achieved by administering 100% oxygen via the mechanical ventilator and increasing the oxygen in the membrane lung for 10 min prior to testing.
4. Some patients on ECMO may not be mechanically ventilated. In these patients oxygenation will depend upon providing 100% oxygen via the sweep gas. If oxygenation cannot be maintained satisfactorily, the test must be aborted and probably replaced by ancillary testing.
5. Once arterial blood gas pH reaches less than 7.30 and $PaCO_2$ 60 mmHg (or 20 mmHg above the baseline $PaCO_2$ in patients with pre-existing hypercapnia), mechanical ventilation must be restarted and ECMO sweep gas flow rate be returned to the starting value.

14.10 Ethical, Legal, and Religious Aspects of Brain Death

Diagnosing death by neurological criteria is a relatively new concept in the history of medicine. The advancement in critical care medicine has made it easier to sustain and maintain metabolic and cellular homeostasis after brain death. This makes it difficult for general public and family members of the patient to accept the concept the death when defined by neurologic criteria. Despite most legal systems and religions all over the world generally accepting the concept of brain death public awareness and understanding remains inadequate and because of this conflict often arise between clinicians and family members regarding continuation of organ support.

Such issues are more common in paediatric practices [23]. A survey of 201 neurologist in the USA concluded that up to 48% of clinicians reported encountering situations in which family requested continuation of organ support. In this survey 48% of the respondent also stated that they will continue support due to fear of litigation [24].

The situation is further complicated by presence of inadequate legal mandate accommodating the such requests. In the USA alone, despite adoption of the uniform determination of death act by all 50 states recognising the brain death, there is a wide variation in the language of actual statute [25]. This results in confusion, reduced public acceptance and fear of litigation amongst clinicians when declaring death by neurological criteria.

Many religions and cultures also do not recognise brain death. In some community death is defined solely by absence of heartbeat [26] which only comes after withdrawal of organ support in brain dead. To some withdrawal of organ support may be seen as equivalent to actively killing the patient [27]. There is also a wide variation in local and national policies regarding the logistics of accommodating continuation of organ support after declaration of brain death. Also, such policies remain silent on clear end points of such continuation of organ support.

Beyond the medical and scientific rationale involved in the determination of brain death and its complex relationship between legal and religious systems doctors face another ethical dilemma. This is the dilemma of stewarding expensive and limited provision of critical care resources. Directing resources to someone who is likely to survive as opposed to a brain-dead patient who has no chance of recovery [28].

To satisfactorily overcome ethical, legal, and religious issues related to brain death a great deal of joint up effort is required from various stakeholders all over the world.

Without a doubt there is a need for uniformity in institutional, legal, and religious mandate for determination of brain death. There is also a need for consistency and uniformity in training of clinicians who are involved in determination of death by neurological criteria [29]. This later initiative will ensure a greater objectivity and accuracy in diagnosis eliminating erroneous declaration.

14.11 Donor Management

The number of people awaiting organ donation remains an all-time high with a wide gap between the supply and demand. World health organization's (WHO) global observatory on donation and transplant reported that 146,800 transplants occur annually worldwide. However, this figure represents a mere 10% of the global needs.

Maximal rate of organ donation remains low at 50 donors per million [30] population with significant regional and national variation.

A great majority of potential organ donors fail to become actual donors due mainly to one of the three reasons. Firstly, there is the family refusal to consent for organ donation. Secondly, even when the family does consent for donation, many donors are lost secondary to extreme physiological changes that follow brain death, resulting in cardiovascular collapse and cardiac arrest. Thirdly some donors are deemed unsuitable due to end-organ injury resulting from post-brain death physiological changes [31].

The process of brain death induces considerable haemodynamic, metabolic, and hormonal changes, which if left untreated will result in somatic death of the patient. Standardising the donor optimisation of physiology results in a decrease in loss of donors due to circulatory collapse [32]. Papworth programme for organ donation in the UK showed that 84% of donors who were well outside the acceptance criteria could be optimised to yield organs with useful graft functions [33].

14.11.1 Pathophysiology of Organ Failure After Brain Death

A precipitous increase in intracranial pressure (ICP) usually precedes the process of brain death. This leads to a set of systemic physiological changes that occur as the ischaemia spreads in an orderly fashion from cerebral hemisphere to the spinal cord.

Ischaemia of the pons causes Cushing's reflex, a state of mixed sympathetic and parasympathetic activity manifested by severe hypertension and bradycardia. This period is followed by a spread of ischemia to vagal nuclei in rostral medulla resulting in a state of "catecholamine storm" marked by hypertension and tachycardia due to unopposed sympathetic activity [34].

In the final moments of the process, the ischemia spreads to the upper cervical spinal cord due to herniation of cerebellar tonsils through the foramen magnum, resulting in a state characterised by severe hypotension, bradycardia and a rapid cardiovascular collapse, leading to a state akin to spinal shock [34].

14.11.1.1 Cardiovascular Effects of Brain Death

Catecholamine storm caused by the herniation process results in cardiotoxicity via catecholamine excess in patients who are brain dead. Myocardial necrosis is often seen during histological examination of the heart in brain dead patients with cardiac dysfunction. These histological findings are similar to those observed in experimental animals with catecholamine excess and prevented by a total cardiac sympathectomy before the cerebral insult [35, 36]. The magnitude of catecholamine response and myocardial injury seems to be related to the pace at which the intracranial pressure rises after an intracranial event causing brain death. In experimental animal models, a steep rise in ICP results in a 750-fold increase in plasma epinephrine and a 400-fold increase in norepinephrine levels which a gradual increase results in 175- and 40-fold increase only [37].

Indeed, these experimental findings are further substantiated by the presence of sudden death and cardiac arrest after spontaneous subarachnoid haemorrhage (SAH). A meta-analysis of 18 population-based studies reported the combined overall risk of sudden death for aSAH was 12.4 and 44.7% for posterior circulation aneurysm [38]. It is possible that cause of the ECG abnormalities and cardiac involvement in SAH patients can be attributed to a sudden rise in ICP [39].

Another group of investigators using a canine model demonstrated that haemodynamic instability in experimental brain-dead animals was attributed to vasodilation and reduction in afterload, which leads to reduced coronary perfusion and decrease in preload. These investigators concluded that myocardial injury caused by brain death could be reversed or avoided by correction of preload and afterload and the haemodynamic collapse noticed after the brain death is due to afterload reduction rather than primary myocardial dysfunction [40].

14.11.1.2 Pulmonary Changes

Only 20% of lungs retrieved from donors are brain death are used for transplantation [41]. There are many factors before and after the brain death, which may affect the condition of the lungs such as contusions, pneumonia, volumetrauma, infection, volume overload, and neurogenic pulmonary oedema [42].

Neurogenic pulmonary oedema may occur soon after the brain injury and during the event of brain death. It is mediated by catecholamine storm induced systemic vasoconstriction and an increase in cardiac afterload, which in turn increases the left ventricle and atrial pressures. The resulting pulmonary oedema is caused by the combined result of elevated hydrostatic pressure and structural damage to the capillary endothelium [43].

Neurogenic pulmonary oedema is defined by bilateral pulmonary infiltrates on chest X-ray and hypoxemia after exclusion of other causes. One study identified the incidence of neurogenic pulmonary oedema to be 23% in patients with SAH who survived to reach the hospital, and it was life-threatening in 6% of the patients [44].

14.11.1.3 Endocrine Changes

The disruption of blood supply to the pituitary and stress response during the process of brain death results in a significant alteration of the hormonal milieu of the human body.

Thyroid Hormones

In brain-dead patients, the decline of T3 plasma levels is heterogeneous.

Subnormal level of T3 occurs in 60–80% of patients, but very low values are seen only in 15% of the patients. However, this decline in T3 is also mirrored by an increase in reverse T3 levels. Free T4 levels are decreased only in one-third of the patients. Thyroid-stimulating hormone levels remain unchanged in these patients. The pattern of thyroid hormonal alteration is indicative of the sick euthyroid syndrome, an adaptive response to stress rather than of the neuroendocrine failure [42, 45].

The supplementation of thyroid hormones after brain death remains controversial. A randomised controlled trial in 80 potential cardiac donors, low T3 levels were not associated with worse haemodynamic indices, and the supplementation of the hormone did not affect the retrieval rate beyond that achieved by other components of the donor management [46].

Cortisol

Plasma cortisol levels remain within normal limits in most brain-dead patients. However, the rise of cortisol in response to ACTH stimulation is blunted. In a study of a total of 37 patients with 17 brain-dead patients, cortisol levels were found to be significantly lower in brain-dead patients. Also, in the majority of brain-dead patient, the cortisol levels failed to increment in response to ACTH stimulation, implying a suppression of the hypothalamic-pituitary-adrenal axis. Diurnal variation of cortisol was also lost in these patients [47].

Pituitary Hormones

Anterior pituitary hormones are usually detectable in the peripheral blood within the normal range.

In contrast to that, posterior pituitary hormonal functions are lost or severely diminished in 80% of the patients [48]. As a consequence, most of the brain-dead patient develops diabetes insipidus with resultant hypovolemia, electrolyte disturbances, and haemodynamic instability.

14.11.1.4 Inflammatory and Immunological Aspect of Brain Death

The process of brain death triggers an inflammatory response involving pro-inflammatory cytokines and upregulation of major histocompatibility antigens (MHC). The consequences of this inflammatory state are apparent in all transplantable organs. These inflammatory changes and immunological activation eventually result in end-organ damage and reduced graft survival.

The blood levels of tumour necrosis factor (TNF)-alpha, interleukin (IL)-6, IL-8, IL-1b, and IL-2R are elevated after brain death [49]. These cytokines activate leukocytes populations and adhesion molecules like selectins and intracellular adhesion molecules (ICAM-1). The adherent leukocytes in turn release pro-inflammatory lymphokines such as TNF alpha and interferon-gamma which mediates the upregulation of major histocompatibility complex (MHC) class I and class II. MHC upregulation results in graft immunogenicity via T-cell recognition [50].

In renal transplantation, both short- and long-term results of unrelated living transplants are superior to well-matched cadaveric donor and the difference may be attributed to the increased cytokine levels in the blood and kidney of brain-dead donors [51–53].

The origin of this cytokine activation is not well studied but could be explained by catecholamine storm and subsequent haemodynamic instability that occurs after it. Haemodynamic changes if left untreated may cause hypoperfusion and ischemia in various organs leading to activation of the cytokine cascade. These changes can be mitigated experimentally by the use of alpha antagonists and haemodynamic optimisation by volume loading and noradrenaline infusion [54–56].

14.11.2 Clinical Management

Once a patient is identified as a potential donor, every attempt must be made to optimise physiology to preserve the functions or organs. Diagnosis of brain death marks the shift of paradigm from lifesaving to organ preserving.

14.11.2.1 Haemodynamic Management

Haemodynamic management after brain death can be challenging.

The goal of haemodynamic management should be to maintain euvolemia and adequate cardiac output to ensure optimal oxygen delivery to the tissues. The aftermath of the catecholamine storm leads to systemic hypotension, and sustained hypotension is associated with impaired graft function. Hypovolemia is common due to diabetes insipidus caused by posterior pituitary dysfunction, and fluid resuscitation is the first step towards optimization. There is no consensus on what fluid is best for resuscitation. However, recently published Canadian practice guidelines have recommended using crystalloids in favour of colloid for optimisation of fluid status in organ donors [57].

Adequate fluid resuscitation may not be enough to restore blood pressure and cardiac output. Majority of donors will require additional ionotropic or vasopressor support. In this situation, vasopressin should be the first vasopressor of choice [57]. Vasopressin has a dual effect in these situations, an antidiuretic via V2 and a vasoconstrictive effect via V1 receptors [58]. Practically vasopressin is useful not only for lowering the requirements of catecholamines but also protects organs for transplantation.

Vasopressin is recommended as first-line vasoactive agent for hypotension after brain death [57].

Noradrenaline is recommended as a second-line agent for vasopressin refractory hypotension [57]. Caution should be exercised with the use of high dose catecholamines. Higher concentrations of catecholamines are associated with primary nonfunction of the heart after the transplantation [59].

14.11.2.2 Haemodynamic Monitoring

Routine haemodynamic monitoring in the form of invasive arterial blood pressure, central venous pressure (CVP) should be routinely employed in all donors. Also, if the patient requires vasopressin or noradrenaline, the use of a cardiac output monitor is desirable. Routine use of a pulmonary artery catheter is not recommended. However, serial Echocardiograms can also be used to assess cardiac functions [57].

14.11.2.3 Thyroxine Supplementation

The evidence for thyroxine supplementation after brain death is not robust. Four randomised control trials did not show any improvement in the number of transplantable hearts following supplemental of thyroid hormone in brain-dead donors [46, 60–62]. Another large retrospective cohort study from United Network for Organ Sharing (UNOS), reported a favourable association of T3/T4 supplementation on heart recovered, patient and graft survival after 1 and 12 months. However, thyroid hormone was given with other hormones as a part of therapy bundle, thereby firm conclusion could not be drawn about the exclusive effect of the thyroid supplementation on the outcome [63].

Given the absence of proven benefits on heart retrieval rate, cardiac functions and post-transplantation patient and graft survival, the routine use of thyroid hormones is not recommended at the present time. However, as there is no published evidence of physiological harm of thyroid hormone supplementation, the decision to use it must be based on local guidelines and merits of individual situations [57].

14.11.2.4 Pulmonary Care

The wide gap between demand and supply of organs available for donation is most serious for patients awaiting lung transplantation. The procurement of lungs remains low, and a recent longitudinal audit reported a lung procurement rate of 20% in a cohort of 2359 eligible lung donors [64].

Lung-protective strategies should be practised in all actual and potential donors. Lung-protective strategies are defined as low tidal volume 6–8 mL/kg of predicted body weight, PEEP of 8–10 mmHg and recruitment manoeuvre after any disconnection from the ventilator [57].

A randomised control trial of lung-protective strategies in potential organ donors after brain death has shown to increase the number of eligible and harvested lungs compared to the conventional strategy [65].

Bronchoscopy is advisable initially as a diagnostic and therapeutic tool to aspirate secretions, to detect evidence of active bronchitis or aspiration, and to obtain a bronchoalveolar lavage specimen for culture [66]. The inhaled beta-2 adrenergic agonists can also be given to decrease excessive alveolar fluid by increasing its clearance [67].

14.11.2.5 Immunosuppressive Strategies

Brain death triggers a pro-inflammatory state that leads to an increase in immunogenicity of the organs are suitable for donation by upregulation class 1 and class 2 MHC antigens [50].

Intravenous corticosteroids can be used for donors needing vasopressor support [57]. High dose Methylprednisolone when given to brain-dead donors can reduce the serum and tissue expression of pro-inflammatory cytokines comparable to that of living donors [68]. Pratschke and colleagues demonstrated in a randomised control trial in 100 brain-dead patients that use of methylprednisolone resulted in significant down-regulation of MHC class 2 expression, ameliorating ischaemic reperfusion injury, and incidence of acute rejection after liver transplantation [69]. A retrospective review of records of thoracic organ procurement from the California transplant donor network showed that the use of corticosteroid and clear breath sounds were two independent predictors of successful lung donation in a multivariate analysis [70].

A single bolus dose of 15 mg/kg body weight should be considered in all donors soon after brain death [71].

Therapeutic Hypothermia

Therapeutic hypothermia or targeted temperature management is used commonly in most critical care units. Hypothermia may offer protection to donor kidneys by reducing metabolism and reduction of free-radical production. A randomised control trial on 394 brain-dead patients studied the impact of mild hypothermia (34–35 °C) on the delayed renal graft functions. Patients were randomised to mild hypothermia and normothermia (36.5–37.5 °C). The primary outcome was delayed graft function (the requirement for dialysis during the first week after transplantation). Delayed graft function occurred in 29% of the 280 patients in the hypothermia group compared 39% of 286 patients in the normothermia group [72]. Recently published Canadian clinical practice guidelines on donor management recommended the use of mild hypothermia in all patients unless kidneys are ruled out for donation [57].

14.11.3 Conclusion

Even though the concept of brain death was first introduced 50-years ago, wide variations in practice, criteria and standards exist globally. The tests are performed chiefly by intensive care physicians. However, most physicians involved in the testing learn to perform these on the job rather than a formal structured training process. Although national guidelines exist to standardise the process for the diagnosis of brain death, they do not address the current variations, inconsistencies, and training gaps in the performance of the clinical tests. These training inconsistencies with many pitfalls of clinical examination and ancillary tests can lead to errors or delays in diagnosing brain death. Therefore, international consensus is necessary to standardise physician training, pre-conditions, procedures for clinical examination, and the apnoea tests.

References

1. Cushing H. Some experimental and clinical observations concerning states of increased intracranial tension. Am J Med Sci. 1902;124:375–400.
2. Mollaret P, Goulon M. [The depassed coma (preliminary memoir)]. Rev Neurol. 1959;101:3–15.
3. Beecher HK, Adams RD, Barger AC, Curran WJ, et al. A definition of irreversible coma. JAMA. 1984;252(5):677–9.
4. Ave ALD, Bernat JL. Inconsistencies between the criterion and tests for brain death. J Intensive Care Med. 2018;35(8):772–80.
5. An appraisal of the criteria of cerebral death: a summary statement. JAMA. 1977;237(10):982.
6. Colleges A of MR. A code of practice for diagnosis and confirmation of death [Internet]. 2008. p. 41. https://www.aomrc.org.uk/reports-guidance/ukdec-reports-and-guidance/code-practice-diagnosis-confirmation-death/.
7. Greer DM, Shemie SD, Lewis A, Torrance S, Varelas P, Goldenberg FD, et al. Determination of brain death/death by neurologic criteria. JAMA. 2020;324(11):1078–97.
8. Spittler JF, Wortmann D, Düring MV, Gehlen W. Phenomenological diversity of spinal reflexes in brain death. Eur J Neurol. 2000;7(3):315–21.
9. Shlugman D. Abnormal pupillary activity in a brainstem-dead patient. Br J Anaesth. 2001;86(5):717–20. http://bja.oxfordjournals.org/content/86/5/717.
10. Posner JB, Saper CB, Plum F. Plum and Posner's diagnosis of stupor and coma. 2007. p. 401. http://books.google.com/books?id=Otivdh2ZoVwC&printsec=frontcover.
11. Murphy PJ, Patel S, Marshall J. The effect of long-term, daily contact lens wear on corneal sensitivity. Cornea. 2001;20(3):264–9.
12. Wijdicks EFM. The diagnosis of brain death. N Engl J Med. 2001;344(16):1215–21.
13. Sawicki M, Bohatyrewicz R, Walecka A, Sołek-Pastuszka J, Rowiński O, Walecki J. CT angiography in the diagnosis of brain death. Pol J Radiol. 2014;79:417–21.
14. de Freitas GR, Andre C. Sensitivity of transcranial Doppler for confirming brain death: a prospective study of 270 cases. Acta Neurol Scand. 2006;113(6):426–32.
15. Kuo J-R, Chen C-F, Chio C-C, Chang C-H, Wang C-C, Yang C-M, et al. Time dependent validity in the diagnosis of brain death using transcranial Doppler sonography. J Neurol Neurosurg Psychiatry. 2006;77(5):646–9.
16. Huang AH. The hot nose sign. Radiology. 2005;235(1):216–7.
17. Munari M, Zucchetta P, Carollo C, Gallo F, Nardin MD, Marzola MC, et al. Confirmatory tests in the diagnosis of brain death: comparison between SPECT and contrast angiography. Crit Care Med. 2005;33(9):2068–73.
18. Heckmann JG, Lang CJG, Pfau M, Neundörfer B. Electrocerebral silence with preserved but reduced cortical brain perfusion. Eur J Emerg Med. 2003;10(3):241–3.
19. Buchner H, Schuchardt V. Reliability of electroencephalogram in the diagnosis of brain death. Eur Neurol. 1990;30(3):138–41.
20. Practice parameters for determining brain death in adults: (summary statement). Neurology. 1995;45(5):1012–4.
21. Sonoo M, Tsai-Shozawa Y, Aoki M, Nakatani T, Hatanaka Y, Mochizuki A, et al. N18 in median somatosensory evoked potentials: a new indicator of medullary function useful for the diagnosis of brain death. J Neurol Neurosurg Psychiatry. 1999;67(3):374–8.
22. Nakagawa TA, Ashwal S, Mathur M, Mysore M, Pediatrics S of CCM Section on Critical Care and Section on Neurology of American Academy of, Society CN. Guidelines for the determination of brain death in infants and children: an update of the 1987 task force recommendations. Pediatrics. 2011;128(3):e720–40.

23. Lewis A, Adams N, Chopra A, Kirschen MP. Organ support after death by neurologic criteria in pediatric patients. Crit Care Med. 2017;45(9):e916–24.
24. Lewis A, Adams N, Varelas P, Greer D, Caplan A. Organ support after death by neurologic criteria: results of a survey of US neurologists. Neurology. 2016;87(8):827–34.
25. Lewis A, Cahn-Fuller K, Caplan A. Shouldn't dead be dead?: The search for a uniform definition of death. J Law Med Ethics. 2017;45(1):112–28.
26. Rosner F. Definition of death in Jewish law. N Y State J Med. 1983;83(7):973–8.
27. Loike J, Gillick M, Mayer S, Prager K, Simon JR, Steinberg A, et al. The critical role of religion: caring for the dying patient from an orthodox Jewish perspective. J Palliat Med. 2010;13(10):1267–71.
28. Biel S, Durrant J. Controversies in brain death declaration: legal and ethical implications in the ICU. Curr Treat Option Ne. 2020;22(4):12.
29. Hocker S, Schumacher D, Mandrekar J, Wijdicks EFM. Testing confounders in brain death determination: a new simulation model. Neurocrit Care. 2015;23(3):401–8.
30. Gortmaker SLP, Beasley CLM, Brigham LEM, Franz HGR, Garrison RNM, Lucas BAM, et al. Organ donor potential and performance. Crit Care Med. 1996;24(3):432–9.
31. Nathan HM, Jarrell BE, Broznik B, Kochik R, Hamilton B, Stuart S, et al. Estimation and characterization of the potential renal organ donor pool in Pennsylvania: report of the Pennsylvania Statewide Donor Study. Transplantation. 1991;51(1):142–9.
32. Salim A, Velmahos GC, Brown C, Belzberg H, Demetriades D. Aggressive organ donor management significantly increases the number of organs available for transplantation. J Trauma Inj Infect Crit Care. 2005;58(5):991–4.
33. Wheeldon DR, Potter CD, Oduro A, Wallwork J, Large SR. Transforming the "unacceptable" donor: outcomes from the adoption of a standardized donor management technique. J Hear Lung Transplant. 1995;14(4):734–42.
34. Schrader H, Hall C, Zwetnow NN. Effects of prolonged supratentorial mass expansion on regional blood flow and cardiovascular parameters during the Cushing response. Acta Neurol Scand. 1985;72(3):283–94.
35. Novitzky D, Rose AG, Cooper DKC. Injury of myocardial conduction tissue and coronary artery smooth muscle following brain death in the baboon. Transplantation. 1988;45(5):964–6.
36. Novitzky D, Wicomb WN, Cooper DKC, Rose AG, Reichart B. Prevention of myocardial injury during brain death by total cardiac sympathectomy in the Chacma baboon. Ann Thorac Surg. 1986;41(5):520–4.
37. Shivalkar B, Loon JV, Wieland W, Tjandra-Maga TB, Borgers M, Plets C, et al. Variable effects of explosive or gradual increase of intracranial pressure on myocardial structure and function. Circulation. 2018;87(1):230–9.
38. Huang J, van Gelder JM. The probability of sudden death from rupture of intracranial aneurysms: a meta-analysis. Neurosurgery. 2002;51(5):1101.
39. Skrifvars MB, Parr MJ. Incidence, predisposing factors, management and survival following cardiac arrest due to subarachnoid haemorrhage: a review of the literature. Scand J Trauma Resusc Emerg Med. 2012;20(1):75.
40. Sebening C, Hagl C, Szabo G, Tochtermann U, Strobel G, Schnabel P, et al. Cardiocirculatory effects of acutely increased intracranial pressure and subsequent brain death. Eur J Cardiothorac. 1995;9(7):360–72.
41. Venkateswaran RV, Patchell VB, Wilson IC, Mascaro JG, Thompson RD, Quinn DW, et al. Early donor management increases the retrieval rate of lungs for transplantation. Ann Thorac Surg. 2008;85(1):278–86.
42. Bugge JF. Brain death and its implications for management of the potential organ donor. Acta Anaesth Scand. 2009;53(10):1239–50.
43. Novitzky D, Wicomb WN, Rose AG, Cooper DKC, Reichart B. Pathophysiology of pulmonary edema following experimental brain death in the Chacma baboon. Ann Thorac Surg. 1987;43(3):288–94.
44. Solenski NJM, Haley ECJM, Kassell NFM, Kongable GR, Germanson TP, Truskowski LM, et al. Medical complications of aneurysmal subarachnoid hemorrhage. Crit Care Med. 1995;23(6):1007–17.
45. Masson F, Thicoïpe M, Latapie MJ, Maurette P. Thyroid function in brain-dead donors. Transplant Int. 1990;3(1):226–33.
46. Venkateswaran RV, Steeds RP, Quinn DW, Nightingale P, Wilson IC, Mascaro JG, et al. The haemodynamic effects of adjunctive hormone therapy in potential heart donors: a prospective randomized double-blind factorially designed controlled trial. Eur Heart J. 2009;30(14):1771–80.
47. Dimopoulou I, Tsagarakis S, Anthi A, Milou E, Ilias I, Stavrakaki K, et al. High prevalence of decreased cortisol reserve in brain-dead potential organ donors. Crit Care Med. 2003;31(4):1113–7.
48. Howlett TA, Keogh AM, Perry L, Touzel R, Rees LH. Anterior and posterior pituitary function in brain-stem-dead donors. Transplantation. 1989;47(5):828–33.
49. Birks EJ, Burton PBJ, Owen V, Mullen AJ, Hunt D, Banner NR, et al. Elevated tumor necrosis factor-α and interleukin-6 in myocardium and serum of malfunctioning donor hearts. Circulation. 2000;102(Suppl 3):III-352–8.
50. Pratschke J, Neuhaus P, Tullius SG. What can be learned from brain-death models? Transplant Int. 2005;18(1):15–21.
51. Bugge JF, Hartmann A, Osnes S, Bentdal O, Stenstrøm J. Immediate and early renal function after living donor transplantation. Nephrol Dial Transpl. 1999;14(2):389–93.
52. Hariharan S, Johnson CP, Bresnahan BA, Taranto SE, McIntosh MJ, Stablein D. Improved graft survival after renal transplantation in the United States, 1988 to 1996. N Engl J Med. 2000;342(9):605–12.

53. Stangl M, Zerkaulen T, Theodorakis J, Illner W, Schneeberger H, Land W, et al. Influence of brain death on cytokine release in organ donors and renal transplants. Transplant Proc. 2001;33(1–2):1284–5.
54. Avlonitis VS, Wigfield CH, Golledge HDR, Kirby JA, Dark JH. Early hemodynamic injury during donor brain death determines the severity of primary graft dysfunction after lung transplantation. Am J Transplant. 2007;7(1):83–90.
55. Rostron AJ, Avlonitis VS, Cork DMW, Grenade DS, Kirby JA, Dark JH. Hemodynamic resuscitation with arginine vasopressin reduces lung injury after brain death in the transplant donor. Transplantation. 2008;85(4):597–606.
56. Barklin A, Larsson A, Vestergaard C, Koefoed-Nielsen J, Bach A, Nyboe R, et al. Does brain death induce a pro-inflammatory response at the organ level in a porcine model? Acta Anaesth Scand. 2008;52(5):621–7.
57. Ball IM, Hornby L, Rochwerg B, Weiss MJ, Gillrie C, Chassé M, et al. Management of the neurologically deceased organ donor: a Canadian clinical practice guideline. CMAJ. 2020;192(14):E361–9.
58. Nakagawa K, Tang JF. Physiologic response of human brain death and the use of vasopressin for successful organ transplantation. J Clin Anesth. 2011;23(2):145–8.
59. Schnuelle P, Berger S, de Boer J, Persijn G, van der Woude FJ. Effects of catecholamine application to brain-dead donors on graft survival in solid organ transplantation. Transplantation. 2001;72(3):455–63.
60. Jeevanandam V. Triiodothyronine: spectrum of use in heart transplantation. Thyroid. 1997;7(1):139–45.
61. Mariot J, Jacob F, Voltz C, Perrier JF, Strub P. Intérêt de l'hormonothérapie associant triiodothyronine et cortisone chez le patient en état de mort cérébrale. Ann Françaises D'anesthésie Et De Réanimation. 1991;10(4):321–8.
62. Randell TT, Höckerstedt KAV. Triiodothyronine treatment in brain-dead multiorgan donors—a controlled study. Transplantation. 1992;54(4):736–7.
63. Novitzky D, Mi Z, Collins JF, Cooper DKC. Increased procurement of thoracic donor organs after thyroid hormone therapy. Seminars Thorac Cardiovasc Surg. 2015;27(2):123–32.
64. Israni AK, Zaun D, Hadley N, Rosendale JD, Schaffhausen C, McKinney W, et al. OPTN/SRTR 2018 annual data report: deceased organ donation. Am J Transplant. 2020;20(s1):509–41.
65. Mascia L, Pasero D, Slutsky AS, Arguis MJ, Berardino M, Grasso S, et al. Effect of a lung protective strategy for organ donors on eligibility and availability of lungs for transplantation: a randomized controlled trial. JAMA. 2010;304(23):2620–7.
66. Miñambres E, Pérez-Villares JM, Chico-Fernández M, Zabalegui A, Dueñas-Jurado JM, Misis M, et al. Lung donor treatment protocol in brain dead-donors: a multicenter study. J Hear Lung Transplant. 2015;34(6):773–80.
67. Ware LB, Fang X, Wang Y, Sakuma T, Hall TS, Matthay MA. Selected contribution: mechanisms that may stimulate the resolution of alveolar edema in the transplanted human lung. J Appl Physiol. 2002;93(5):1869–74.
68. Kuecuek O, Mantouvalou L, Klemz R, Kotsch K, Volk HD, Jonas S, et al. Significant reduction of proinflammatory cytokines by treatment of the brain-dead donor. Transplant Proc. 2005;37(1):387–8.
69. Kotsch K, Ulrich F, Reutzel-Selke A, Pascher A, Faber W, Warnick P, et al. Methylprednisolone therapy in deceased donors reduces inflammation in the donor liver and improves outcome after liver transplantation. Ann Surg. 2008;248(6):1042–50.
70. McElhinney DB, Khan JH, Babcock WD, Hall TS. Thoracic organ donor characteristics associated with successful lung procurement. Clin Transplant. 2001;15(1):68–71.
71. Wood KE, Becker BN, McCartney JG, D'Alessandro AM, Coursin DB. Care of the potential organ donor. N Engl J Med. 2004;351(26):2730–9.
72. Niemann CU, Feiner J, Swain S, Bunting S, Friedman M, Crutchfield M, et al. Therapeutic hypothermia in deceased organ donors and kidney-graft function. N Engl J Med. 2015;373(5):405–14.
73. Busl KM, Greer DM. Pitfalls in the diagnosis of brain death. Neurocrit Care. 2009;11(2):276–87.
74. Hall CA, Chilcott RP. Eyeing up the future of the pupillary light reflex in neurodiagnostics. Diagnostics. 2018;8:19.